THE
PUBLIC-PRIVATE
HEALTH CARE
STATE

THE
PUBLIC-PRIVATE HEALTH CARE STATE

Essays on the History of American Health Care Policy

ROSEMARY STEVENS

Transaction Publishers
New Brunswick (U.S.A.) and London (U.K.)

Library of Congress Catalog Number: 2006044484
ISBN: 978-0-7658-0349-8
Printed in the United States of America

Library of Congress Cataloging-in-Publication Data

Stevens, Rosemary, 1935-
      The public-private health care state : essays on the history of American
   health care policy / Rosemary Stevens.
         p.   cm.
      Includes bibliographical references and index.
      ISBN 0-7658-0349-6 (cloth : alk. paper)
   1. Medical policy—United States—History.

RA395.A3S817   2007
362.10973—dc22   2006044484

Contents

IV. The Medical Profession: Between Government and Market?

V. The American Health Care State

Acknowledgments

Putting this collection together has made me realize how many individuals deserve thanks for stimulation, helpful criticism, feedback, good suggestions, and—not least—practical and emotional support over a longish (and continuing!) career. I would like to acknowledge every single one of the mentors, colleagues, students, and friends who spurred me on to research and write the essays published here. Irving Louis Horowitz deserves special appreciation for suggesting and encouraging this book. Robert B. Stevens generously gave me permission to include and edit the original material for chapter 5, which was coauthored. David A. Pearson was similarly courteous with respect to chapter 8, which I wrote with him and the late Beverlee Myers.

My wonderful husband, Jack D. Barchas, M.D., is in a category all his own. As neuroscientist, psychiatrist, and academic administrator, he deals with the mixed results of American health policy, coping with its conflicts, costs, and complexities in real time, every day. Thank you, Jack, for sharing your experiences and critical skills with me, and for suffering with kindness, understanding, and grace the frequent trials of living with a scholar in the throes of work.

As befits a book on the public-private healthcare state, much of the work presented here was funded through government and private sources. In some instances federal government sources directly influenced what I wrote. Chapters 7, 8, and 9 were written specifically for policy as defined by government agencies. I would not have missed these opportunities for a moment, and hope that similar interchanges (and the spirit of "public" and "private" give-and-take illustrated in these chapters) will be similarly available to social scientists in the future. On the "private" side, I would like to thank in particular the Commonwealth Fund, the Robert Wood Johnson Foundation through its Investigator Awards in Health Policy Research, the School of Arts and Sciences at the University of Pennsylvania, and the Department of Psychiatry at the Weill Cornell Medical College, where I am currently a DeWitt Wallace Distinguished Scholar in Social Medicine and Public Policy.

Grateful acknowledgment is made for permission to reprint the following copyright material:

"Sweet Charity: State Aid to Hospitals in Pennsylvania, 1870-1910," *Bulletin of the History of Medicine*, 1984, 58: 287-314, 474-495.

"'A Poor Sort of Memory': Voluntary Hospitals and Government before the Depression," *Milbank Memorial Fund Quarterly/Health and Society*, 1982, 60 (4): 551-584.

"Can the Government Govern? Lessons from the Formation of the Veterans Administration," *Journal of Health Politics, Policy and Law*, 1991, 16 (2): 281-305.

"Letter from America," *The Hospital* [Great Britain], October 1961: 623-25.

"Medicaid: Anatomy of a Dilemma," *Law and Contemporary Problems*, Health Care, Part I, 1970, XXXV (2): 348-425. Coauthored with Robert Stevens.

"Governments and Medical Care," in Gordan McLachlan, ed., *Medical Care: A Scottish-American Symposium* (London: Oxford University Press for the Nuffield Provincial Hospitals Trust, 1977), pp. 157-175.

"Preface," *Health Care in a Context of Civil Rights, Report of a Study*, Institute of Medicine, publication IOM 81-04 (Washington, D.C.: National Academy Press, 1981), pp. vii-x.

"Goals, Values and Equity in Health Care: A U.S. View," in T. B. Binns and M. Firth, eds., *Health Care Provision under Financial Constraint*. Royal Society of Medicine International Congress and Symposium Series No. 115 (London: Royal Society of Medicine Services, Ltd., 1988).

"Trends in Medical Specialization in the United States," *Inquiry*, 1971, VIII (1): 9-19.

"The Future of the Medical Profession," in Eli Ginzberg, ed., *From Physician Shortage to Patient Shortage: The Uncertain Future of Medical Practice* (Boulder: Westview Press, 1986), pp. 75-93.

"Public Roles for the Medical Profession in the United States: Beyond Theories of Decline and Fall," *Milbank Quarterly*, 2001, 79 (3): 327-53.

"The Changing Hospital," in Linda H. Aiken and David Mechanic, eds., *Applications of Social Science to Clinical Medicine and Health Policy* (New Brunswick, NJ: Rutgers University Press, 1986), pp. 80-99.

"Preface, 1999," in *In Sickness and in Wealth: American Hospitals in the Twentieth Century* (1989) on its reissue in 1999 (Baltimore and London: The Johns Hopkins University Press), pp. xi-xxxvi.

Introduction

American health policy advocates often talk about the public and the private sectors, or government versus market, as if these were separate entities. This is a culture that loves the dualities of "for" and "against": winning or losing, socialism or capitalism, us or them. The practical world does not, however, so clearly differentiate. Calvin Coolidge made his famous remark that the "chief business of the American people is business" (to the American Society for Newspapers in 1925), but included an important, if less catchy, parallel phrase: The "chief ideal of the American people is idealism." The twin themes of commerce (or market) and idealism (or charity, altruism, or what is best for the "public") coexist in the history of social policy as balancing themes. Yin and yang. In Coolidge's day as in our own, public and private actions are necessarily entwined and interdependent.

This book explores the interweaving of public and private enterprise in health care in the United States as a basis for thinking about health care in terms of its history and also as it continues to evolve today. Ideas about charity, entitlement, and equity have long had public *and* private valence. Not-for-profit hospitals and professions have claimed public responsibilities and private roles. Government (state and federal) has shored up one gap after another in the medical marketplace in attempts to provide services to deserving members of the American public; and has helped maintain the viability of private health care organizations, suppliers, biotechnology, employer-based insurance benefits, and private health insurance. In turn, private corporations may serve as government's agents. The title of this work, *The Public-Private Health Care State*, emphasizes my primary theme: the distinctive mixing and continuous remixing of public and private roles as a defining feature of health care in the United States. I have borrowed the term "health care state" from Michael Moran's *Governing the Health Care State* (1999) and others who have used the term in Europe.

I have selected the chapters from my published and unpublished work. The individual pieces were written between 1961 and 2001. Since I am an historian, in addition to writing about health care organization and policy in the rolling present (typically in the role of observer-participant), the subject matter ranges more widely than this, from 1870 through the twenty-first century. The subject matter of the essays represents my own research interests over time, and in some cases my involvement with policy questions at a specific time (including health services research, health maintenance organizations, physician workforce policy, and medical specialty certification). This is not an analysis of the entire, sprawling health care system but a set of idiosyncratic, illustrative windows onto public-private issues as I have observed and thought about them in specific roles and settings. I have tried to capture the spirit of public-private enterprise that distinguishes the health care system in the United States, how it has been justified and explained over time, and, not least, how it works.

Common themes abound—more than I had initially expected from a collection of papers written at different times for different purposes. Three recurring themes are good examples. First, the terms "public" and "private" have no fixed meaning. Indeed, as is easy to see through the examples given in the essays, each term has multiple meanings—and these terms are all the more useful as a result. American policy has been (and is) remarkably fluid, demanding a continuing process of renegotiation and reinterpretation in which a flexible vocabulary is invaluable. The definition of a public or a private act varies at different times according to the force of circumstance. Not-for-profit hospitals, which are still the great majority of American hospitals, can be described as public, as private, as both, and as neither (part of a third domain, outside of government and commerce), depending on specific economic and political contexts, and in light of the usefully fuzzy meaning of those terms. Five of the essays focus on hospitals, in which I have had a special interest.

Second, ideology serves as a vehicle for getting agreed-upon things done rather than as a ruling strategy for change. Hence the value of fugitive terms that serve as rallying rhetoric, generating enthusiasm and (too often, alas) the illusion that there are simple solutions to system-change. On the subservient role of ideology, for example, I note how the United States justified, on reasonable and practical grounds, the establishment of a "socialized" system of hospitals for veterans not long after the Russian revolution (chapter 3). Section III, on buzzwords, rationality, and dreams, describes some of the rhetoric for change and attending enthusiasm that I experienced firsthand as a participant-observer in the policy process in the 1960s and 1970s. Similar observations apply equally today.

Third, people behave very much the same in the face of pecuniary opportunity, no matter what the time period or whether funds flow via the private or the public sector. The mutual interests of Pennsylvania legislators and prominent private citizens who sought state tax funds for local hospitals in the 1870s and 1880s, described in chapter 1, were little different from those of later public-private coalitions. Similarly, the actions of (quasi-public) professional groups and not-for-profit hospitals to money flowing from Medicare and Medicaid in the late 1960s (see chapter 5) were little different from those of any marketplace player, earlier or later.

Words like "lurching," "weaving," "groping," and "trading" can be applied to the process of policy change in government, the nonprofit/professional and the for-profit sectors, as each redefines itself in relation to the others and adjusts to problems and opportunities. But as these essays illustrate, there is also yearning for an ideal, consensus-based solution to whatever is seen as the major health policy problem of the day. Negotiations typically lead to partial solutions and short-term changes. The public-private health care enterprise has become enormously complex. Overall there have been slow but real gains toward more humane treatment of the public. Over the years, too, medicine has become extraordinarily more effective. It is worth remembering the gains as a basis for further changes in the face of today's concerns about runaway expenditures.

Structure of the Book

Looking back over one's own work is a salutary experience. It is also to some extent an exercise in autobiography. Not only are there questions of what to include and how much to edit but also of the context in which each piece was written: for what purpose, and for which intended audience. Some of the chapters are historical articles; some deal with historical material but address themes that were important in health policy discussions at the time the piece was written; some focus purely on contemporary material. In putting this book together I have sometimes found myself writing from one time (the early twenty-first century) about a piece I wrote in another time about events in a third time. Chapter 1, for example, published in 1984, looks at events that took place between 1870 and 1910. Integrating diverse approaches and time warps into a new form as part of a collection was (mostly) fun. I have written introductions to each section to set each piece in the context in which it was written, and provide explanatory information. The section introductions provide thematic continuity and can be read serially as an extension of this introduction.

Section I, Inventing Public-Private Policy for Hospitals in the United States, describes early and close relationships between state government, private interests, and hospital provision that are now largely subsumed under Medicaid. Section II, Negotiating a National Government Role, takes the story further ahead in time and focuses on government's role at the national level: in the establishment of veterans hospitals in the 1920s, the coming of Medicare, the implementation of Medicaid, and comparative observations with Great Britain, as seen in 1977. In Section III, Buzzwords, Rationality, and Dreams, I have selected mostly short pieces to illustrate perceived rhetorical and organizational levers for changes in parts of the health care system, as I have experienced them at specific times. These include the early days of federal participation in health services research and HMOs, the potential (or, rather, lack of potential) to use regionalization as change-agent in the 1970s, the power and limitations of civil rights legislation, and problems in the concept of equity as a rallying cry for change. Section IV considers the role of the medical profession as a public-private social and organizational entity, and Section V deals with somewhat comparable issues faced by not-for-profit hospitals. Inbuilt tensions in the implied, if unstated, social contract between society and professions, and between society and not-for-profit institutions are an intrinsic element in the public-private health care mix.

I chose the articles and other pieces that form the chapters here with two criteria in mind: first, that they help illuminate the history of the American health care system as a public-private enterprise, and second, that they add something new, outside of my published books. I have excluded much of the work I have done on the medical profession, which focuses on the history and character of the British and American professions and their institutions, international physician migration, and standard-setting organizations, since these topics can be better organized elsewhere under the theme of medical professionalism. The exceptions (chapters 12-15) are included because they address more general public-private themes.

Disciplinary and Autobiographical Contexts

This is the most personal book I have done. Some disciplinary and autobiographical comments may be helpful to set the stage. First, as is made abundantly clear from this collection, I am a comparative, applied social scientist with a strong historical perspective. The cultural disorientation of being an immigrant, arriving as I did in the United States from England in 1961 (actually by boat, not so easy to do today) certainly honed my comparative instincts. A comparative perspective has marked all of my work, with two of the chapters in this volume (chapters 4 and 6) having overtly transatlantic themes.

Members of my scholarly generation were fortunate to enter the history and sociology of medicine when these and related social science fields were emerging—and were fluid enough to encourage generalization across disciplinary boundaries, tackle new areas, and engage large themes. I have professional affiliations in the history of medicine, health care management and policy, public health, and health services research, and have written for each of these groups.

My work has benefited enormously from the ideas and interpretations of political analysts and social theorists over the years, including Charles Lindblom, Aaron Wildavsky, Lawrence D. Brown, Talcott Parsons, Renée C. Fox, Eliot Freidson, Max Skidmore, Robert Alford, George Rosen, and many others. But by inclination and preference I am not primarily a theorist. There was actually little useable theory to apply to past and evolving health policy when I began my career in 1957. There was, however, a great opportunity to undertake new historical and policy-related research.

Extraordinary, historically minded individuals were then working to improve health care on each side of the Atlantic. I cannot think of better mentors than the ones I had. Theodore E. (Teddy) Chester, an Austrian lawyer by background and an acute policy and management analyst, ran the health care program at Manchester University, where I did two years of graduate work in applied social science in the late 1950s as an intrinsic part of the national training program for hospital administration in Great Britain. (Teddy was later credited as a founder of business studies at Manchester.) Apart from being an influential figure in British health care, he was an inspired teacher and an enthusiastic purveyor of provocative adages and quips. Delivered in his compelling Viennese accent, they came with the punch of Freudian revelation. "It's not what you know, it's who you know" has stuck with me through the years.

In London, Richard Titmuss and Brian Abel-Smith became mentors and friends. My first job, at the age of twenty-five, was as administrator of a 100-bed general hospital, the Princess Beatrice Hospital, part of the National Health Service. Brian was chair of the board; we toured the hospital together with aplomb on Christmas Day, 1960. Abel-Smith's books on the history of nursing and the history of hospitals have become classics, and indeed history pervades all his work. Richard Titmuss chaired a committee surveying health care for the government of Tanganyika (now Tanzania) in 1961. I served the committee as statistician and drafted two chapters of the report. On two occasions I held visiting appointments at the London School of Economics and Political Science in the department of social administration (later social policy), headed at different times by Titmuss and Abel-Smith. Titmuss, too, saw history as an integral part of effecting change. His work on the history of social welfare infused the advice he gave to the Labour government after World War II, and his major study of blood policy, *The Gift Relationship*, sought to explain the different cultural attitudes he saw in social policy in Great Britain and the United States. Each was an accomplished and committed scholar who saw history as a fundamental skill for policymaking.

At Yale, where I did a Master of Public Health degree and Ph.D. in the 1960s, Isidore S. Falk and John D. Thompson were equally important mentors. John's interests were expressed in studies ranging from operations research, through community studies, to history. Later to be well known (somewhat to his chagrin, as this was merely one of his research interests) as inventor of the "diagnosis related group" or DRG, which became the basis for hospital payment under Medicare in the 1980s, John was a serious student (and published scholar) of the life, work, and influence of Florence Nightingale. She, like himself, was interested in standardization of information, statistics, organization, and efficiency.

Ig Falk's professional life was itself a microcosm of the history of health care in the United States—from his early writings, before 1920, on the case for compulsory health insurance, through his work as research director of the privately funded, blue-ribbon Committee on the Costs of Medical Care in the late 1920s and early 1930s, through a long career in the Social Security Administration (from which he retired to his professorship at Yale), and on to his instrumental role late in his life in setting up a health maintenance organization in New Haven.

Teddy Chester was, I think, philosophically a pragmatist, and so I would characterize John Thompson. Titmuss and Abel-Smith were Fabian socialists. Isidore Falk was an American progressive, who saw evolutionary logic in the long arguments for social insurance in the United States, with Medicare as an intermediate step toward health insurance coverage of the entire population. Each was an exceptional individual whose life and work continue to be important for the study of health care history in the two countries. I was truly blessed by the opportunity of knowing and working with each of them.

My graduate work at Yale included the traditional fields of public health, to which I had not been exposed before, as well as health management and policy from the American perspective. (A good reality check on how policy works on the ground occurred in 1961 when I was a witness in New Haven in the birth control case that eventually led to the Supreme Court as *Griswold v. Connecticut*). For the Ph.D. I fortuitously chose fields that would serve well in the future: sociology, chronic disease epidemiology, and health administration. Ig Falk, my dissertation adviser, suggested the topic of medical specialization before I embarked on the Ph.D. and was principal investigator of the grant that then happily provided me with a salary. That grant, which I wrote (it reads persuasively), had enormously unrealistic ambitions: no less than a historical comparison of the history of health care in Great Britain and the United States, and all to be accomplished, as I recall, in eighteen months! In any event, I published my first book on specialization in British medicine in 1966, and on American medicine (the topic of my dissertation) in 1971. By then I was a faculty member in public health (health administration) at Yale, where I stayed until 1976.

During the 1970s I studied the implementation of Medicaid (see chapter 5 in this volume) and, with Louis Wolf Goodman and Stephen S. Mick, worked on a series of studies of physician migration to the United States (not included here). I was also increasingly involved in national policy evaluation (see, for example, chapters 8 and 9), working with an array of different groups, including the Institute of Medicine. Moving to Tulane University in 1976 as part of a two-career professional family, I returned more forcefully to health systems management, becoming the chair of the department of that name in 1977.

In 1979, I moved to the University of Pennsylvania and remained happily there until taking emeritus status in 2002. This move allowed me to take up full-time intellectual practice as an historian. I was a professor (with two stints as chair) of history and sociology of science, with time out as dean of arts and sciences from 1991 through 1996. I owe much to my distinguished colleagues at Penn after my arrival, particularly Charles E. Rosenberg and Thomas P. Hughes; not least, they persuaded me that I was actually a professional historian of medicine. Charles and I both embarked on (complementary) histories of American hospitals, his published in 1987, mine in 1989. Tom and I taught a memorable (at least to us) course where he began with the view that health care was a technological system like other such systems (such as power systems), while I argued otherwise, namely that health care was unique and different; and we ended the course with each having switched views to the opposite position. At the time of writing, I am a DeWitt Wallace Distinguished Scholar at Weill Cornell Medical College, pursuing research once more into medical specialization, the history of veterans hospitals, and other questions.

How I would my own characterize my own political philosophy for this book? As a pragmatist, I think. You be the judge. As an historian, I have been acutely aware of the problems of imposing theory, narrative structure, and agency too rigidly on the messy, changing, and constantly surprising stuff of history. As a policy analyst, one needs to be finely tuned to the possibility of change. As someone who has lived through seven decades (and in two countries) I am also well aware of how difficult it is to escape the ruling narratives, theories, political, social, and economic messages and other often-unexamined beliefs that constitute the dominant cultural messages of the time—whatever that time happens to be. I have tried to be a watchful and open-minded critic—a skeptic and sometimes a contrarian. Riding the crest of one policy wave does not imply that the next wave will be the same, or even flowing in the same direction.

During my career as student, historian, and analyst of American and British health care, from the late 1950s through the early 2000s, expectations and approaches to health care have passed through a veritable kaleidoscope of expectations and beliefs. Here are seven illustrative examples of the perceptual environments I have (so far) moved through in my own history:

First, belief in the virtue of nationalized enterprises in Great Britain, ranging from health care to railroads and electricity, mostly touted as efficient in the late 1950s when I was a graduate student in health management (then tellingly encompassed within a program of social administration) at Manchester University.

Second, belief in the overriding virtue of privately organized and funded health care, strengthened by fear of any taint of "socialized medicine" (an American phrase), which was readily observable in my role as a new immigrant to the United States in 1961, when I once again became a graduate student in health management, this time at Yale, where the program was, interestingly, part of public health.

Third, the rhetoric of social justice and federal responsibility for equal opportunity that distinguished the Great Society programs in the 1960s, including the passage of Medicare and Medicaid, which greatly expanded the federal government's financial commitments to health care. The programs fulfilled those commitments through privately owned institutions and professional practices—thus, in turn, encouraging not-for-profit hospitals to drop their roles as "charities" and become competitive, profit-oriented businesses, and stimulating the economic growth of American health care as one of the nation's largest businesses.

Fourth, attempts to curb some of the expansionary effects of public and private programs through legislation for federally-sponsored health planning in the 1960s and 1970s, built on principles of private "community" responsibility at the local level, with the exercise of oversight by the states—followed by the abandonment of both policy and principle when local responsibility largely failed, and games-playing was apparent at every level.

Fifth, in the 1970s and 1980s, scholarly and public concern about the political and economic self-interest and social "dominance" of the medical profession, whose members were newly dubbed as behaving in an excessively "private" or commercial manner as participants in the "medical-industrial complex," and seemed to have drifted away from the broader, "public" spirit supposedly subsumed in the profession's social contract.

Sixth, beliefs in the superior managerial efficiency, nimbleness, and financial flexibility of private enterprise in the 1970s, and a full-fledged movement toward market "solutions" to health care in the 1980s and 1990s. Managed care insurance corporations tried to rationalize and curb the costs of health care through negotiated contracts with providers, rules for allowable services, and "gatekeepers" to oversee the use of medical specialists; however, private regulation by insurers proved little more appealing to the public (or "consumers" or "taxpayers," depending on context) than had federally-sponsored local health planning.

Seventh, in the first years of the twenty-first century, a sense of confusion, demoralization, and helplessness, even anomie, crusted over by a thin layer of hope in a rather vague doctrine of consumer-centered care. Cost control was a more important message than adding value in health care. Doctors felt themselves imprisoned in bureaucracy without having the advantage of working in a bureaucratic structure. No single set of beliefs served as mobilizing ideas.

The eighth will come along in its own good time...

Most of these ideas and beliefs can be held at once, even where they logically conflict for, as I note elsewhere in this volume (see Section II), at any particular period there are numerous consensus-building beliefs available for the taking. This is, in part, what makes health care policy so dynamic in the United States, where a consistent ideology has never ruled policy directions. Commitment to a welfare state in Great Britain and other European countries required them to rethink social principles on a large scale when those welfare states proved too expensive to sustain. In the United States, with the most expensive health care system of all, the public-private mix described in these essays allows spontaneous and often scattered change, depending on shifting social, economic, and power agendas.

For example, the Medicare legislation (1965) and its early implementation appeared to commit the United States to three important principles: 1) social insurance to provide hospital care to the sixty-five-plus population; 2) non-intervention by government in the free operation of the largely private health providers; and 3) reimbursement for services given to Medicare beneficiaries at similar rates to those charged for the privately insured. All of these principles have been breached to some degree. Medicare "reform" in the early twenty-first century hinges, pragmatically, on cost and tax agendas, and on the divided interests of different constituencies.

This is a system run not by ideology but by opportunity and interests. Herein lies both its strengths and weaknesses—both of which I have tried to show in these essays. While the ability to change may be counted as a strength, lack of consistent social and strategic goals has been and remains a major weakness.

* * *

Three final introductory comments are in order. First, ambiguity in the roles of all major players marks the history of American health care. That, to me, is what makes it so fascinating to observe, if sometimes infuriating to engage with. Sometimes it seems as if health policy, as implemented, has subverted the strong points of every player represented here. Nevertheless, with each change, each new idea, each legislative proposal, all rise energetically to the fray again. The enthusiasm of would-be reformers (and their critics) matches the opportunistic energy of players in the system.

Second, and strikingly, the United States has not provided the standards one might expect for one of its major private enterprises. Health care is far less regulated than, for example, the banking industry. Hiding behind the public-private health care state is the anomaly in that it vacillates in intention. American health care is neither one thing nor the other, nor wholly successful as a mixed public-private enterprise. The health care state is controlled neither by the market nor by effective government regulation. Meanwhile, its large middle ground of not-for-profits, for-profit providers, and professions struggle, often unsuccessfully, to find advantage in the shifting mud of circumstance.

Third, and by no means least, America remains committed to both of the principles adumbrated by Calvin Coolidge in the 1920s: both to the market and to idealism. There are honestly held differences in view as to what would constitute an ideal system, but there is little question that everyone should have reasonable access to good quality health care. Some see an ideal system emerging from a less regulated, others from a differently regulated, health care market. Some see government as the only organization capable of rationalizing and guaranteeing care. Some may favor single payers in different areas, which might or might not be governmental. Some believe that individuals could learn to act effectively as prudent buyers of health care, given appropriate incentives. And so on. However, all of these "ideals" are focused on means, not ends; on vehicles for change, not desired results. It is more important to decide what results should be achieved than who should achieve them in the public-private health care state. Given the will, the means will be found.

I present these essays to you in the hope that they will cast a useful, even colorful, light onto some of the public-private workings of American health care as a basis for provoking thought about the future.

I. Inventing Public-Private Policy for Hospitals in the United States

Introduction to Section I

Sometimes—not as often as one would like—research projects come through serendipity. In 1979, I moved from Tulane to the University of Pennsylvania, with a sharp change in academic environment from health systems management to the history of science and medicine. Writing about the history of American hospitals seemed a challenging next step. My office at the School of Public Health at Tulane had been a few steps from the huge Charity Hospital, state-owned and used for medical teaching by Tulane and LSU. I had long mulled over the idea of "charity," and admired the sonority of the word. But how congruous was it to anything in health care now that Medicare and Medicaid paid hospital bills for the elderly and poor? Tulane was also a leader in changing perceptions toward for-profit enterprise in the health care community in the late 1970s, and for recognizing hospitals as business enterprises that would rise or fall through application of skills in finance, financial management, and marketing, rather than charitable intent. Maybe charity was dead.

Most hospitals were, however, nonprofit institutions in the terminology of the day, charitable or benevolent in legal form, and tax-exempt. Many had religious foundations. At board meetings at Presbyterian Hospital in Philadelphia in the 1980s we started our meetings with a prayer. As a group, tax-exempt hospitals, otherwise known as voluntary hospitals (founded by voluntary associations, owned by not-for-profit corporations, and run by unpaid boards of trustees), claimed a special, if unspecified, social mission or voluntary "spirit." They still do to some extent today. The developing relations between government, not-for-profits, and for-profit organizations demanded historical as well as policy attention, and the interplay of public and private roles in the American polity became a primary—and continuing—theme of my research. But I was also interested in understanding the American history of hospitals more generally—as a national movement, social enterprise, or industry, as if one were writing about the history of railroads or of steel. This work resulted in my book *In Sickness and in Wealth: American Hospitals in the Twentieth Century* (1989).

The two chapters in this section represent separate though related studies. As a new resident of Pennsylvania, I decided to look at the history of hospitals in that state as a reality test before moving to national exploration. Serendipity visited one day at the Library of Congress, where I hunkered down to leaf through the card catalog under "Hospitals." (Yes, there were still card catalogs in libraries, and hard on the fingers they were, too.) To my delight and surprise, I found a printed table of figures on hospital expenditures and state grants to hospitals in Pennsylvania, prepared for tax hearings in that state in 1910. This find alone showed that Pennsylvania was heavily subsidizing voluntary hospitals with tax funds; to such an extent that hospital subsidy had become an issue for tax policy in the state. One third of the combined income of voluntary hospitals came from state taxes in 1910, while state grants to hospitals represented 11 percent of total state expenditures. Follow-up research unearthed a fat printed volume of the testimony given at the 1910 hearings: a goldmine of contemporary views about charity, the government (state) role, and the nature of voluntary institutions. Further research into the history of charitable subsidy, industrial conditions, tax policy, census data, hospital reports, and related subjects laid the foundation for "Sweet Charity" (chapter 1), and for the extension of the history in "A Poor Sort of Memory" (chapter 2).

"Sweet Charity" traces the development of hospitals in Pennsylvania at the end of the nineteenth century and into the twentieth, including the highly political maneuverings for state funds. In 1870 the state-aided hospitals could be seen as fulfilling public roles as quasi-governmental (or at least public) enterprises. By 1910, they were more clearly private institutions, struggling to keep government subsidy without strings attached; that is, without government regulation. Hospital leaders positioned their institutions as both charities and businesses, and were adept at changing the hospital's image as circumstances changed. All sides, though, inside and outside government, were reluctant to strengthen government's role as payer, except on an ad hoc, developmental, or residual basis. This history plays out recurring and continuing themes: on the fuzzy meaning of both "public" and "private"; the interdependence of government and not-for-profits in the American system; the mix of religious and nonsectarian organizations and confusion as to how to deal with them; and advantage-seeking behavior on all parts. Pennsylvania's state-aid system went through various transitions in subsequent years, eventually morphing into today's state program for Medicaid. Not surprisingly, despite a very different environment for hospitals and for the provision of health care as "welfare," many of the same questions confront policy today.

"Sweet Charity" was written for medical historians, and is thick in historical detail. It tells a story: A network of individuals and associations negotiated tax-supported health care for the poor in a significant U.S. state, leading to a system that was widely recognized as notorious by 1910. "A Poor Sort of Memory" takes a national perspective on the history of government aid to hospitals, and extends it in time, through the 1930s. The audience was also different; the essay is geared toward readers in the social sciences and policy fields.

In "A Poor Sort of Memory" I describe a long history of government involvement in paying for hospital care, well before the 1930s. Government involvement was not, in short, an invention of the Depression and New Deal, as seemed to be the message of the early 1980s. New policies often create new histories, mythological though these may be. By 1982, when "A Poor Sort of Memory" was published, for-profit entrepreneurship was becoming the new hope for health care change. Efficiency and effectiveness were now to be sought through corporate innovation and the nimbleness of competition. Viewing the new market orientation as an overdue reaction to New Deal (and even progressive) policies had some strategic, political appeal. At the same time, this revised history threatened the not-for-profit hospital by assuming the superiority (and presumably, more successful future) of investor-owned institutions. (The medical profession, relabeled as a business, also found itself stumbling to reinvent itself, a process that continues; see chapters 12-15.) The idea of the not-for-profit voluntary hospital as a successful organizational chameleon, both public and private, charity and business, did not fit contemporary messages. Not-for-profits promised to become a definitional and organizational casualty of pro-market policy, no longer sure of occupying firm ground as the partner of government or acting as a legitimate third force between the "market" and government.

I argue, then, for a more nuanced, less partisan history, based on the story and evidence I present here. Now, as then, it is important to recognize the social and political utility implicit in the long, intertwining history of public and private roles in health care in the United States—including that "distinctively American practice" of public support of private, not-for-profit hospitals. That history plays out an array of roles that government might take, and has taken in the past: as venture capitalist, silent partner, grant-giver, and buyer of services in the private sector. "A Poor Sort of Memory" shows, too, the permeability of boundaries between public and private roles, the shifting meanings of terms like "private," the mythology vested in such terms, and the historical strangeness of lumping both not-for-profit and for-profit (or investor-owned) hospitals into one, undifferentiated "private" category.

Despite all the rhetoric from the 1980s on, and the growth of investor-owned enterprise, voluntary hospitals continued to thrive (see chapters 16 and 17). Tax funds, represented primarily by Medicare and Medicaid, accounted for a much larger proportion of hospital expenditures in the first five years of the twenty-first century than in 1903, 1922, 1935, or 1958. For needy individuals seeking health care—signaled most decisively in the passage of Medicaid as a program of federal grants to states in legislation in 1965 (described in chapter 5)—charity was a bureaucratic, governmental function, streaming funds to private institutions.

1

Sweet Charity: State Aid to Hospitals in Pennsylvania, 1870-1910

"You can not put doctors and ministers who are en-
gaged in the distribution of sweet charity in the line
of men who are managing Standard Oil and the
Sugar Trust." "I think human nature is the same."[1]

Between 1870 and 1910 the American hospital was transformed from an asylum for the indigent into a modern scientific institution. In the same period hospitals, collectively, developed from the scattered handful of institutions that existed in the early 1870s into a widespread, multimillion-dollar enterprise. By 1910 there were more than 4,000 hospitals in the United States. Many of these were small, proprietary institutions owned and operated by physicians. More important were the "benevolent" hospitals, established and run by religious groups, by voluntary boards of trustees, or by government (usually local government). There were 1,918 benevolent hospitals and sanitaria in the United States in 1910; 184 of these were in Pennsylvania. Hospital property in Pennsylvania was valued at well over $50 million.[2]

Social, industrial, and medical interests in the founding of hospitals interconnected; the establishment of a hospital became the goal of every civic-minded community. Cities and factories provided the population base to support new institutions, a hierarchy of would-be philanthropists, new money, and the need for somewhere to send the accidentally maimed and sick. Immigration emphasized ethnic and religious distinctions, which impelled, in turn, the creation of hospitals for Swedes, Lutherans, Germans, Baptists, Roman Catholics, blacks, Jews, Episcopalians. The development of professional nursing, acceptance of the germ theory of disease, and concurrent changes in bacteriology, pathology, and surgery provided an ordered, clean institutional environment and an attractive, scientific ethos for hospital care, while reforms in medical education created a demand by medical schools for hospital patients as "teaching material."[3] In Pennsylvania, however, another important factor intervened, for much of the initial investment in the construction and maintenance of the new hospitals came directly from the state. Indeed, many of the institutions came into being expecting state aid for construction and maintenance. Of the 167 religious and voluntary hospitals in Pennsylvania in 1910, 141 received state aid.[4]

This chapter examines the politics, economics, and growing wealth of the hospital business in Pennsylvania in light of the important and unusual role played by the state. The role of government in the history of hospitals is only beginning to be explored. Yet, long before 1910, Pennsylvania's subsidies had become famous, even notorious, among hospital trustees, government reformers, and other observers of organized charity inside and outside of Pennsylvania. In 1910 an estimated one-third of the total income of religious and voluntary hospitals in Pennsylvania came from government, chiefly from the state—more than their income from endowments and contributions, and only a little less than their income from paying patients.[5] For the hospitals such "charity" was sweet indeed.

In parallel, hospitals developed their own collective, lobbying interests. Participating in a large-scale system of state grants-in-aid, hospital representatives became shrewd observers of the scene in Harrisburg and sensitive political manipulators. Pennsylvania hospitals emerged collectively as a state-supported private service industry. Whether their activities were to be viewed as self-serving and manipulative or as noble and benign was a matter of opinion—and of heated debate. By 1910 the hospitals in Pennsylvania were an entrenched system of vested interests.

Quite apart from Pennsylvania's visibility as the second largest U.S. state (after New York) in this period, Pennsylvania is of special interest for at least three reasons. The first is, of course, the unusually strong role, though not a unique role, played by state government in subsidizing the construction and maintenance of general hospitals. For the most part, these hospitals were independent, not-for-profit institutions, operated by volunteer boards of trustees (i.e., voluntary hospitals). As Pennsylvania's hospitals looked to the state for continuing appropriations, they provided a well-publicized model for hospitals elsewhere in seeking government assistance.

A second reason is to illuminate a scarcely-touched element of medical history: the involvement of hospitals in politics in the nineteenth and early twentieth centuries. State government in Pennsylvania was notoriously sloppy and corrupt for almost the entire period 1870 to 1910; but while critics of the time might claim that little comprehensive decision-making was evident in the legislature, the hundreds of deals and decisions made each session on individual appropriation bills—for there was typically a separate appropriation bill for each institution—added up to a policy of legislative approval and appeasement: approval, that is, of general hospitals as a public good, deserving subsidy via taxation, and appeasement of numerous, worthy, local lobbying groups that came earnestly to Harrisburg year by year. Well before 1910, Pennsylvania grants to hospitals were a major element in the more general system of subsidies to private charities in the state. In turn, grants to private charities formed a significant segment of the state's general appropriations. Excluding psychiatric hospitals, the state's expenditures on hospitals represented 11 percent of all state expenditures in 1910, almost all of which went to voluntary hospitals.[6] Since appropriations were the vehicle for manipulating political power in the legislature, the hospital lobby was an important aspect of policymaking in the state.

A third reason for studying Pennsylvania is its value as a case study of wider questions, debated between 1870 and 1910 (and since), about the nature of charity, the role of government in medicine, and the definitions of public and private enterprise. State grants to voluntary hospitals assumed that the hospitals performed public functions. In the 1870s and 1880s, these functions could be justified as delegatory functions of the state: that is, the voluntary hospitals were providing services that, arguably, might otherwise have had to be provided by state or local government institutions. But such arguments could only prosper in the earlier, small-scale years of grants-in-aid. With the great burst of specialized charitable and eleemosynary institutions of all kinds in the late nineteenth century came criticism of government involvement and praise for charitable enterprise. Philanthropists engaged in strategic, "scientific" charity, together with many municipal and state reformers, argued for a divorce of function between governmental and private institutions. While some would keep charity-giving, as far as possible, in private hands, others would increase the accountability of government agencies by concentrating social services in government institutions. Amos Warner's well-known book, *American Charities*, continued to recommend in its various versions between 1894 and 1919, "consistent opposition to any and all public [i.e., governmental] subsidies to private charities."[7] By the 1890s, at the latest, subsidy of voluntary hospitals could no longer be justified without question as a delegated function of the state. By 1910, with state subsidies running at between two and three million dollars a year, the voluntary hospitals were more clearly private organizations, offering services for purchase by paying patients and government agencies alike and pursuing their own institutional agendas. The question remained, on what principle—and how far—government should be involved in the provision or subsidy of hospital care, and how far the hospitals were to be regulated as private businesses.

Beginnings of the State-Aid System

The state-aid system in Pennsylvania, an early ancestor of today's Medicaid program, began before the Civil War, but only sprang into prominence in the 1870s and 1880s. State appropriations to worthy institutions were generally accepted before the war as a natural function of state government. It was not unusual for states to work in partnership with private organizations, using essentially a private corporate model for developing a public service, and it was on the basis of this model that state aid to charities developed. Governor William Fisher Packer cited as examples of Pennsylvania's state-aided institutions in 1859 the State Lunatic Hospital at Harrisburg, the Western Pennsylvania Hospital at Pittsburgh, the House of Refuge at Philadelphia and Pittsburgh, the Pennsylvania Training School for idiotic and feeble-minded children, asylums for the blind and deaf and dumb at Philadelphia, and the Northern Home for friendless children, Philadelphia.[8] State governments gave money to academies as a way of sponsoring education, a system that ended when public high schools began, and state aid to colleges and universities was common before the Civil War. Great hospitals, including the Pennsylvania Hospital (established 1751) and Massachusetts General Hospital (1811), received state aid on their foundations. While general responsibility for public welfare was vested in local government, the states maintained a general economic and benevolent role, initiating and developing institutions for industry, education, shelter, and punishment that met the perceived needs of a growing industrial economy and contributed to the social stability of the state. As a result, there was no clear distinction as to what was properly a "public" function and what was "private."[9]

The Commonwealth of Pennsylvania had a long tradition of working cooperation with private groups in the establishment of essential services, including roads, canals, railroads, and banks. Pennsylvania also subsidized ten charitable institutions, of all kinds, in 1860: four owned and operated by the state, and six private institutions. State subsidy to care for the dependent and the sick in private institutions increased rapidly during the war; twenty-six private charities were subsidized in 1865 alone. It was not surprising that immediately after the war, in Pennsylvania as in other states, serious concern should be expressed about the nature and principles of charitable aid.

Debates at Pennsylvania's Constitutional Convention in 1872-73 elicited an array of views. One speaker stated flatly that it was "not the business of the Commonwealth to be the public almoner to distribute charity";[10] another argued that it was important to keep "bad men" from polluting religious charities with money out of the public treasury;[11] another warned of the favoritism, gross inequality, and religious dissension that could result if every charity in the state thought itself eligible for appropriations;[12] while others favored state aid to charities without exception. New York cut off its aid to hospitals in 1872. In Pennsylvania, in contrast, appropriations to charitable institutions moved rapidly upward from the early 1880s. Many of these new state-aided charities were new hospitals. By 1898, Pennsylvania could boast 113 benevolent or not-for-profit hospitals, of which sixty-nine were aided by the state; and all but six of these had been established after 1870.[13]

The disruptions of the Civil War, the development of the manufacturing, railroad, and mining industries, and an increasing focus on clinical teaching in medical education, provided incentives for hospital development and subsidy. The war disrupted existing hospitals, created others, and underscored the importance of hospitals in treating wounds and injuries. War left a legacy of hospitalized soldiers in temporary federal hospitals and in private institutions, and of a large number of influential citizens with experience in and outside the army (notably those who had worked with the U.S. Sanitary Commission, which was active throughout Pennsylvania), with experience in hospital establishment, utility, and logistics.

In times of war, public and private roles are intermixed; cooperative patterns develop that may suggest precedents for times of peace. Thus, Mercy Hospital, a Roman Catholic institution in Pittsburgh, cared for soldiers and was reimbursed by the Union government for doing so with little concern about the principles of separating church and state. Catholic sisters also cared for soldiers at the Western Pennsylvania Hospital in Pittsburgh and at Stanton Military Hospital. Some private institutions became government facilities for the duration of the war.[14] Other hospitals received state aid. Mercy Hospital, Pittsburgh, received $4,000 from the state in each of the years 1864 and 1865. Protestant Episcopal Hospital, Philadelphia, received $5,000 from the state in 1864 and again in 1865.[15] There was no overall plan for such aid. Where a need was seen, it was met. As before the war, state aid to charities was given on a pragmatic basis.

In strictly legal terms, the state could only move to subsidize private charities where the need served was statewide rather than local, and where the institution was open to all members of the public who fell into a particular category of care. In most states, the provision of psychiatric hospitals (and the segregation of such patients from the general population) was seen as serving statewide interests and the statewide population. However, general hospital care, like public assistance, was demonstrably more a matter of local or parochial interest. Nevertheless, where the will to act existed—as in Pennsylvania—the principles on which practice rested were fuzzy and flexible. Given the wheeling and dealing of machine politics in the legislature, a strong legislator could persuade his peers that both statewide and public needs were served for almost any charity in which he was interested—given, of course, the clout to steer proposals through to legislation and appropriation. Pennsylvania was famous for political deals and legislative toadying to powerful interests.[16] But while governors might complain that "this matter of charity is fast running into a great abuse," or that "special legislation is the great and impure fountain of corruption, private speculations and public wrongs,"[17] there was no clear or firm definition of responsibility for the development of charities and no specific guidelines for policy as to which institutions might be eligible for state aid. The system was open for currying of favor and exploitation.

Pennsylvania in the 1870s was rapidly industrializing. In 1874, Pennsylvania produced about half of the country's pig iron. Anthracite production was increasing rapidly; bituminous coal came into general use after 1860. The oil, lumber, textile, and other industries were expanding rapidly, and prospects for further economic growth seemed excellent. As in other states, the population was also increasing, largely through immigration: from 3.5 million in 1870, to 5.3 million in 1890, to 7.7 million in 1910. In each of these years, Pennsylvania followed New York as the second most populous state. In the expanding mining and manufacturing centers, immigrants were an important presence by 1870. More than one-fourth of the inhabitants were reported as "foreign" in Luzerne County (Wilkes-Barre), Allegheny County (Pittsburgh), Schuylkill County (Pottsville), Philadelphia County, and Carbon County (Mauch Chunk).[18] Politically, the state was dominated by the concentrations of population, wealth, and influence in Philadelphia and Pittsburgh.

The Republican Party became dominant in Pennsylvania during the war, under the extraordinary influence of Simon Cameron, self-made businessman turned national and statewide politician, and remained powerful through the political machine Cameron left behind when he retired from public life in 1879. The Pennsylvania Republican Party was predominantly the party of business. But the political machine was effectively an alliance of municipal and county organizations, with strongholds in Philadelphia and Pittsburgh. This pattern, continuing well into the twentieth century, could not have been better designed for the promotion and success of local applications for state aid. The political system supported vote-trading, logrolling, and back-scratching among state legislators as each promoted local projects; it upheld Philadelphia's strong medical interests and promoted competitive interests in medicine in Pittsburgh; it stimulated concern in cities such as Erie or Scranton that they, too, get their "fair share" of state largesse. Business interests behind the local Republican machines benefited both practically and symbolically by the appearance of hospitals and other charitable institutions: practically, as providing places for sick, injured, and dependent employees; symbolically, as a visible expression of the cooperation of capital and labor at a time of uneasy tension, high accident rates, and violent strikes. The mix of public and private efforts in "public charities" before and during the Civil War, as well as growing interest in hospitals and in charitable institutions in general, were to lead the creative minds of prospective founders increasingly to government aid. The political party system, geared up for economic expansion and local interests, was "the steam that drives the machine."[19]

Pennsylvania had no budget category for charities; indeed, it had no state budget. Income and expenditures were reconciled on a pragmatic basis, with the governor pruning as he saw fit. Each request for funds for an institution was incorporated into a separate bill, sponsored by the legislator in whose constituency the proposed charity rested (and for which he would get due local credit). Each request for an appropriation was separately considered by the legislature in no particular order of priority; the bills for charities interwove with other business. At the end of the legislative session, all the appropriations were bundled together and rushed to the governor, sometimes on the last night of the session, leaving little time for overall review. Following the example of several other states, Pennsylvania established a State Board of Public Charities in 1869 to impose some order and to collect information. The Board inspected hospitals, as well as other charities, and made recommendations to the legislature about the value of funding requests, but its advice could be, and often was, ignored. The power of appropriation rested squarely with the legislature: a power susceptible to special interests, deals, and logrolling even in the relatively low-budget 1870s. However, the governor had the power of veto.

A blatant early example of the process—and of the confusion over the principles of state aid—was the proposal in the 1860s for state funding for a Marine Hospital at Erie. It was common practice for the federal Marine Hospital Service to use private hospitals on a contract basis and the prospect of success at Erie must initially have seemed good. Pennsylvania's Committee on Ways and Means opposed the proposal on the grounds that such a hospital was ineligible for aid because it was a "private charity" and, with some perspicacity, that an appropriation would open the door to "a hundred such amendments."[20] Nevertheless, in 1868, under the pressure of a powerful senator, an appropriation of $10,000 was granted to establish the new hospital, conditional on local matching funds. Among arguments for its support were the large amount of state funds flowing into Philadelphia and Pittsburgh, the desirability of competing with other prominent ports on the lakeshore, and the need to protect this entry to the state from alien contagions.[21] The state also donated 100 acres of land. Once started, however, state aid proved difficult to stop. By 1871, the state had appropriated a total of $90,000 for the Marine Hospital at Erie. A substantial brick and stone building had been erected, but there was an embarrassing hitch: The hospital was not opened, allegedly because of problems of title to part of the land. Legislators were quite open as to why the appropriation had been granted in the first place: It was a "steal" by the former senator from Erie in return for his vote on other issues.[22] The legislature tried to get rid of the building by granting the land to Erie County for a workhouse, but the Erie commissioners refused to take it.

Given the considerable flexibility of principle, other more plausible applications for state aid might be expected. One successful applicant of this period was the Philadelphia Orthopaedic Hospital, established in 1867. By 1875, it had received $25,000 from the state, accompanied by a glowing press. The hospital had obvious advantages as a candidate for funding. It focused, first, on treatment, most notably of cases of "bent spines," club foot, and nervous disorders (on the assumption that many deformities, such as palsy, were originally due to nervous diseases), and reported a high rate of improvement. It met a need not dealt with anywhere else in the state, and thus could claim a statewide, rather than a local, interest. It used technology, including appliances and electricity. And it had the particular appeal of treating children. And finally, it was argued that subsidizing the hospital saved the state from supporting many persons who, untreated, would otherwise rely on charity.[23] Hospital representatives were attuned to the political process. It can have been no coincidence that a page in the House of Representatives at Harrisburg in 1871 was a boy who had lost both legs and who had been provided with artificial limbs by the Philadelphia Orthopaedic Hospital (at a reported cost of $170). Lobbyists know the value of such visibility. The hospital encouraged members of the Board of Public Charities to visit and witness operations. While such visits may not have appealed to the squeamish, members were reportedly impressed by the "perfect restoration" of patients.[24]

The interplay between members of the legislature and citizens interested in hospital care, both at the local and statewide level, is apparent in both the Erie and the Philadelphia cases. It was a principle heeded by many in the years ahead. The unpaid members of the Board of Public Charities were part of the same network of charitable organizations as hospital boards of trustees. These interests, joined with those of local legislators, formed a potent stimulus for hospital development. By 1875, "medical hospitals" appear as a recognized classification for charitable aid, if still relatively small in total funding. A study done for the Board of Public Charities concluded that the state had appropriated, in all, over $7 million for public benevolent institutions and private charities from the years of the Provincial government up to 1875. Of this, $1.5 million was appropriated for reformatories; $2.3 million to institutions for the deaf and dumb, blind, and feeble-minded; $2.8 million to hospitals for the insane; and $645,166.67 for seventeen "medical hospitals."[25] Most of this latter sum had been appropriated in the previous five years. The most notable exception was the sum of $70,667 appropriated for the Pennsylvania Hospital in the eighteenth century, negotiated by the canny Benjamin Franklin, but this was, in many ways, an aberration in what was to emerge as a new funding system.[26] Apart from the abortive Marine Hospital, Erie, the largest recipients were hospitals connected with medical schools in Philadelphia. Here was a challenge for other groups throughout the state—and a headache, in terms of precedent, for the legislature.

Medical Schools Take the Lead

The role of leading medical schools as expert lobbyists for state aid set a tone of respectability on charitable appropriations. In 1871, plans were underway in Philadelphia for the establishment of two large hospitals: Presbyterian Hospital and the Hospital of the University of Pennsylvania. Presbyterian Hospital, richly endowed, did not need or seek state aid.[27] But the University of Pennsylvania was immediately successful. Its spokesmen spoke eloquently before the legislature, assuring the new hospital's promises to assuage pain and to minister to the wounded and the sick, irrespective of distinctions. Under the leadership of noted physician Dr. William Pepper, then chairman of the University's Finance Committee, and of Cadwalader Biddle, secretary of the University's Board of Trustees, the University obtained $100,000 for its hospital from the legislature in 1872 and a further $100,000 in 1873. In return for the state's aid, the hospital was required to raise privately the sum of $350,000 and to maintain 200 beds free, in perpetuity, for the injured.[28] The City of Philadelphia donated the land. Governor John F. Hartranft opened the University Hospital officially in June 1874.

The University of Pennsylvania, providing educational and scientific leadership to the idea of grants-in-aid for hospitals, could draw on its previous experience in gaining state appropriations for higher education. As its hospital lobbying campaign rolled smoothly into gear—and as additional appropriations were sought from the legislature—its lessons were perceived by other institutions. Spokesmen for the new hospital were well aware of the political importance of describing the institution as providing service to the state as a whole and not merely being of local interest, of being nonsectarian at a time of deep concern about the separation of church and state, and as responding to the needs of industry, including the railroads.[29] A "Dear Doctor" letter sent to medical school alumni by the University in November 1874 urged alumni, inter alia, "earnestly and confidently to make it your special care to secure a favorable consideration of [an appropriation] from the Senator and Member of the House of Representatives from your district."[30] Thus the news of the appropriation spread to every part of the state and physicians were corralled as lobbying agents. In turn, the legislature gained powerful supporters and the gratification of supporting a worthy, scientific institution.

Good relations between the University hospital and the state, once started, continued. This was fortunate, since the hospital soon fell into financial difficulties, accumulating a debt of over $33,000 by 1890, despite "more watchful zeal" over costs, including efforts to limit the length of stay in the charity wards and the number of ward admissions, and increasing the number of paying patients.[31] However, the appointment of the astute Dr. John Shaw Billings as director of the hospital led to state money again being made available: $35,000 in 1891-92. Thus, the state was instrumental in both the founding and the bailing-out of the University's hospital. (It undoubtedly helped that Cadwalader Biddle had become general agent and secretary of the State Board of Charities, a position he held from 1884 until his death in 1906.) Billings described the new appropriation not only as "gratifying," but as pointing to further state assistance in the future.[32] Between 1871 and 1911 the Hospital of the University of Pennsylvania received $1,190,000 from the state, mostly for general maintenance. It was one of six hospitals to receive over $1 million from the state by 1911. The others were Jefferson Medical College and Medico-Chirurgical Hospital in Philadelphia, Homeopathic Medical and Surgical Hospital, Pittsburgh, Western Pennsylvania Hospital, and Allegheny General Hospital.

With state aid granted to the University of Pennsylvania, Jefferson Medical College, Philadelphia, was not slow to see the possibilities. By December 1872, Jefferson's campaign for its own new hospital was in high gear. At a meeting that month, the Jefferson Alumni Association agreed to try to raise

$250,000 by private subscription by mid-1874, and to appeal to the state for at least $100,000. Dr. Samuel Gross, Jefferson's nationally eminent surgeon, was prominent in these requests.[33] Jefferson secured its first state appropriation of $100,000 in 1873; its second $100,000 in 1878. The first surgical operation in the new hospital was performed, in August 1877, on a significant patient, politically speaking. Dr. F. F. Maury amputated the middle finger of the left hand of Malcolm Meyer, son of the Speaker of the House of the Pennsylvania legislature.[34] Both Jefferson and the University Hospital were small by modern standards; both were expensive. Jefferson's hospital, with thirty-eight occupied beds in 1878, including twenty-five paying patients, cost $188,000 to build, including ground, buildings and equipment. The state had been extremely generous.

With such precedents, other medical schools were bound to follow, and did. Women's Hospital, Philadelphia, received grants for building in the 1870s. The incorporators of a new homeopathic hospital in Philadelphia (Hahnemann) sent out a letter to well-wishers in 1880, "to ask your influence in furthering the application they are now about to make to the Legislature of the State," and the State Homeopathic Medical Association urged homeopathic physicians to lobby members of the legislature.[35] These pleas, too, were successful. Governor Robert E. Pattison was present at the cornerstone ceremonies for Hahnemann in 1884. Women's Homeopathic Hospital in Philadelphia received its first appropriation in 1885; Medical-Chirurgical Hospital in 1887; the Philadelphia Polyclinic in 1889. The process of lobbying for state aid was becoming widespread and well-accepted.

The medical schools were the most fortunate recipients of aid in these early years of state appropriations, but they were by no means the only such recipients. The seventeen hospitals that had received state aid by 1875 represented a range of sponsorship and interests.[36] The rationale for aid also varied. Money might be given for construction, for maintenance, or for general purposes. The amounts given by the state were not tied to expectations that any set amount of care would be given to the state's poor without charge, nor were there searching studies of the institution's financial needs. Many, if not most, of the new hospitals were not predominantly "charitable," if the term is limited to the provision of free care. At the University of Pennsylvania, as at Jefferson in the 1870s, a majority of inpatients were paying patients. The gauge of an appropriation was persuasiveness. Successful lobbyists were those who could convince their legislators, the Board of Charities, the governor, and the party machine that their institution was worthy of support, their purpose serious. In a sense, the state acted as if it were a modern foundation. It acknowledged the public role of hospitals and a willingness to fund requests. However, it took no responsibility for the provision of hospital care throughout the state. The legislature was a granting agency and grants were given with few strings attached. There was no incentive to plan, to control, or to regulate.

Accidents and Industry

The beginnings of a new pattern were also evident in the 1870s in the founding of hospitals in industrial strongholds outside the two major cities: in Scranton, in Wilkes-Barre, in the Lehigh Valley, in Harrisburg. State appropriations enabled small hospitals to grow from tenuous beginnings into established institutions. Lackawanna Hospital, Scranton, is a good example. It was established on a shoestring in 1871 by a group of local citizens, including the mayor and a local physician, first in an old church, then in a hotel. Originally, it had only fifteen beds; its seven physicians and surgeons cared for patients without charge. Lackawanna received its first state appropriation in 1873: $10,000 to purchase real estate, with an additional $10,000 the following year. By 1898, this hospital had received a total $232,000 from the state, allowing it to expand to sixty beds, add operating rooms and a morgue, and to open a nursing school (in 1893).[37] Lackawanna Hospital, predominantly an accident hospital in a major center for coal, iron and steel was unusual in that it became so dependent on the state that it was transferred to state ownership in 1901. [When this article was published in 1984, it was the State Hospital of the Northern Anthracite Coal Region of Pennsylvania.] But the general progression of subsidy held true for many other institutions.

Wilkes-Barre Hospital, another accident hospital (with twenty beds) was opened in 1872 through the support of local physicians, a ladies' committee, and voluntary contributions, to provide care for workers in industry and in mining, after several "thrilling occurrences" in 1870 and 1871, including a man dying with a crushed skull in the station house, since there was nowhere else to take him. This small hospital received its first $5,000 from the state in 1874. By 1898, this hospital had received $272,000 from the state.[38] By then, the hospital could accommodate seventy-five to one hundred patients. Its buildings commanded an extensive view across spacious, landscaped grounds; it had a separate fever building, a stable (for the ambulance), and modern steam heating. Like most of the new hospitals of the late nineteenth century, it had established a nurse training school. Like most of the other recipients of state aid, Wilkes-Barre Hospital remained a private, not-for-profit, voluntary institution.

The need for a hospital in the Lehigh Valley was discussed from 1871. St. Luke's Hospital, South Bethlehem, opened in 1873; it received $58,000 from the state between 1873 and 1898.[39] Williamsport Hospital in Lycoming County, which opened in 1877, was on its fourth site by 1898, but clearly well-established. This predominantly male, surgical hospital of sixty to seventy-five patients had an ophthalmologist, a pathologist and microscopist, two resident physicians and an active outpatient clinic. State aid ($95,000 by 1898) could thus be seen to serve scientific interests.[40]

Harrisburg Hospital was opened in 1872 by a group of businessmen, and included J. Donald Cameron, son of political boss Simon Cameron, on its roster of planners. This connection undoubtedly helped to pass state legislation in 1874, during the general economic depression, which fitted Harrisburg's needs with a neatness so obvious as to be suspect. Authority was given to hospital managers in cities of more than 20,000 inhabitants to requisition county commissioners for up to $5,000 for the care of poor patients, provided the hospital had no encumbrances on its property or received no more than $5,000 a year from its endowments.[41] This legislation was declared unconstitutional in 1877 but by this time general economic conditions were improving, donations and contributions could be expected to increase, and the hospital could look forward to state appropriations.[42] For all of these hospitals, experience of state appropriations, even in the 1870s, proved that hospitals and politics do mix.

With no explicit expectation that state-aided hospitals would treat a relatively large number of patients without charge, state charity was charity to *the institution*, rather than charity to specific patients. It assumed that these hospitals were playing public roles; that they were worthy institutions in a benevolent network of social commitment. The institutions, not the state, identified the poor: that is, those who were worthy of charitable treatment. The institutions also opened their doors to pay patients. The absence of guidelines for making appropriations opened the door to any group that considered itself "worthy." Those groups with private funds, the greatest industrial accidents problem, or the most political influence, were most likely to move ahead. However, it would be misleading to imply that the demand for, and growth of, hospitals in Pennsylvania was solely the result of medical and political interests and the accident rates of modern industry. Charitable appropriations increased as well *because the money was available*, through Pennsylvania's peculiar pattern of state taxation and the sensitivity of the political system to business interests.

The Commonwealth of Pennsylvania was a pioneer in diversified corporation taxes; of $7.1 million raised by the state in 1873, $2.9 million came from railroad, canal, and other transportation companies and over $660,000 from coal, iron, mining, and manufacturing companies.[43] By 1883 corporations contributed over half of all state revenues. Moreover, not only did the state draw heavily on taxes of business, but the revenue sources of state and local government were separated to an extent unknown in other states. Local government relied largely on property taxes. Potential conflict between state and local government (i.e., competition for taxes such as property taxes) was thus reduced in Pennsylvania, compared with the situation in other states. As corporate enterprises blossomed after 1870, so did the tax money available to the state. Total state expenditures grew from less than $7 million a year in the late 1870s to over $15 million in the late 1890s. Appropriations to charity grew in tandem. State-aided hospitals were thus the beneficiaries of involuntary contributions by business.

However, accident hospitals also served corporate interests. The direct damage inflicted on workers through industrialization was evident in the state's own statistics. In 1875, in the collieries of Schuylkill County alone, there were ninety-two deaths and 308 persons maimed and injured. In the Pottsville district twenty-eight coal workers died in 1875; in Shenandoah, twenty-six; in Shamokin, thirty-eight. Swings in the economic cycle forced thousands of workers on and off the job market year by year. In 1875-76, 5,000 mechanics were reported unemployed in Philadelphia and forced to seek public charity; and there was an increasing army of tramps. Such conditions were the breeding grounds not only for anticorporate sentiment but for violent strikes and, in turn, both for sympathy for the strikers and armed suppression by the state.[44] Expenditures on hospitals could be seen as a palliative measure; partial, it is true, but representing a fair contribution from the state (and thus indirectly from the corporations) for the improvement of laboring conditions at a time when miners' wages had collapsed and struggles for unionization continued. At the very least, state aid could turn back money collected from corporations as taxation to the areas in which corporations were located, providing services that the corporations might otherwise have been advised to fund directly—but that might have been regarded by the workers as suspect.

The fact that thousands of state dollars were flowing to institutions in Philadelphia and Pittsburgh, where the interests in charities were organized and the lobbyists strong, emphasized through stark contrast the terrible medical conditions in the coal mining areas. With notable exceptions (such as in Wilkes-Barre), there was little organized private charity in these areas on to which state appropriations could be piggybacked—or even to stimulate grant requests. The coal mining industry rested, moreover, on numerous small firms that had little interest in joining in unprofitable activities. Not surprisingly, proposals appeared in the legislature in 1879 for the erection of a *state-owned* hospital for injured miners in the anthracite coal region, if only to redress the imbalance of funds flowing to hospitals across the state. One representative pointed out: "We have been paying some five hundred thousand dollars a year [in taxes on anthracite coal] for the last few years, and now we ask only sixty thousand dollars in return."[45]

While state funds were flowing into new teaching hospitals in Philadelphia, injured miners typically lacked any care whatsoever. The injured man was carried home on a jolting coal wagon or a stretcher, without first-aid, often to a chilly tenement room shared with others. Local surgeons were not only poorly trained, they were reported as unwilling to deal with some of the very injuries mines inflicted, those caused by burns and explosions.[46] Trained nurses were virtually nonexistent. Representatives from the anthracite regions were quite clear about the need for a hospital. Their arguments included the need for scientific medical skill, for professionals to give proper care, for proper shelter for the injured, saving workers' skills and corporate disability payments, and rescuing families of injured wage earners from becoming a burden on the rolls of local public assistance. Overlying all of these arguments was the natural interest of local representatives in securing state aid for the mining areas.

There was some opposition in the legislature to this first state accident hospital, and there was some question as to whether this was a local bill (i.e., not of statewide significance), whether employees in other industries, such as the iron industry or railroads, would be eligible, and which counties would be included as eligible to send patients; nevertheless, the measure was approved.[47] The first state medical and surgical hospital in Pennsylvania, at Ashland, was opened in 1883. It was understood that the reception, care, and treatment of injured persons took precedence over the care of paying patients.[48] The land (eighteen acres), donated to the state, was accessible by turnpike road from all the coal mines in the Schuylkill County area. The new hospital, described as a pleasing frame structure, sat on a commanding site upon the brow of a hill, overlooking the valley of Mahanoy Creek. Five other state general hospitals for the mining areas were to be built in the 1890s, and there were eventually to be eleven.

The role of an emergency hospital in industrialized areas can be illustrated in four cases admitted to the Ashland Hospital in 1890:

Andrew Galusky, aged thirty, injured at Shenandoah on a railway siding. Several coal cars passed over him and crushed both his legs and his right arm "into a pulp." He arrived at the hospital nine hours after the accident suffering from shock. His right arm was amputated near the shoulder and both of his legs below the knees. However, the patient died of diarrhea one month and eight days later, reportedly due to defective water closets.

Salvator Quell, aged thirty-five, laborer on a gravel train, injured near Louisburg. Several cars passed over his legs. He arrived at the hospital twelve hours after the accident in good condition, made a rapid recovery and was fitted with artificial legs. He was reported as walking "remarkably well."

Arthur G. Stickler, aged seventeen, injured in a coal mine by a trip of cars which passed over his legs. He arrived at the hospital four hours later. The legs were amputated. He made a quick recovery and was given a job as watchman at the entrance of the hospital grounds, walking with artificial legs.

Rafalle Colipatre, aged thirty-one, railroad laborer, injured by a train of coal cars which crushed both his legs. He arrived at the hospital a few hours later. His left thigh was amputated and his right leg below the knee. A good recovery was reported.[49]

By 1890, the accident hospital, whether state-owned or state-aided, was regarded as an important element of the industrial economy of Pennsylvania. Indeed, as far as state aid was concerned, the state could be seen as a small-scale partner of corporate enterprise. But the amounts spent on hospitals by the state were small when compared with the direct costs of accident and disability incurred by major industrial enterprises. By 1890, all the more important railroad companies in the state had relief associations or "friendly societies" to which employees contributed on a compulsory or voluntary basis. The Baltimore and Ohio Railroad's employees' relief association alone incurred a total of 2.4 million dollars in surgical expenses and other benefits between 1880 and 1890. The Pennsylvania Railroad in 1890 had enrolled over 24,000 employees (40 percent of all its employees); these benefits, too, included surgical attendance.[50] Where subsidy of hospitals, either state-owned or privately-owned, allowed for the provision of adequate hospital care, some of these payments might be avoided. With the acceptance of aseptic surgical techniques in the 1890s and the widespread development of nursing schools (and trained nursing staffs), such arguments were strengthened.

The voluntary accident hospitals that developed throughout the state in the 1880s and 1890s eclipsed in numerical importance the modest contributions of the state hospitals in the mining areas. But these, too, served both public and business interests. Typically, the voluntary hospitals were sponsored by business and other influential leaders, by women's groups, by physicians, and sometimes by groups of employees. Altoona Hospital, for example, received regular contributions from 1888 from employees of the machine and car shops of the Pennsylvania Railroad. Columbia Hospital was developed in the 1890s to serve railroad employees. McKeesport Hospital was established through pressures from the Board of Trade to provide care for the injured in railroads and in coal mines in the area. Oil City Hospital followed a terrible fire and flood in 1892, which necessitated the opening of rooms for patients in a vacant building and the employment of ladies of the "best families of Oil City" to nurse the accident cases. Phoenixville Hospital received its first money at a meeting of the Johnstown Flood Relief Association of 1889.[51] All of these hospitals were voluntary hospitals. All were established outside the major cities of the state. Almost all of the new hospitals were beneficiaries of state aid. Typically, they accepted paying as well as charity patients. All developed into general hospitals serving both medical and surgical patients.

Politics and Principles

By 1898, there were 113 hospitals in Pennsylvania; sixty-nine of these were receiving state aid for construction, maintenance, or both.[52] Because tax money was available, Pennsylvania's hospital system was largely the product of state aid. Some of the larger institutions—including the Hospital of the University of Pennsylvania, Jefferson, Hahnemann and Medico-Chirurgical in Philadelphia, Homeopathic in Pittsburgh, Wilkes-Barre Hospital and Lackawanna Hospital, Scranton, each of which had received over $200,000 in state aid by 1898—would probably have been developed without state aid, if perhaps on a more modest basis. However, many of the smaller hospitals outside the major cities might not have been able to develop without state aid, or at least not to develop at the time, and to the extent they did. Thus, while both large and small hospitals benefited from state appropriations, a major effect was on the establishment of small hospitals throughout the state. The politics of state appropriations meant automatic interest in hospitals from representatives from every county. For everyone concerned, the appropriations process was intensely political and apparently entrenched.

The rapid expansion in state subsidy of hospitals, from a grand (cumulative) total of seventeen in 1875 to sixty-nine state-aided hospitals in 1898 alone, and on to 141 in 1910, was accomplished by a connected process of special interests and legislative drift. The expansionary hospital wishes of medical schools and other large urban institutions joined with the demands for accident hospitals by industrial and labor groups, and the righteous claims for general hospitals of civic-minded citizens. When tax funds were available, such claims were irresistible; notions of science, industry, and humanity could be linked. There was still no cohesive or comprehensive hospital policy for the state. As the increased interest in the founding of hospitals generated increasing applications for state aid, the state's role continued to be responsive rather than directive, responsive, that is, to each individual hospital request. However, from the 1870s on, there were serious reservations about state aid to private charities as a matter of principle.

Pennsylvania's Constitutional Convention Debates of 1872-73 provided a major forum for debate over state aid to private charities.[53] The resulting Constitution of 1873 was designed to curb state aid to private charities in two significant respects. Under Section 17, appropriations to private charitable institutions required a vote of two-thirds of all members elected to each house of the legislature. Section 18 forbade the granting of appropriations to any person or community, or to any denominational or sectarian institution, corporation or association. It would appear that serious barriers had been imposed on future applications for state aid in Pennsylvania, as in many other states. But appearances were deceptive. First, the machine politics of the legislature meant that virtually any appropriation favored by the party leadership could receive a two-thirds vote. Second, sectarian institutions were to reorganize their boards and claim, successfully, that they were no longer sectarian. Third, local interests insured that applications for state aid would continue to be made. While critics might continue to complain that thousands of dollars were being given to purely private hospitals with no state patients, that Philadelphia, at least, *"needs no more hospitals"*[54] and that even hospitals such as the state accident hospital at Ashland served local rather than statewide interests, state subsidies were well on the way to becoming a system.

Future patterns—and their problems—were apparent in Pennsylvania by 1880. Quite apart from the politics and traditional machinations of the legislature, and even apart from Pennsylvania's rapid industrial expansion from the 1870s, two circumstances combined to make Pennsylvania a special case. The first was the dominant role of medical schools and of leading physicians in the hierarchy of institutions in Philadelphia, and thus the state. The second and probably more significant was Pennsylvania's corporate system of taxation.

The problems of imposing order on the state-aid system were illustrated in the experiences of Robert E. Pattison, the young, reforming standard-bearer of the Democratic Party who served as governor from 1883 to 1887, in a brief change from Republican administration. Pattison was faced, in 1883, with appropriations for charitable purposes, including hospitals, other charities, and penitentiaries, amounting to over two million dollars. While he might complain that a private charity, once funded, "becomes a perpetual pensioner," the charities were serving needy individuals who might be much worse off if appropriations were turned down, and were sponsored by upright citizens.[55] There were, in short, no villains. It was difficult to find a clear-cut principle on the basis of which particular appropriations could be vetoed, once the system was in place. Thus even Pattison, a critic, signed all the bills recommended for state aid by the Board of Public Charities that year—and the majority of those not recommended.

Governor after governor vetoed part of the appropriations to charities on an ad hoc basis. With no overall plan for appropriations, the legislature tended to throw the decision to the governor. Thus, a situation could be reached where, for example, Wilkes-Barre Hospital received approval from the Board of Public Charities in 1885 for an appropriation of ten thousand dollars; the legislature appropriated twenty thousand; and the governor (Pattison) disapproved the whole.[56] Governor Beaver, who succeeded Pattison, cited lack of funds rather than questions of principle in the large cuts he made in appropriations in the late 1880s.

Political Momentum, Decisional Drift

As more groups considered founding hospitals in the 1880s and 1890s, the prospect of state aid for prospective grantees turned from a hope to an expectation. Lobbying in Harrisburg became a necessary aspect of hospital development. Hospitals were only one among many other types of charitable organization, but they were becoming increasingly important applicants for aid. By the early 1880s, the politics of appropriations had spread rapidly throughout the state.

Altoona, Blair County, then the tenth largest city in Pennsylvania, provides a good example of what was necessary. Colonel Theodore Burchfield, a member of the House of Representatives and one of the organizers of the Altoona Hospital, introduced a bill in the 1883-1884 session for an appropriation for erecting and furnishing a hospital. In March 1883, a deputation from Altoona visited Harrisburg to attend hearings of the appropriations committee. In May, the Altoona bill passed the House by 150 votes to 16, and in June it passed the Senate 41 to 1. The two-thirds rule for passage was thus easily achieved. A second deputation then went to lobby the governor (Pattison) for the bill's approval and the bill became law in July 1883. Fifteen thousand dollars was appropriated. Together with local funds of $15,000, a twenty-four-bed hospital was built, incorporating the "very best experience in hospital architecture."[57] From this time Altoona, like other towns and cities, had a vested interest in charitable appropriations—and Colonel Burchfield had demonstrated his political success.

One hospital deputation after another visited Harrisburg in the 1880s and 1890s. Ideally, the lobbyists visited the governor, the Board of Charities, and the Appropriations Committees of House and Senate. With luck a major contribution could be assured. York Hospital and Dispensary, York County, gained $7,000 in state appropriations in 1881-82 to establish a hospital, when they had only $2,000 of their own in the kitty.[58] Shenango Valley Hospital, Lawrence County, opened in 1893, cost $35,000 to build, of which $19,500 was appropriated by the state.[59] Other hospitals were less fortunate with their political clout or finesse, but if they were sensible, they tried at least.

Some proved successful in comebacks or negotiations. Pittston Hospital, Luzerne County, is a good example. The legislature approved a grant of $25,000 to Pittston Hospital in 1890, requiring only $2,000 to be raised locally; but this appropriation was vetoed by Governor Beaver. A new bill was drawn up by Pittston's representative. In 1891, the hospital gained an appropriation of $15,000, with the provision that $5,000 be secured locally. The Pennsylvania Coal Company was asked to donate the land.[60] The hospital opened, with state aid instrumental.

Excluding the University of Pennsylvania (whose hospital grant was included with the larger university appropriation), sixty-eight hospitals requested funds totaling more than one million dollars for the biennium 1897 and 1898. The largest beneficiaries of state aid were the major teaching institutions of Philadelphia and Pittsburgh. However, the most striking feature of state aid, politically, was that the tentacles of appropriations spread right across the state. Cities and towns such as Allentown, New Brighton, Carbondale, Easton, Reading, McKeesport, Meadville, York, and Sayre, with other towns and cities outside the major commercial centers, were sensitive to the voting patterns of the Appropriations Committee, and ultimately to the governor's power of veto.

Reliance on state funding spread rapidly. Allegheny General Hospital, which was to become a major beneficiary of state aid, opened in 1886 and applied almost immediately to the state for an appropriation for maintenance and to liquidate its mortgage debts.[61] Even the Cambria Iron Company, urged on by an enthusiastic company surgeon, presented a proposal to the legislature in 1885 for $15,000 for the erection of a hospital in Johnstown. The Company pledged itself to subscribe a matching amount and to agree to open the hospital to the general public. This bill passed the legislature. Governor Pattison vetoed it, but in 1886 the Company subscribed the entire amount, thus providing one of the few company-owned hospitals in the state. Virtually all other industries were able to rely on the voluntary hospitals that were springing up everywhere in the 1880s and early 1890s, or on the state accident hospitals. Cambria's hospital was probably typical of the new hospitals in the 1880s: a good-looking frame structure with a well-equipped operating room employing the "latest antiseptic methods," a modern ventilating system, a reading room for patients, a convalescent verandah with a southern exposure, rugs on the asphalt floor, and white fringed bedspreads.[62]

Criticism of charitable appropriations on grounds of principle had not, however, gone away. A critical report of a special committee of the legislature in 1891 complained that managing officials seemed to develop "almost a mania to get possession of and disburse public funds."[63] Many hospitals appeared to regard state aid as an entitlement. Harrisburg Hospital, for example, was allegedly so confident that it constructed covered ways to a nonexistent central kitchen and dining room, in the anticipation that state aid would be available for the actual building.[64] (It was.) But while the committee stated that "Charity is not a proper function of government…," accused the legislature of being "socialistic," complained about lack of fiscal standards and public accountability, and urged the state to turn over responsibility for the sick poor entirely to local government,[65] these conclusions fell on deaf ears. Hospitals had attracted a network of benevolent interest. Built on hills, in well-groomed, landscaped grounds, their wards neatly furnished and their shelves stocked with food and linens contributed by local women's committees or church groups, the hospital of the 1890s was a symbol of community pride and commitment. When Pittston Hospital was opened for public inspection in 1893, it received 8,000 curious visitors.

The state had opened six state miners' hospitals by mid-1891. These hospitals, too, engendered local pride.[66] State-owned hospitals remained, however, an aberrant example of state aid for medical and surgical care. They lacked the glamour, status, and self-justification of private charitable effort—and, outside the mining districts, the partisans for their development. The state hospital, even with its private contributions and paying patients, was still a residual institution. There was no incentive for voluntary hospitals or their physicians to lobby in favor of limiting state aid to state-owned institutions—quite the reverse—and little incentive for business to decry state aid on principle.

In any event, statements of principle, so often made in politics, were useful to ratify rather than control the Pennsylvania appropriations system. In vain, as far as Pennsylvania was concerned, might Illinois, New York, and other states outlaw state aid to private hospitals on grounds of principle. Such views could hardly jibe with those of the hospital raisers in Pennsylvania or, if they wished reelection, with those of their political representatives. The barriers imposed by the Pennsylvania constitution proved weak. While some major sectarian hospitals in the state chose not to apply for state aid—the then well-endowed Episcopal Hospital, Philadelphia, was one major case—others were beneficiaries.[67] State subsidy of sectarian hospitals in Pennsylvania was not seriously challenged until the 1920s, when the courts finally ruled it was unconstitutional.

While Pennsylvania's system of state aid was vulnerable to criticism on grounds both of practice and of principle, the coalitions in favor of aid held firm into the twentieth century. A state survey of Pennsylvania's charitable institutions in 1898 noted the development of hospitals with pride. Despite the depression years of the early 1890s, the growth had, in fact, been spectacular. German (later Lankenau) Hospital, Philadelphia, is a good example of the rapid development of large institutions. Originally opened as a Civil War hospital, this hospital was a huge, imposing structure in the 1890s, with its own artesian wells, a complete electrical plant, electric lights throughout, an elevator, and a large cellar for storing coal. Tunnels connected the engine house and the hospital. There were separate laundry buildings and a separate operating pavilion designed as a model of aseptic and antiseptic practice. The ambulance stable was connected to the hospital by electric call. There was an isolation building, a pathological museum, a mortuary with a postmortem room attached, and laboratories for urinary work, microscopical and bacteriological studies. The hospital had an accident reception room, a medical library, a hydrotherapy department (including the "needle, rain, bidet, cold and hot water, steam and dry hot air baths, and the various douches"), a specialized staff of attending physicians, and a nursing staff of forty-three sisters. Accompanying this technological splendor, the hospital stressed fresh air (it was located on a high site) and comfortable, homelike rooms for private patients, some with connecting rooms for relatives.[68]

Other urban hospitals, too, showed rapid development. Pictures chosen to illustrate the hospitals of 1898, largely of operating rooms, laboratories, and equipment, celebrated hospital medicine as modern science and technology. Gynecean Hospital in Philadelphia was described in 1898 as one of the most complete institutions for gynecology in the country.[69] Hahnemann had opened new buildings in 1890, following ceremonies attended by the "best people of Philadelphia."[70] Jefferson, also with a new hospital (for 125 patients), an amphitheatre for operations, and a thoroughly modern plant, had installed the new Roentgen X-ray apparatus, to "meet the call for the latest appliances."[71] Medico-Chirurgical Hospital in Philadelphia, which in 1886 was a small room rented on the southwest corner of Broad and Market Streets, with two beds, a few necessary appliances, and a trained nurse, had become a massive, monumental building with two projecting wings by 1898. Its amphitheatre was thought to be the best, as well as the largest in the United States and Europe.[72] This hospital, like other teaching hospitals in the city, included a large number of private rooms and thus appealed to the rich, both as donors and as patients. Again, like the other larger hospitals, it saw a substantial number of accident cases and ran extensive, specialized outpatient clinics.

By the late 1890s even small hospitals boasted well-equipped, marble-coated operating rooms, and a cadre of physicians anxious to use them. On the horizon, however, were clouds of criticism of the operation of, and necessity for, the state-aid system.

Cracks Appear in the System

Pennsylvania's state aid to charities in the 1890s was distinguished organizationally and philosophically in two important respects from the small, idiosyncratic pattern of subsidy of the early 1870s. First, with growth, subsidies had become a recognized system. Phase one of grantsmanship, the individualized, ad hoc effort, had given way in phase two to a generalized program with built-in local expectations. Second and simultaneously, as the program grew, the relationship between the state and charities subtly changed. In 1870, the legislature and the recipients of state aid saw themselves, in moral and political terms, as being on the same side of the fence. The state, granting aid to institutions, and the charities, the recipients of such aid, were part of one undifferentiated charitable network. State-owned institutions and state-subsidized private institutions were seen as differing in particulars, not in essence. Donald Cameron's role as a planner for the voluntary Harrisburg Hospital was similar to Simon Cameron's role as an organizer of the state miners' hospital at Ashland. A combination of circumstances attacked the assumption of a single set of benevolent interests just as the system itself was being roundly criticized.

The urge to differentiate private from governmental roles was evident in numerous general discussions by the 1890s, by no means limited to Pennsylvania, nor indeed to the administration of charities. Yet the Pennsylvania system continued to assume that private charities were responsive, in all senses, to the public good; in short, that the single network of benevolence continued. It was convenient to think of each worthy applicant for state aid as contributing independently to the public good, irrespective of the existence of other state-aided institutions in an area or the total outlays on charities by the state. As a result, charitable aid was a system by the 1890s but it was a system without a plan or any clear principle, maintained through the momentum of a political system characterized by expediency.

Yet the financing system in Pennsylvania, unwieldy and wasteful, was eminently vulnerable to criticism. The president of the Board of Public Charities noted rather sadly in 1894 that "this Board has no report made to it whereby it can form any idea of the amount of aid which may be given to charitable institutions..."[73] The Board, forced to make its recommendations in a vacuum, appeared both discouraged and overwhelmed. Expectations were accelerating. As they did, a routine game of budget padding developed. For example, for the biennium 1907-08 the hospitals applied to the state for $10.0 million; the Board recommended $4.5 million and the legislature appropriated $4.6 million.[74] Everybody gained from these maneuvers. Hospitals could claim they received only a fraction of what they needed; the Board of Charities could justify its existence; and the legislature could blame the Board and show itself as generous as it saw fit.

Once appropriated, there was minimal accountability for these expenditures, and no direct obligation to provide free care. An editorial in the *Medical News* of Philadelphia in 1895 pointed out that state appropriations to hospitals were far less constricted than private contributions:

When an individual endows a bed in a hospital he has a right to send anyone there, at any time, to occupy such a bed. When the state gives a grant of $50,000 it virtually endows ten beds, yet does not possess any right to such beds. The only place a poor incurable tuberculosis or other invalid needing the attention a hospital can give has a right to go is the Philadelphia [municipal] Hospital and here, alas, there is but little room for him.[75]

The editorial concluded with the by-no-means unpopular view, that "strong lobbying" by the hospitals should be resisted, that institutions receiving state aid should be under state direction, and that state subsidies should be linked with some form of state planning. But the problem was where those decisions should be made. The legislature thrived on deals made among local interests; it was not geared up to be a statewide planning agency. The governor's veto remained the most powerful vehicle for decisions, but the governor could only chip at the edges of appropriations already approved by the legislature, not recast the system altogether.

Problems at the margin are illustrated in the action by Governor Daniel Hartman Hastings in 1897 in vetoing an appropriation of $30,000 to Titusville Hospital. Before he made his decision, the governor asked a member of the Board of Charities to visit Titusville to see what, if anything, was going on. The visitor reported that nothing was happening there at all; there was no building and no fundraising effort. Moreover, there were already two hospitals in nearby Meadville, one at Corning (twenty-eight miles away) and one at Oil City (seventeen miles).[76] The governor's veto was thus quite reasonable. For the Titusville group the veto was regarded, however, as only a temporary setback. Titusville Hospital was not only established, it received $42,000 in state aid by 1911. Without a statewide plan—or any effective means or wish to enforce it in the legislature—such maneuvers were inevitable.

Over the years feeble efforts were made to tie subsidies to specific expectations. For example, when Wilkes-Barre Hospital received an appropriation of $10,000 in 1879, it was required not to discriminate in its admissions in respect to color, nationality, religion, or residence; and not to refuse a case of recent injury on account of ability to pay. (No evidence about subsequent practice is available.) More systematic concerns were even harder to address, so long as private charities were regarded as natural public agents. The statement by the State Board of Public Charities in 1879, that Philadelphia "needs no more hospitals" was to be repeated over the years, yet nothing was done.[77] The establishment of major hospitals in the 1880s exacerbated such over-bedding. In 1910 it was claimed that, at times, 3,000 hospital beds were lying vacant in the state.[78]

Nevertheless, the lack of any rule for making appropriations and the lack of any effective planning agency became increasingly frustrating to those administering the subsidies and those criticizing their effect. General Isaac Wistar, president of the State Board of Charities, resigned his office in 1902, reportedly in protest against the methods of subsidy.[79] Meanwhile, speakers at national gatherings, including the National Conference on Charities and Corrections, spoke more generally about the relationships between private institutions and government supervision. Debate ranged from the views of the "voluntarists" (my term) who would see the state as a universal provider, which must, however—in traditional fashion—leave autonomy to the voluntary institution as the "moral family of the dependents," to those of the "regulators," who were recommending the establishment of a federal bureau for charity and correction parallel to Agriculture, Education, and Labor.[80] Ideologically, the critical question was whether private charities (and their representatives) were to continue to be seen as selfless, paternalistic servers of the poor, which could be trusted to work for the public interest, or whether they were, instead, self-serving, entrepreneurial private agencies. By the early 1900s the latter view was quite frequent. A second question was public accountability. It could be held persuasively that government money ought to go only to government-operated institutions.

To those concerned with aid in Pennsylvania the immediate questions were practical rather than philosophical. The system was felt to be corrupt at all levels. It was an accepted fact that hospitals with the most political "pull" usually received the largest amounts. Hospitals receiving state aid were required to submit itemized accounts and patient statistics to the Board of Public Charities. However, cheating was allegedly common, in the form of double-counting of cases. Some hospitals "admitted" any dispensary patient who reportedly needed a whiff of ether and remained for three or four hours to recover. Philadelphia remained over-bedded yet new hospitals continued to appear, and to be given state money. Lip service was given to the idea that the purpose of state aid was to serve the poor. Yet, state aid was not given to provide medical care for the poor through clinics or dispensaries in the poorest parts of the city. When asked why this was, a member of the Board of Charities reportedly told the administrator of the Polyclinic Hospital in Philadelphia (one of the state's major beneficiaries) that "we do not approve of dispensaries." Why? "Because the doctors do not approve." Another member added, "nor the druggists...don't forget the druggists."[81] Self-interest was apparent at all levels.

Though there was not planning in the overt sense of developing norms and guidelines for hospitals in the state, there *were* clear policies apparent in the distribution of state aid. State funding served directly to stimulate voluntary hospitals over government hospital development, hospital outpatient care over independent dispensaries, and acute over chronic hospital care. For chronic cases in Philadelphia the Philadelphia General Hospital, run by the city, provided the residual place of treatment.

The management of state aid by a coalition of charity-givers and legislators responsive to dominant local interests (including members of voluntary boards and physicians) stimulated the idea of voluntarism as the proper vehicle for hospital organization in Pennsylvania. While the voluntary ideal, rather than government control, was, indeed, the dominant ideology for benevolent hospitals throughout the United States at the turn of the century, except for the provision of care to the unwanted poor, Pennsylvania's state-aid system raised the question of voluntarism in concrete form. Given the large sums of tax money involved, the state legislature could have developed a statewide program for independent dispensaries (general and special clinics) and/or hospitals for chronic diseases, both of which might have reduced the need for general hospital care. The state was, indeed, to establish a unique network of state-operated tuberculosis clinics in the early twentieth century. Quite apart from the entrenched interests involved, the tax-support system sent out a clear message: The voluntary form of organization was preferable to government provision.

Hospitals and Government in the Early Twentieth Century

When the U.S. Census conducted its first survey of benevolent institutions in 1904, Pennsylvania had 145 hospitals, excluding hospitals that were part of almshouses, psychiatric hospitals, and small private hospitals run by physicians. Among the states, only New York could claim more hospitals (194) and more hospital admissions.[82] As in other states, most of Pennsylvania's hospitals were new; many were struggling to make ends meet; and most were, in today's terms, quite small (the average size was seventy-eight beds). Of the 145 hospitals, 112 were private and nonsectarian, and another eighteen were church-associated. (The others were under state or local governments.) Here was the network of voluntary hospitals benefiting from and expecting state appropriations. It would be unrealistic to expect the trustees and staffs of the major beneficiaries to decide, on principle, that state aid should be diminished or eliminated—whatever the general rhetoric about charities or concurrent developments in other states.

In any event, the ad hoc development of state and local government aid in different states suggested no clear line of development, although it was clear that Pennsylvania stood out, together with Maryland and the District of Columbia, in its general willingness to subsidize private charities as a group. Taking public aid to all types of charities in 1903, including hospitals, homes for children, institutions for the deaf, and so on, Pennsylvania and Maryland gave more tax funds to private than to government-run institutions.

In terms of dollar amounts, the state of Pennsylvania and the city of New York spent many times the amount of tax funds on voluntary hospitals as did other jurisdictions (see Table). Since their methods of appropriations were quite different by 1900, the two areas provided a showcase, and to some a cautionary tale, for discussions on the pros and cons of subsidizing hospitals, as distinct from the more general questions of public and private charitable interests. New York City had revised its subsidy program in 1899 as part of a more general movement to centralize and enforce municipal administration. A per capita, per diem reimbursement system for eligible patients, with substantial controls, replaced the older grants process. In effect, in Rosner's phrase, the municipal administration "took control"; government was no longer willing to delegate all

Annual Subsidies to Private and Ecclesiastical Hospitals from Public Funds, Ranked by Percent of the Cost of Hospital Maintenance, by State, Selected States, 1903

	Annual subsidies from public funds	Percent of cost of maintenance of all hospitals in the state
District of Columbia	$97,286	33.4
North Carolina	23,233	24.5
Georgia	33,900	22.3
Connecticut	93,349	20.1
Pennsylvania	725,554	20.0
Alabama	13,600	17.8
Maryland	126,002	17.5
Rhode Island	38,382	16.4
Maine	33,000	14.3
New Jersey	99,449	12.4
Arizona	11,171	12.4
Mississippi	3,430	10.8
New York	712,129	10.6
Vermont	5,294	7.7
New Hampshire	8,641	7.4
Virginia	9,575	5.5
All other states	242,341	
Total	$2,276,336	8.1

Table includes all states where 5 percent or more of the cost of hospitals was met by public funds in 1903. Profit-making hospitals were not included in the census.

Source: U.S. Bureau of the Census, *Benevolent Institutions*, 1904, p. 35.

responsibility to private, voluntary institutions.[83] In New York City, buttressed by the more general movement for municipal reform, regulation was accepted to an extent unheard of (and politically impossible) in Pennsylvania.

But if Pennsylvania was a special case by virtue of its size, its large-scale commitment of state revenues to voluntary hospital development, and its block grant appropriations system, its problems were not unique. It represented in exaggerated form, for all to see, the problems of transition from an older, oligarchic view of charity as part of the governing structure of the community to one in which the charities could be seen as separate, private, vested interests.

This newer, skeptical view of hospitals as selfish, self-seeking organizations—in short, as quasi-businesses—added a new dimension to the debates over hospital appropriations in Pennsylvania. The contrast between the older view and the new is nicely encapsulated in the exchange (quoted at the beginning of this paper) at state tax hearings held in Philadelphia in 1910, between establishment lawyer Francis Shunk Brown for the legislative committee on taxation, adherent of the older view of charity, and feisty medical newsman Henry W. Cattell, watchful critic. Brown took an aristocratic, *noblesse oblige* view of charity. Cattell, in contrast, saw profit-seeking and collusion in the operation of the state-aid system. The exchange is a catechism of ideological positions:

> Q. [Brown] You can not put doctors and ministers who are engaged in the distribution of sweet charity in the line of men who are managing Standard Oil and the Sugar Trust.

> A. [Cattell] I think human nature is the same...

> Q. I can not understand it. These men and women do care for the sick and the poor, are engaged in the noble work of saving lives and fighting disease, and are giving up hours and hours of their time.

> A. And they are getting money out of the private patients in the rooms.[84]

Cattell claimed that the new clinical wing of the University of Pennsylvania Hospital, paid for by state funds, was for the benefit of the rich. He said the University would not let his accountant examine its books to see how state money was being spent, asked why every hospital needed to be equipped with an X-ray plant, and complained that the "great middle class" received no benefits from state appropriations. He raised questions, in short, of undue influence, accountability, fairness, and the democratic purposes of taxation. Such comments might have been dismissed by the patricians involved in charities as bourgeois, or even as socialistic, disaffection with the American class system, if other aspects of the appropriations process were not buttressing such views from other directions.

The president of the Pennsylvania Bar Association, hardly dismissible as socialistic, made charitable appropriations the topic of his presidential address in 1902. Estimating that between 1862 and 1901 the population of Pennsylvania had increased by 117 percent, while appropriations to charities of all kinds had increased by over 4000 percent, he argued for stopping the system of appropriations in its tracks; but, if this were impossible, for at least strengthening the supervisory power of the Board of Public Charities.[85] These two alternative approaches, abolition of the system of state aid or regulating the existing system, formed two continuing themes for debate between 1902 and the late 1920s.

The days of easy money were over. Business enterprises were eyeing the rising tax bill with distaste. In 1910, state expenditures to general and special hospitals reached $3.1 million out of a state budget of $27.7 million: 11 percent of the budget. Expenditures on hospitals for the insane added another $2.0 million, making a total commitment to hospital care of 18.5 percent of Pennsylvania's budget.[86] Hospitals, well-organized and expensive, had become the most important element in the category of charitable appropriations. It was thus logical that the hearings on corporate taxation, following discussion of a new excise tax on corporations and other organizations in 1909, should focus on how these revenues were being spent and particularly on how they were being spent on hospital care. With trade unsettled, general concern about rising local taxes, and criticism of big business in the form of regulation of the trusts on the national scene, much "unrest and anxiety" was reported among business corporations in the state at the prospect of additional taxation.[87] Inevitably came the countervailing claims from business that government programs were marked by fraud, mismanagement, and waste. The old coalitions were disappearing.

As hospitals became more important to the practice of medicine, physicians without hospital appointments were increasingly critical of state appropriations, which funneled money to their competitors with hospital appointments. It was probably true that state-aided hospitals were managed, as frequently claimed, in the interests of their attending physicians and that surgery was restricted to those on the attending staff.[88] Kitchen-table surgery was no longer the norm. As hospitals captured and expanded the surgical business, private surgical fees were captured too. Elite physicians in the medical schools and on hospital staffs could afford to favor state funding, but others raised their complaints to the philosophical plane. In supporting hospitals with closed (restricted) medical staff systems, state funding could be seen as undemocratic and monopolistic.

Recommendations made at the Philadelphia County Medical Society in 1909 reveal deeply-felt deficiencies in the existing system: Hospitals should be inspected; appropriations for maintenance should take into account what the hospital had received from private sources; appropriations should not be determined by political and social influence; a per diem system of payment might be introduced, with indigency "rather rigidly determined" (to preserve fee-paying practice where possible); no money should actually be given for maintenance until the hospital had been built (!); the state should not buy sites nor put up expensive structures, and if the buildings were sold later the state should be repaid; new hospitals should be prohibited; the House and Senate should not be allowed to raise the sum appropriated beyond that recommended by the Board of Charities; public hospitals should be properly maintained before other appropriations were made. In brief, the medical profession "should to a man insist that specious claims of philanthropy should no longer be permitted to hide from the public the fact that the State's treasury is being looted under the guise of charity." More tellingly perhaps, at a time of acknowledged surplus of both doctors and hospital beds in Pennsylvania, the "multiplication of hospitals over the country beyond the need is taking away the legitimate income of the physician and requiring the State to pay for hospital treatment of people who are able to pay for their own treatment."[89]

For progressive reformers, as well as other interested parties, the most serious and damaging criticism lay in the political process itself. With each new biennium of the legislature, a new round of lobbying and deals began. The flavor was of accommodation, if not of cooption of the legislative process by special interests. It was estimated that kickbacks to lobbyists and favors to legislators represented 10 or 15 percent of all appropriations. In the legislature, the appropriation system continued to demonstrate the dominance and inefficiency of the party machine; the two-thirds rule for appropriations to charities was still being circumvented by a tradition of general approval of almost all requests. Allegedly, the charitable appropriation system had reached such a point that it shackled the legislature on general issues.[90] But now the secrecy of Appropriations Committee decisions was criticized, as well as the expectation that all members would go along with whatever the Committee suggested. One member exclaimed, "Go along with what? Go along to let things run haphazard, galley-west and crooked."[91]

Frustration among legislators was evident. The ridiculous situation had been reached whereby a legislator felt he had no choice but to sponsor appropriation bills for his district, whatever the merits of the case. In 1913, for example, Senator McIlhenny of Philadelphia found himself introducing a bill for an appropriation to a new hospital in Germantown to which he said he was opposed, on the ground that Germantown had enough hospitals and another was unnecessary.[92] Nevertheless, the appropriation received its two-thirds approval. In the Senate, there were only two votes against.

Politically, then, the growing movement to modernize the Pennsylvania subsidy system was a product not of radical reform (as in New York City) but of general frustration with existing arrangements from private practitioners, lawyers, newsmen, legislators. But in the long run, practical economics would prove the most potent factor for change. Despite the fact that almost a third of the income of voluntary hospitals in Pennsylvania came from government sources in 1910, the days of uncritical largesse were coming to an end. The capacity (or incapacity) of government was a given. A municipal reform group in Philadelphia suggested in 1913 that state aid should be used to force hospitals to develop as quasi-public institutions, each serving a defined population.[93] Yet in a sense, the appropriation system had been too successful to force such radical changes. Hospitals throughout the state, relying to greater or lesser extent on government funds, provided potent resistance. Hospitals had, indeed, become a self-conscious industry.

Hospitals as Vested Interests

Tables of statistics circulated at the State's tax committee hearings in 1910 underlined the size of the hospital enterprise in Pennsylvania as well as the major commitment of state funds. More than 1.5 million inpatient days were given to patients without charge in the reporting hospitals. State appropriations were the equivalent of more than half of the cost of these "free days."[94] Whatever the rationale for state aid, tax money was an important part of the growing system of hospital care in Pennsylvania.

In Philadelphia, state appropriations to the medical school hospitals represented between 30 percent and 56 percent of each hospital's receipts.[95] Medical school interest in state aid continued, therefore, to be intense. But in terms of the proportion of hospital budgets, tax funds continued to be a bonanza to community hospitals outside the major cities. Thirty-five voluntary hospitals received at least half of their budgets from government sources in 1910, and most of these were small community hospitals with an annual budget of less than $50,000: hospitals like York Hospital; Mary Ann Packer Hospital, Sunbury; Nason Hospital, Roaring Spring; Coatesville Hospital; or Lock Haven Hospital. Funds to sectarian hospitals also continued. Nineteen hospitals in Pennsylvania were supervised or conducted by ecclesiastical groups in 1910, mostly by Roman Catholic sisters. Fourteen received government appropriations, totaling $218,613. The network of interest in favor of hospital appropriations thus continued to be wide: a combination of large teaching institutions that could argue scientific and educational advancement, local hospital boards, physicians jealous of the dominant role of Philadelphia and Pittsburgh, who could argue for the equitable geographical distribution of tax funds, and religious interests.

Legislators from small towns had little interest in seeing their appropriations rationalized away, in a tide of Progressivism, toward the large hospitals of Philadelphia and Pittsburgh, where the bulk of poor people were treated. Sectarian hospitals had no wish to see the enforcement of the constitutional prohibition of aid to sectarian institutions. Representatives of the larger hospitals might favor—as some did—moving from lump sum appropriations to a reimbursement system more like that of New York City, with a flat rate, per diem, tied to the number of poor patients seen; but both the Philadelphia and the small-town hospitals would have suffered substantially if state aid were withdrawn altogether. Many hospitals were in the midst of major expansion. Jefferson Medical College Hospital, for example, shifted from an annual budget of $64,000 in 1899 to $277,000 in 1916, the result of opening a completely new hospital in 1907.[96] Like many other institutions, it had come to depend on and to expect its annual state appropriation. Smaller hospitals around the state were rebuilding and expanding in the same period.

As a group, the voluntary hospitals had learned to defend their financial interests and to adapt, strategically, to the political ideology of the day. Leading hospital spokesmen were eloquent apologists for the value of state subsidies to the welfare of the state. And, as prevailing values and notions of the nature of government shifted, so did the rhetoric of the recipient institutions. By the early twentieth century, charity, once the paternalistic expression of the state as a family, was justified by the hospitals as advancing science, technology, and education. A good example is the public testimony of Dr. John M. Baldy, a canny medical reformer in the state for many years, on behalf of Gynecean Hospital, Philadelphia, a major recipient of state aid. In 1898, Baldy had praised the state appropriations for their humanitarian impulses in serving the poor: the "hundreds of poor women with suffering and death written on their faces" who, before Gynecean was established, had dragged themselves to the door of the Philadelphia Dispensary only to be told that the surgical relief they needed could only be obtained in a proper institution.[97] By 1910, the emphasis had changed from a place of relief to a place of expertise. In his testimony, Baldy now emphasized the great contributions of individual institutions in advancing the cause of medical science, particularly surgery, and in bringing down mortality rates; and he praised the state for helping to train expert surgeons for every county in the state—it "would have taken one hundred years to have accomplished what was accomplished in fifteen or twenty years had the state not stepped in with its assistance." In the main line of progressive thought, Baldy made the connections between charity, social organization, and science explicit. State funds had advanced medical science so that both rich and poor had benefited; and in so doing had stimulated an attitude of social reform and the numbers of those who were "charitably inclined."[98]

However, even Baldy, an enthusiast, could not ignore the rising tide of criticism of appropriations that existed by 1910. The most telling, because the most precise, were the complaints about the lack of any fixed rule for making charitable appropriations and the lack of any guarantee that the money would benefit needy patients. The tax committee found twenty-one hospitals receiving from the state more than they apparently spent on free treatment, while at the other end of the scale, thirteen hospitals received no appropriations, among them the Pennsylvania Hospital and Episcopal Hospital, Philadelphia. Representatives of these two hospitals at the hearings noted that they did not need state aid because of their substantial endowments. However, both hospitals were lobbying vigorously for a different form of state relief: repeal of the collateral inheritance tax on charitable bequests.[99] Virtually all hospitals in the state were thus involved in government to a greater or lesser extent.

Even among the state-aided hospitals there were, however, great variations in the amount received from the state compared with the amount spent on charity patients or the number of free days given. Hospital daily costs also varied enormously, from $0.63 to $3.70 a day. It was not clear how these figures reflected differences in clientele (case mix), in quality of care, in services, in efficiency, or in cost-accounting methods. However, it was clear that the leading hospitals would not favor a flat-rate reimbursement system applicable to all hospitals in the state; the system, for example, that was in effect for hospitals in New York City. Available cost figures did not take into account the large amount of free outpatient work being done by some hospitals, especially large city hospitals, nor whether hospitals were engaged in medical teaching. In 1910, hospital outpatients in Pennsylvania outnumbered inpatients by five to one. Medico-Chirurgical Hospital in Philadelphia reported giving nearly $30,000 worth of care to free inpatients, while receiving $60,000 from the state.[100] But it was difficult, without guidelines, to say whether this was good or bad policy, given this hospital's large outpatient service and its general functions as a teaching institution.

It was perhaps not surprising that reform in the air in 1910 circled around such administrative questions rather than shifts in the philosophy of aid. Strategically, change could only be achieved through cooperation between government and hospitals rather than through government regulation or confrontation. The joint legislative committee on taxation in 1910 approved state aid to private institutions as a general policy. However, it advised a shift to a fixed per capita, per diem reimbursement system, with a daily rate negotiated separately for each institution; and such arguments were repeated for years. The committee also called for the creation of a relatively strong Department of State Charitable Institutions to replace the Board of Public Charities. Neither recommendation was immediately successful, but the patterns of eventual reform were set. Pennsylvania achieved its State Department of Welfare in 1921, by which time several other states had already moved in this direction. (Dr. Baldy became the first director.) In 1923 the system of individually negotiated block grants was changed into a system based, loosely, on the volume of free care given in each hospital, a system more nearly approximating a per diem reimbursement system.

Meanwhile, hospitals had become a recognized bloc of vested interests, committed to tinkering with state aid as a palatable alternative to stronger changes. Most of the hospital representatives at the 1910 tax hearings favored making the mechanism through which state funds were apportioned more efficient, but not centralizing control over hospitals by the state. The general notion of efficiency was, indeed, useful as a diversionary tactic, averting more dangerous criticisms, including the abolition of state aid altogether. It was used, perhaps, as the same kind of rallying cry for reform as much later cries to rid Medicaid of fraud and abuse; neither effort challenged the basic assumptions on which the program was based.[101] Hospitals in Philadelphia organized themselves into a hospital association in 1902, providing a combined front for discussions and debates about state aid and the potential uses of state aid to control the type and distribution of beds.[102] There was little disagreement that there were too many hospitals in Pennsylvania by 1910; nor that, ideally, hospitals should be consolidated, just as industrial firms and medical schools were consolidating in the same period. The problems, then as now, lay in how bed reductions might be achieved. Major city hospitals were most willing to consider tighter regulation, but they had the most to gain from reforms designed to tie state aid to the volume of free care given, since these hospitals served most indigent patients. Thus the large Pennsylvania hospitals protected their own interests, both individually and collectively. As the beneficiaries of a massive program of grants-in-aid, it was naturally to be expected that they would. The state aid system continued, though major increases in the program were not seen after 1910.

The Role of Government Aid

By 1910 the subsidy system represented twentieth-century, rather than nineteenth-century patterns and practices. Pennsylvania's system in 1910—and the behavior of the various actors involved in policymaking—was more akin to Medicaid, its eventual descendant, than to the beginnings of the system in the 1870s.

One major shift in view between 1870 and 1910 was the idea that the purpose of state appropriations was to reimburse hospitals for care given to the indigent, rather than to support benevolent institutions *because they were benevolent*, that is, for general purposes. A second shift resulted from the differentiation and specialization characteristic of charitable institutions as a whole between 1870 and 1910. Hospitals were clearly differentiated from other charities by the turn of the century; it no longer made sense to discuss charitable subsidies to residential homes and hospitals as if they were part of a single group. The ability of hospitals to sell their services to paying patients emphasized the gap still further. How far the twentieth-century hospital was, indeed, a "charity" was a matter of confusion by the early twentieth century, as hospitals aggressively sought private patients.

Two broader circumstances were to change the context of state aid, making the year 1910, in retrospect, the high point of the hospital block grant system. Social policies are more often dictated by the pocketbook than by principle; and both these questions were financial. First, tax funds were becoming severely limited; there was increasing competition for state tax dollars and a disinclination by corporations to accept more taxation. The state ran a surplus in four of the years 1906 through 1911, years in which charitable subsidies increased. However, from 1912 through 1918, annual state expenditures remained more or less stationary, while demands for other services increased: for education, state highways, tuberculosis prevention and treatment, a new mothers' assistance program, state workers' insurance. The momentum of hospital appropriations led to no immediate decline in state aid to hospitals, but rather to the expectation of no (or minimal) increases. Voluntary and miners' hospitals together received approximately $3 million a year between 1910 and 1918, representing between 8 percent and 11 percent of the state budget, as the totals fluctuated year by year; in 1910 the percentage was the greatest. The system had reached a steady state. Governors' vetoes were thus to be taken very seriously and hospitals' lobbying changed to accommodate a no-growth grants system.

The second financial circumstance concerned the hospitals themselves. After 1910, state aid became relatively less important to hospitals as their budgets swelled with fees from private patients. Luxurious and comfortable private accommodations, gleaming operating rooms, a trained and disciplined nursing staff (the product of numerous new hospital schools), and the mystique of pathological and X-ray laboratories combined into a potent image. The modern hospital had come to stay. Appendectomies, tonsillectomies, and maternity care created a new middle-class clientele; there were almost twice as many births as deaths in Pennsylvania's state-aided hospitals by the mid-1920s.[103] In short, hospitals could be seen as private enterprises that were largely self-sustaining. In turn, the state's role was diminished to the limited purpose of contracting with private institutions, solely for the care of indigent patients.

Outside the major cities, Uniontown Hospital Association was merely the most striking example of this change, reporting over two-thirds of its income from tax funds in 1910, but 90 percent from private patients by 1924. Hospitals lacking the large endowments of, say, Episcopal Hospital, Philadelphia were heavily dependent on tax funds in the late nineteenth century. This dependence increased in the first decade of the twentieth century but then fell off rapidly as a proportion of budget as the contributions of private patients rose. By the mid-1920s, most hospitals were getting the great majority of their income from patients, with the pattern most marked outside Philadelphia and Pittsburgh. As they became increasingly proficient at selling their services in the new market for hospital medicine, hospital budgets also expanded rapidly. At Jefferson Medical College Hospital, for example, annual state subsidies remained relatively constant between 1900 and the early 1920s; but the hospital expanded steadily on all fronts. Thus, state funds represented 42 percent of that hospital's income in 1908, but only 17 percent of a much larger budget in 1923.

The hospitals were nimble and adaptive in the face of changing financial conditions: many of them dependent on state aid as they became established, but moving from dependence with the ability to attract private patients. Nevertheless, to the hospitals concerned, state aid was continuous and by no means trivial. Despite efforts to downplay the state's role in the 1920s, Pennsylvania's commitment to hospitals was well entrenched. The Department of Welfare claimed in the late 1920s that Pennsylvania had the "best known system in operation anywhere."[104] State subsidy for the indigent had come to stay.

In the process, the hospitals, individually, had shown their expertise in playing the political system and had found a collective interest and a collective voice. The committee set up by reform mayor Blankenberg in Philadelphia to develop a comprehensive plan for charities, along "modern and scientific lines," noted in 1913 that: "[A] lobby at Harrisburg or a friend in powerful political circles has been more efficacious in procuring appropriations than an epidemic."[105] While it was easy to conclude, as this committee did, that hospitals were "quasi-public institutions" that should be licensed, inspected, and audited, and that there should be hospital planning enforced through the state appropriations system, there was little danger of such proposals being put into effect. Cooperation, rather than regulation, became the order of the day. By the 1920s, the hospitals were working with the Department of Welfare to develop mutually agreeable regulations for state aid.

By 1910 there was a patchwork of government involvement in hospital care throughout the country. Maryland, Connecticut, and Maine provide other notable, if less important, examples of state subsidies to voluntary hospitals, while West Virginia, like Pennsylvania, developed state-owned hospitals in the mining areas, and the state-owned Charity Hospital in New Orleans was one of the largest hospitals in the country. Local governments within many states owned and operated county or city general hospitals. New York City was the single most prominent example, with its string of "public hospitals," but the city or county general hospital was an important focus for care of the indigent in other major cities, including Chicago, Los Angeles, and Philadelphia. San Francisco had a string of accident hospitals. Government hospitals were receiving a special emphasis by 1910 as a provider of "clinical material" for medical school teaching. For similar reasons, state university medical schools were developing their own hospitals in the early twentieth century in states such as Iowa, Colorado, and Kansas.

Many local governments also provided money to voluntary hospitals for the care of the indigent, money that in Pennsylvania was provided almost entirely by the state. Though New York City was the outstanding example in terms of the program's size, this practice was followed in cities as geographically diverse as Charleston, Wichita, Terre Haute, and Houston.[106] Yet in general, as in Pennsylvania, there was no clear-cut rationale for government involvement in hospital care. Governments became involved in different places for different reasons: to provide a hospital where there was none, to subsidize care to indigent immigrants, to respond to the demands of persuasive groups. Conversely, government might not be involved at all, because of a lack of local government interest or taxes, the existence of self-supporting voluntary hospitals, or the absence of lobbies. In most states, voluntary hospital provision was abundant by 1910 and the prospect of private fees suggested an expansionary, entrepreneurial future. Voluntary hospitals had established their place in American society as independent, if not yet indispensable, institutions.

Conclusions

Seven general conclusions flow from this study. First, the role of the state in Pennsylvania between 1870 and 1910 reflects a general ambivalence as to the proper role of government in providing social services on a massive scale. The shifting characterization of the role of the charity givers (the hospitals) and the pragmatic characteristics of decision-making, when decisions to fund were made, underline this reluctance to accept government responsibility for medical care on anything but an ad hoc, developmental, or residual basis, and the readiness to spend tax money on private organizations, however inefficient, rather than on government-owned institutions. Pennsylvania operated seven state general hospitals in the coal mining areas in 1910, but even these were to be regarded as unfortunate encumbrances by the early 1920s; the Commonwealth was still trying to divest itself of these institutions in the 1980s. Despite a growing disaffection with the way the subsidy system to voluntary hospitals worked—its lack of public accountability, its administrative sloppiness, the absence of criteria for making grants, the corruption inherent in the lobbying system—there was no major lobby for the state (or for that matter local government) to develop government-owned institutions as an alternative form for middle-class or fee-paying care.

Instead, and second, tax funds were used to stimulate and advance the private sector. In one sense the model of aid in Pennsylvania was one of corporate development; The state provided the seed-money for hospitals to become established throughout the state, in much the same way as it had been instrumental in the development of banks, communications, and industry in the late eighteenth and early nineteenth centuries. When aid was no longer necessary, it was reduced in importance, or jettisoned. However, it can also be argued that state money in Pennsylvania, drawn as it was largely from corporate taxation, was an indirect form of corporate philanthropy. Business was a major beneficiary of the new hospitals, where accident cases could be neatly parceled away under the ministrations of modern medicine. Industry was also obviously the major cause of accidents and thus seemed to have some responsibility, either directly or through the state, for caring for those harmed in its machinery.[107] Whatever the justification, state money benefited business enterprise throughout the state.

A third conclusion is that government played a large role in the establishment and early development of hospitals in at least one major U.S. state. Hospital histories of the past tend to leave the impression that voluntary hospitals were largely the products of individual philanthropy.[108] In Pennsylvania, the second largest state, this was not the prevailing pattern—and it may not have been the pattern elsewhere. Reinventing hospital history to conform to modern notions of the importance of the "voluntary idea" in America is wishful thinking. Patterns of hospital development in Pennsylvania between 1870 and 1910 show a cozy collusion among political, medical, and corporate interests.

Fourth, the nature of corporate taxation in Pennsylvania made state (rather than local government) appropriations a logical vehicle for hospital subsidy. Whether, without state aid, Pennsylvania hospitals would have been more successful, earlier, in marketing their services to private patients is a matter for speculation."[109] In 1904, Pennsylvania voluntary and government hospitals together drew 30 percent of their income from paying patients; New York, 29 percent. At the other end of the scale Illinois hospitals reported 63 percent and California 56 percent. The evidence, including the abundance of beds and the large number of vacancies by 1910, suggests that the market for private patients was less robust in Pennsylvania than, for example, in California, and that Pennsylvania, like New York, with a large industrial work force, repeated waves of unemployment, and massive immigration, had special problems that made some form of government assistance essential. But it can also be argued that the hospital enterprise was sufficiently strong to create its financial sources, and that in Pennsylvania government was a ready target.

Fifth, the subsidy system, once started, developed its own organizational momentum. The history of the state-aid system is an illustration of classic organizational behavior by legislative bodies and private agencies in response to the availability of large-scale, government grants-in-aid. The subsidies grew by a process of drift from the first ad hoc arrangements in the 1870s, which served (as it were) as "demonstration grants," to a widespread system of expectations whereby almost every institution thought it had a legitimate claim—if not a right—to state aid. As a result of this phase of development, the total cost of the appropriations escalated. The rapid expansion of the 1880s was thus followed from the 1890s by reaction in the form of charges of hospital waste and mismanagement, by attempts to slow or stop further expansion of the system, and by discussions of rules and standard setting. Reimbursement mechanisms were eventually to be modified, but the system promised to remain. While the setting is different, the process is similar to the development of the Medicare and Medicaid programs between 1965 and 1980.

A sixth conclusion is that voluntary hospitals tend to behave like other successful systems: They redefine their goals as conditions change. In 1910, with an acknowledged surplus of hospital beds in Pennsylvania, state aid could no longer be justified as institutional development. Nor, indeed, could it be claimed that hospitals were charities, in the sense that they ministered freely to the public good. By gradual metamorphosis, hospital days given to persons who could not pay, originally the responsibility of hospitals, were redefined as the responsibility of the state. Where the state provided, on average, for only half of the cost of such "free care," the state could be said to be *underpaying* hospitals, and the hospitals described as either extremely generous or on the brink of ruin if state aid did not increase. Either way, both partners to the enterprise benefited, the legislature by being apparently generous to the poor and frugal in its appropriations, since it paid for only part of the cost, the hospitals by stressing their public responsibilities.

Voluntary hospitals of the early twentieth century competed with each other openly for patients, for physicians, and for funding. With empty beds and overlapping services and with at least some hospitals giving favors to legislators in the hope of additional tax funds, hospitals could hardly be justified as serving solely the public good; many appeared to be greedy and wasteful. The move by leading hospitals toward a more efficient reimbursement system in the twentieth century was in part to counter more radical suggestions for regulation or consolidation. A concomitant of this change was the shift from the idea of subsidy as grant-in-aid to worthy institutions to that of public purchase of care in the private sector. Relationships between government and hospitals were to move, gradually, from that of principal and agent (on the same, morally superior side) to that of buyer and seller of services (on opposite sides of the counter, if not of the bargaining table). These shifts were not completed by 1910, but the ingredients were there for subsequent development.

Finally, Pennsylvania's experience shows how important politics, rather than philosophies, were to such developments. From the 1870s the lobbying system ensured that the hospitals and the legislature worked together. As Colonel William Potter of Jefferson Medical School Hospital remarked in 1910: "I have never gone before the legislature in the position of a supplicant or asking for alms, I have always gone in the feeling of mutual agreement."[110] From the 1890s on, numerous speakers at national and regional meetings of charities and corrections sought the divorce of governmental and private agencies as a matter of principle. Only with the runaway costs of state appropriations—and after decades of frustration over the political shenanigans of aid in Pennsylvania—were attempts made to differentiate the role of the state as guardian of public funds from the expansionist predilections of private agencies. As conditions changed, it became convenient for legislators to look more kindly on reform and for hospitals to cooperate with the state in moving toward grants based on the number of indigent patients, a system finally achieved in 1923. Changes in prevailing ideology followed, rather than foreordained, administrative changes.

But perhaps the most striking aspect of this history is the active role of voluntary hospitals, individually, and later, collectively, in pressing their claims for government aid. This is a study of political sensibility: the sensibility that distinguishes all successful organizations. Far from being reluctant entrants on the political scene, hospital representatives were enthusiastic and skillful lobbyists for aid. Men such as Dr. William Pepper and Dr. Samuel Gross in the 1870s and later Dr. John S. Billings and Dr. John M. Baldy were effective advocates for government aid and for cooperative public and private hospital development.

In Pennsylvania, at least, voluntary hospitals were successful political chameleons. Over the years hospital spokesmen argued that they needed subsidies for construction, for fulfilling good intentions towards the poor, for bearing the "burden" of poverty care (for which many of them were created), for being vendors of care in a medical marketplace, for support as public institutions, and as innovative private institutions, for freedom from government control. The lack of a continuing, overarching theory of state involvement in the care of dependents allowed for shifts in the image projected by hospitals as a group in order to maximize their economic opportunities. Voluntary (not-for-profit) hospitals can still be presented, as the occasion arises, as charities, as quasi-public institutions, as private enterprises. This chameleon-like ability to present themselves and to survive in a political world marked the American voluntary hospital in this period of rapid hospital development between 1870 and 1910. Hospitals showed—and still show—a remarkable ability to adjust to rapidly changing expectations.

Collectively, voluntary hospitals became a unique American enterprise. As their dependence on paying patients developed in the twentieth century, they were to shuck off the traces of their earlier dependence on government aid as if, perhaps, it had never existed. Yet, even though Pennsylvania provided in many ways a special case, government is an important strand in the development of hospital care in the United States. Voluntary hospitals could play it both ways. One enduring legacy was to be the continuing tension in the meanings of the words "public" and "private" attached to not-for-profit hospitals, which can legitimately claim that they are both public and private, and can shift the emphasis depending on the context of debate. A second is the uneasiness and uncertainty infusing debates on the goals and structures of government involvement in hospital care in the United States. Government charity to the charity-givers, nevertheless, has a long, mutually supportive history, a history to be remembered in present day debates.

In the catechism cited at the beginning of the paper, speaker A (Cattell) was correct. Those engaged in the "distribution of sweet charity"—government tax funds such as those now flowing to hospitals under Medicare and Medicaid—can be expected to behave as business operators. Maximizing subsidy or reimbursement is a rational response to the infusion of vast amounts of tax dollars into a decentralized, competitive, private system. So are engagement in politics, lobbying, and cooperation in the development of regulations. Concerns about the commercialization of the medical care system in the United States in the 1980s and since tend to ignore the fact that there are longstanding, fundamental difficulties in creating any lasting balance between private institutions and government responsibility for medical care, especially where large tax subsidies are at stake. Where money is concerned, voluntary organizations are as concerned about growth and survival as any other enterprise.

This chapter was originally published as "Sweet Charity: State Aid to Hospitals in Pennsylvania, 1870-1910," *Bulletin of the History of Medicine*, 1984, 58: 287-314, 474-495. That article, published in two parts, included additional supporting evidence and illustrative materials.

My special thanks to colleagues Thomas Parke Hughes, Michael Katz, and Charles E. Rosenberg at the University of Pennsylvania for their comments on an early draft of this paper. This study formed part of a larger study of the history of hospitals, supported by the Commonwealth Fund, by research grant 5-R01-LM03849 from the National Library of Medicine, and—in academic year 1983-84—by a Rockefeller Humanities Fellowship, and a Francis C. Wood Fellowship in the History of Medicine at the College of Physicians of Philadelphia.

Notes

1. Pennsylvania Legislature, *Report of the Joint Committee of the Senate and House of Representatives...to Consider and Report upon a Revision of the Corporation and Revenue Laws of the Commonwealth, Pursuant to Joint Resolution of May 13, 1909* (Harrisburg, 1910), pp. 343-44 (hereafter Pennsylvania Joint Committee, 1910).

2. Value of property was reported for 161 of the 184 benevolent hospitals at $50 million. This figure represented one-sixth of the total reported property value for all benevolent hospitals in the United States ($306 million). U.S. Department of Commerce, Bureau of the Census, *Benevolent Institutions* 1910 (Washington, D.C.: Government Printing Office, 1913), Table 38, p. 48.

3. For the rationale, and the social and scientific contexts, of the founding of hospitals between 1870 and 1910, see Charles E. Rosenberg, "Inward Vision and Outward Glance: The Shaping of the American Hospital, 1880-1914," *Bull. Hist. Med.*, 1979, 53: 345-91; David Rosner, *A Once Charitable Enterprise: Hospitals and Health Care in Brooklyn and New York 1885-1915* (New York: Cambridge University Press, 1982), and Morris J. Vogel, *The Invention of the Modern Hospital Boston 1870-1930* (Chicago: University of Chicago Press, 1980).

4. Figures referring to the number of state-aided hospitals throughout this paper, unless otherwise noted, are taken from the annual reports of the Pennsylvania Board of Public Charities.

5. Excluded from the data are private psychiatric hospitals (notably, Friends Hospital, Philadelphia) and an unknown number of small, private, profit-making hospitals, run as adjuncts to private medical practice. Bureau of the Census, *Benevolent Institutions* 1910. Calculated from detailed tables, pp. 342-43.

6. *Smull's Legislative Handbook* (Pennsylvania Handbook) 1910, pp. 884-85.

7. Amos G. Warner, *American Charities: A Study in Philanthropy and Economics* (New York: Thomas Y. Crowell, 1894), p. 354.

8. *Pennsylvania Archives*, Fourth Series, Papers of the Governors, edited by George Edward Reed, vol. 8, 1858-71 (Harrisburg: State of Pennsylvania, 1902), pp. 111-12. On general questions of state aid before and after the war, see Robert H. Bremner, "The Impact of the Civil War on Philanthropy and Social Welfare," *Civil War History*, 1966, 12: 293-94.

9. See Louis Hartz, *Economic Policy and Democratic Thought: Pennsylvania 1776-1860* (1948; reprinted, Chicago: Quadrangle Books, 1968). On the more general relations and distinctions between public and private institutions see John S. White-head, *The Separation of College and State, Columbia, Dartmouth, Harvard and Yale, 1776-1876* (New Haven, Conn.: Yale University Press, 1973).

10. Henry Carter, delegate, Pennsylvania, General Assembly, *Debates on the Convention to Amend the Constitution of Pennsylvania* (Harrisburg, 1872-73), vol. 5, p. 277.

11. John M. Broomall, delegate, ibid., p. 280.

12. C. R Buckalew, delegate, ibid., p. 283.

13. Pennsylvania, Legislature, *Charitable Institutions of Pennsylvania*, compiled by Alexander K Pedrick (Harrisburg: State Printer, 1898) (hereafter, Pedrick), pp. 7-8 and passim.

14. Pennsylvania, Commissioners of Public Charities, *Third Annual Report* (Harrisburg: State Printer, 1873), pp. 20-21.

15. Ibid., pp. 18, 25.

16. Bryce described the Pennsylvania and New York legislatures as "such a Witches' Sabbath of jobbing, bribing, thieving, and prostitution of power to private interest

as the world has seldom seen." James Bryce, *The American Commonwealth*, 3rd ed. (1880; reprinted, New York: Macmillan, 1895), vol. 1, p. 540. See also Frank B. Evans, *Pennsylvania Politics, 1872-1877: A Study in Political Leadership* (Harrisburg: Pennsylvania Historical and Museum Commission, 1966), p. 5.

One delegate to the constitutional convention in 1873 described an appropriation of $8,000 to "one denominational institution in the western part of this commonwealth" where only half of the amount actually reached the institution: "[S]ome gentleman who had something to do with the appropriations secured that $4,000." Logrolling was well recognized. See Pennsylvania, General Assembly, *Debates on the Convention to Amend the Constitution* (Harrisburg, 1872-73), vol. 5, pp. 272-73.

17. Cited, respectively, are Governor Andrew Gregg Curtin in his message to the Assembly, 1865, and Governor John White Geary in his message of 1871. *Pennsylvania Archives*, vol. 8, pp. 646-47, 1127.

18. Pennsylvania Board of Public Charities, *Annual Report for 1872* (Harrisburg: 1872), p. lxxiv. State population figures are from U.S. Department of Commerce, Bureau of the Census, *Historical Statistics of the United States, Colonial Times to 1957* (Washington, D.C.: 1960), Table A, pp. 123-80. See also Evans, *Pennsylvania Politics*, pp. 9-13 and passim.

19. The phrase is Bryce's, in his continuing discussion of the "depraved" politics of New York and Pennsylvania. "What is the steam that drives the machine? The steam is supplied by the political parties." *American Commonwealth*, vol. 1, p. 565.

20. Pennsylvania, *Legislative Record*, 27 March 1867, pp. 303-5.

21. Ibid., pp. 326, 329.

22. Ibid., 1 May 1879, 1432.

23. Pennsylvania Board of Commissioners of Public Charities, *Second Annual Report* (Harrisburg, 1872), pp. xl-xlii.

24. Ibid., p. lxiii.

25. "Report by Andrew J. Ourt, M.D., Statistician," Pennsylvania Board of Public Charities, *Sixth Annual Report* (Harrisburg, 1876), pp. 188-89.

26. The Pennsylvania Hospital appears to have received no further state aid. In the early 1870s, this hospital was a well-endowed, self-supporting institution, limiting the number of patients admitted on the charity list, and charging paying patients $7 a week. Pennsylvania, Board of Public Charities, *Third Annual Report* (Harrisburg, 1873), pp. 8-13. See also Benjamin Franklin, *Some Account of the Pennsylvania Hospital* (1754; reprinted, Baltimore: Johns Hopkins Press, 1954).

27. Presbyterian Hospital, incorporated in 1871, was founded as a result of the reunification of two branches of the Presbyterian church in Pennsylvania, and the wish to engage in the "evangelization of the masses." The hospital was an important symbol of the new alliance. Presbyterian Hospital in Philadelphia, *History, Charter and Bylaws* (Philadelphia: Presbyterian Hospital, 1871); Pennsylvania Board of Public Charities, *Third Annual Report*, p. 37.

28. The $350,000 was raised by early 1874. Dr. Pepper took close control of the new building, costs, and equipment, signing (and presumably checking) many of the bills on receipt. The bills themselves give a tantalizing glimpse of the 120-bed hospital, from the relative luxury of its furnishings (there were later criticisms of extravagance) to the nature of treatment: 125 jacquard quilts, ninety white quilts, ten dozen huck towels, six dozen napkins; aconite root, arnica, cinchona, ergot, gentian, ginger, Calabar bean, oil of lavender, bromide, quinine; an electromagnetic machine, electrodes for general practice. University of Pennsylvania Archives, "Hospital of the University of Pennsylvania, General," 1874.

29. That there was, indeed, local industrial interest is illustrated in the early gifts. In return for contributions one free bed was granted, each, to the Mutual Assurance Company, the Philadelphia and Wilmington and Baltimore Railroad Company, the Cambria Iron Company, and J.B. Lippincott and Company; and two, each, to the Philadelphia and Reading Railroad Company, and to Henry C. Lea. Letter from Saunders Lewis to Cadwalader Biddle, 3 June 1874. University Archives, General, 1874.

30. Alumni were urged to act in the joint cause of "humanity, the advancement of medical science, and the prosperity of your Alma Mater." In the copy in the archives Dr. Carson underlined this last point, adding a note on the "usefulness of our Alma Mater" in a handwritten addendum. Printed letter from Joseph Carson, M.D., et al. to Dear Doctor, November [no date] 1874. University Archives, General, 1874.

31. The cost problems were attributed in the 1870s to the depression and in the 1880s to the "extravagance of management in former years." Hospital of the University of Pennsylvania, *Report of the Board of Managers*, year ending 31 December 1889, p. 11; and see other years. Of the total income of $24,860 in 1890, $17,972 (72 percent) came from paying patients, but there was a continuing operating deficit. Most of the patients (60 percent) were surgical cases; and the majority of patients were male. Ibid., for 1890, p. 17.

32. Ibid., for 1891, pp. 11-12.

33. Editorial, "Jefferson College Hospital," *Medical Times*, 28 December 1872: 201-2.

34. Edward L. Bauer, *Doctors, Made in America* (Philadelphia: J. B. Lippincott, 1963), p. 168.

35. Circular letter from W. C. Keehmle et al., 20 December 1880. Cited in Thomas Lindsley Bradford, *History of the Homeopathic Medical College of Pennsylvania: The Hahnemann Medical College and Hospital of Philadelphia* (Philadelphia: Boericke and Tafel, 1898), pp. 463-64.

36. In Philadelphia, for example, Wills Eye Hospital has received $10,500 from the state by 1875; Episcopal Hospital, $10,000; German Hospital, $20,000; St Joseph's Hospital, $15,000. In Pittsburgh, the Twelfth Ward Hospital had received $19,000; the Homeopathic Hospital, $15,000; Mercy Hospital, $13,000; and the Infirmary, run by Protestant Deaconesses, $12,000.

37. Pedrick, pp. 213-14.

38. Ibid., pp. 439-40.

39. St. Luke's was started through a bequest from Asa Packer, requiring care to be given to employees of the Lehigh Valley Railroad. A Ladies' Aid committee was also important in getting the hospital underway, as it was in many of the new hospitals of the late nineteenth century.

40. Pedrick, pp. 447-51.

41. Robert Grant Crist, *Harrisburg Hospital: The First 100 Years; 1873-1973* (Harrisburg: Harrisburg Hospital, 1973), p. 21.

42. Harrisburg Hospital received its first state appropriation in 1881, and had received $68,000 by 1898. Here, too, one of the "greatest factors in the services of the management" was a Ladies' Advisory Board, established in 1888. Pedrick, pp. 149-53.

43. Pennsylvania Bureau of Statistics, *Second Annual Report* for the years 1873-1874 (Harrisburg, 1875), p. 209. See also Richard T. Ely, *Taxation in American States and Cities* (New York: Thomas Y. Crowell, 1888), pp. 452-54. U.S. Department of Commerce and Labor, *Wealth, Debt and Taxation*, Special Reports of the Census Office (Washington, D.C.: Government Printing Office, 1907), pp. 776-79; Leonard

P. Fox, *Taxation for State Purposes in Pennsylvania* (Harrisburg: State Chamber of Commerce, 1925), pp. 36, 144 and passim.

44. Pennsylvania, *Annual Report of the Secretary of Internal Affairs, Part III, Industrial Statistics 1875-76*, pp. 485-86, 815. The governor (Hartranft) estimated in 1879 that the state had paid out an average of over $104,000 per year for the suppression of labor troubles in the previous eight years. He attributed the unrest, including the Molly Maguire incidents, to class antagonisms, which could only be alleviated by elevating the lower classes. Ringing property with bayonets was "the best way to promote the spread of communistic ideas." Pennsylvania Archives, Fourth Series, Papers of the Governors, vol. IX, 1871-1883, (Harrisburg, 1902), pp. 684-85.

45. Pennsylvania, *Legislative Record*, 19 May 1879 (Mr. Welsh), p. 1889, and passim.

46. "When a man is burned, he is in no condition to be hauled to a hospital a long distance off and is in no condition even to be hauled home... I have been burned three times, and I tell you that as soon as a man is burned he becomes deathly cold—he becomes chilly. Now these men live in tenement houses where they are all confined to one room...there is no accommodation for the injured miner... I have seen dozens of them with the maggots running out of them, an inch long. I have seen them so badly burned—with their muscles and flesh and sinews so badly burned, that they were not able to move either hand or foot, and emitting a terrible smell. On this account the doctors will not take hold of them. We have not a doctor in the anthracite region that will take the case of a burned man...you never can accommodate those burned men unless you give them some kind of hospital." Ibid., p. 1889.

47. Ibid., 20 May 1879, p. 1776.

48. By legislation of 1887, priority of treatment was given, first, to workers in and about the coal mines, next to railroad employees, third to persons employed in workshops or other laboring men designated by the trustees, and finally, to paying patients. The hospital was allowed to receive donations. By 1895, the Ashland Hospital had received almost $593,000 from the state. The six miners' hospitals then in existence had received a total of $1 million. Pennsylvania, Legislature, *State Prisons, Hospitals, Soldiers Homes and Orphan Schools Controlled by the Commonwealth of Pennsylvania*, compiled by Amos H. Mylin, Auditor General (Harrisburg, 1896), Part II, pp. 159-72 (hereafter, Mylin).

49. Ibid., pp. 127-30.

50. Pennsylvania, *Annual Report of the Secretary of Internal Affairs, Part III, Industrial Statistics, 1890*, Official Document no. 10, pp. E3-5, E25-29.

51. Pedrick, pp. 29-33, 83-84, 223, 269-73, 301-4.

52. Ibid., pp. 7-8.

53. Pennsylvania, General Assembly, *Debates on the Convention to Amend the Constitution* (Harrisburg, 1872-73), vol. 5, 1873. See especially pp. 276-77, 289 and passim.

54. Pennsylvania Board of Public Charities, *Report* 1879, p. 59. Emphasis in original.

55. Pennsylvania Archives, Fourth Series, *Papers of the Governors*, vol. X, p. 188; and passim. Pattison wrote of the charitable appropriations: "Upon no other bills have I been appealed to so personally, so persistently, so pathetically, and by persons actuated by more disinterested and honorable motives." Ibid., p. 185.

56. Ibid., p. 442.

57. The Altoona organizers also leaned heavily on the Pennsylvania Railroad, which provided financial contributions and over four acres of land; the Railroad maintained

four beds in the hospital in 1891. Additional funds were also raised from 1888 by "voluntary contributions" of ten cents a month from railroad employees in the area. Other business firms also contributed. An arrangement was made with the county for an annual payment of $200 for the poor. From the beginning, therefore, this hospital (like many others of the time) was a joint venture of government and business. Pedrick, pp. 29-33.

58. York Hospital grew out of a meeting of interested persons in 1879, to establish an allopathic hospital in this rapidly growing manufacturing center. Only $2,000 had been raised by early 1881. After the first $7,000 in state funds was spent, the hospital struggled financially, but funds were resumed in 1893. Government funds were clearly essential to the hospital in these early years. Ibid., pp. 477-80.

59. This hospital, a verandahed, Victorian turreted structure, built on a rise, accommodated fifty patients by 1898, including five in private rooms. It had received $53,000 from the state by 1898. Presumably its lobbyists were influential. Ibid., pp. 413-14.

60. A picture of Pittston Hospital in 1898 shows a wooden-framed structure with verandahs, which looks like a cross between a contemporary railroad station and a clubhouse. Local contributions were almost entirely from employees of the local collieries and the railroads. By 1898 the hospital had received $58,000 from the state. The hospital housed, on average, sixteen inpatients in the 1890s. Its beautiful grounds were described as the people's only park, enjoyed by hundreds of visitors. Ibid., pp. 307-10.

61. The hospital imputed its initial financial difficulties to the "want of a sufficient number of rooms for private pay patients," and a lack of a demand for private service; potential private patients were going elsewhere. By 1898 this hospital had received $148,000 in state aid. Allegheny General Hospital, *First Annual Report*, Allegheny City, 1887, p. 4; Pedrick, p. 7.

62. Pennsylvania, *Annual Report of the Secretary of Internal Affairs for 1887, Part III, Industrial Statistics*, The Cambria Iron Company, Official Document no. 12, pp. E17-18.

63. Pennsylvania, Legislature, *Report of the Special Committee on Charities and Corrections* (Harrisburg, 1891), p. 32.

64. Ibid., p. 34. In 1889 the legislature was aiding fifty-seven charities in all, including twenty-three hospitals. Ibid., pp. 40-41.

65. Ibid., pp. 11, 12, and passim.

66. For instance, the description of the state hospital at Hazleton, as a "splendid institution," a "spacious and elegant building on the hill east of town: has two wards, twenty-four beds in each." Hazleton reportedly had received private subscriptions of $15,000, as well as state aid of $60,000 by 1893. H. C. Bradsby, ed., *History of Luzerne County* (Chicago: S. B. Nelson, 1893), p. 530.

67. The select committee of 1891 described efforts made by some sectarian institutions to circumvent the constitution as "more ingenious than praise-worthy." Pennsylvania, Legislature, *Report of the Special Committee on Charities and Corrections*, p. 15. Mercy Hospital, Pittsburgh, with its long history of public service, was able to remain a major beneficiary of the state after rearranging its ownership (originally by the Sisters of Mercy) by incorporating in 1882. It began to receive state aid again ($30,000) in 1883-84 and had received a total from the state of $123,000 by the end of 1898. It may have helped that Thomas M. Carnegie was Mercy Hospital's new president after the 1882 reorganization. Religious and other sectarian hospitals argued that they were open to all and that their purpose was public, not secret or religious. Pedrick, pp. 259-66.

68. Pedrick, pp. 113-19.
69. The hospital had forty surgical beds. It accepted both paying and non-paying patients, and had an outpatient service. Ibid., p. 130.
70. Hahnemann had raised and spent a total of $1 million on buildings by 1898, partly with state aid. Ibid., pp. 139-42.
71. Some idea of the growing technological and industrial imagery for hospitals is the report that in 1895 Jefferson's surgical department used 131 miles of muslin and 1,009 miles of gauze bandages. Ibid., p. 191.
72. Ibid.
73. Pennsylvania Board of Public Charities, *Preliminary Report for 1894* (Harrisburg, 1895), p. 36.
74. Ibid., 1907-08, p. 75; 1908-10, p. 105.
75. Editorial, "State Appropriations for Private Hospitals," *Medical News*, 1895, 46: 273-74.
76. Other similar cases were also cited. Pennsylvania Archives, Fourth Series, *Papers of the Governors, vol. XI 1891-97*, Harrisburg, 1902, pp. 197-98.
77. As note 54, supra.
78. Pennsylvania, Joint Committee 1910, p. 56.
79. Katherine H. Norris, "Reports from the States," *Proceedings of the National Conference on Charities and Corrections*, 1902, p. 93.
80. Good examples are: "The Division of Work between Public and Private Charities," Report by the Committee, ibid., 1901: 118-39; Frank A Fetter, "The Subsidizing of Private Charities," *Amer. J. Sociol.*, 1901-02, 7: 359-85; Alexander Fleisher, "State Money and Privately Managed Charities," *The Survey*, 1914, 33: 110-12; "Pennsylvania's Appropriations to Privately-Managed Charitable Institutions," *Pol. Sci. Quart.*, 1915, 30: 15-36; Robert D. Dripps, "The Policy of State Aid to Private Charities," *Proceedings of the National Conference on Charities and Corrections*, 1915: 458-73.
81. Maud Banfield, "Some Unanswered Questions of Hospital Administration in the United States," *Annals Amer. Acad. Pol. Soc. Sci.*, 1902, 20: 328-55.
82. U.S. Bureau of the Census, *Benevolent Institutions*, 1904.
83. David Rosner, "Gaining Control: Reform, Reimbursement and Politics in New York: Community Hospitals, 1890-1915," *Amer. J. Public Health*, 1980, 70: 533-42.
84. Pennsylvania Joint Committee, pp. 343-44.
85. Alexander Simpson, Jr., "President's Address," *Report of the Eighth Annual Meeting of the Pennsylvania Bar Association 1902* (Philadelphia: Pennsylvania Bar Association, 1902), pp. 5-11.
86. *Smull's Legislative Handbook*, 1910, pp. 884-85.
87. Pennsylvania Joint Committee 1910, p. 88. For example, ibid., p. 53.
89. Philadelphia County Medical Society, meeting of November 24, 1909; *New Jersey Med. J.*, 1910, 91: 666-68.
90. For some graphic descriptions see Samuel B. Scott, *State Government in Pennsylvania* (Philadelphia: Harper Press, 1917), pp. 42-43.
91. Pennsylvania, Legislative Journal, House 1913, 4343 (Mr. Allen).
92. Ibid., Senate 4358-59.
93. Committee on Municipal Charities, *Report of the Committee on Municipal Charities of Philadelphia* (Philadelphia: The Committee, 1913), p. 101, and passim.
94. Pennsylvania Joint Committee 1910, pp. 59-68.
95. U.S. Bureau of the Census, *Benevolent Institutions* 1910, pp. 346-47.
96. Jefferson Medical College Hospital, Annual Reports.
97. Pedrick, p. 139.

98. Pennsylvania Joint Committee, 1910, pp. 371-75.

99. Ibid., pp. 353, 368.

100. Ibid., p. 92.

101. For an illustrative range of views, see ibid., pp. 350-51, 680-83, 750-52.

102. There was considerable dismay when the Pennsylvania Hospital (which had no state aid) declined membership. Hospital Association of Philadelphia, *First Annual Report* for the year ending 28 October 1903.

103. Emil Frankel, *State Aided Hospitals in Pennsylvania*, Bulletin no. 25 (Harrisburg: Pennsylvania Department of Welfare, 1925), p. 39.

104. Commonwealth of Pennsylvania, *Fifth Biennial Report of the Secretary of Welfare 1929-1930* (Harrisburg, 1933), p. 12.

105. In turn, hospitals reciprocated with favors. One hospital in Philadelphia "has been turned upon occasion almost into a home for its political friends." Committee on Municipal Charities, *Report*, p. 82.

106. See S. S. Goldwater, "The Appropriation of Public Funds for the Partial Support of Voluntary Hospitals in the United States and Canada," *Trans. Amer. Hop. Assoc.*, 1912, 11: 242-94.

107. See, for example, the testimony of Judge Edwards, president of the West Side Hospital Association, arguing for a tonnage tax on coal to support charitable institutions. J. Vaughan Merrick, "The Relations of the State to Hospitals Privately Managed," *Third Annual Report of the Proceedings of the Hospital Association of Philadelphia* 1905:14.

108. For a clear impression that American voluntary hospitals were founded without government support, see Mary Risley, *The House of Healing* (London: Robert Hale, 1962), p. 158 and passim. Work by Rosner, Kingsdale, and Vogel is now rectifying this misimpression for historians of medicine; nevertheless, the impression persists among other writers about hospitals, and about voluntary hospitals in particular. See supra, note 3 and J. M. Kingsdale, "The Growth of Hospitals: An Economic History in Baltimore" (Ph.D. dissertation, University of Michigan, 1981).

109. Pennsylvania, despite all the state money flowing to its hospitals, did not outstrip other major states in providing inpatient hospital care. In 1904, for example, Pennsylvania ranked only eleventh among all states in the number of persons admitted to voluntary or government hospitals per 100,000 population. In terms of expenditures per bed, Massachusetts spent almost twice as much as Pennsylvania. State aid may have allowed costs to be shifted to capital, to outpatients, to higher fees for contractors or lower fees for private patients; we do not know. There is potentially a research project here. See U.S. Bureau of the Census, *Benevolent Institutions* 1903, p. 32.

110. Pennsylvania Joint Committee 1910, p. 277.

2

"A Poor Sort of Memory": Voluntary Hospitals and Government before the Depression

"It's a poor sort of memory that only works backwards," the Queen remarked.—Lewis Carroll [Charles L. Dodgson], Through the Looking Glass

Four largely unquestioned assumptions about voluntary, not-for-profit hospitals appear regularly—yet strangely—in the hospital journals of the early 1980s. First, voluntary hospitals are often presented as private institutions that began as self-sufficient, endowed organizations but that have become inappropriately attuned to the competitive marketplace, largely because of perverse economic and political incentives brought about through recent government regulation. The "return" of hospitals and other medical care organizations to unregulated competition is a central motif for congressional bills of the 1980s, and the idea that voluntary hospitals are, have been, and ought to be regarded as businesses resonates through the hospital literature.

Second, there appears to be a general belief that government aid to hospitals started in a big way only during the Great Depression. Thus, government's role can be seen as imposed only because of national emergency—and as only reluctantly accepted. Third, voluntary hospitals present themselves as part of a "private sector" that is clearly differentiated from a "public sector," as if these distinctions had always been well understood. Finally, there is the notion that hospitals are neophytes on the political scene. Trustees and administrators are exhorted to seek out legislators and to use available professional organizations to press for legislative or regulatory change, as if lobbying were a new, unfortunate burden of the late twentieth century.

Yet, as anyone in the health field with a long memory can attest, in important respects each of these assumptions is a myth. The history of hospitals shows a long concern about the publicness of private charitable institutions, particularly in the northeastern states. Voluntary hospitals tended to present themselves as public institutions at least up to the 1930s. The flow of government funds to voluntary hospitals has a long and venerable history. And while there were marked geographical variations in government aid to voluntary hospitals before the Depression, the appropriate relationship between government and the hospitals had been debated for decades. Hospital incorporators and officials have also long been effective lobbyists. Benjamin Franklin's account of the founding of the Pennsylvania Hospital, with a matching grant from the Provincial Assembly, stands as a model for successful lobbying by later generations.[1]

Why, then, is there this "poor sort of memory"? Why do such myths exist? We could remark, dismissively, that each generation invents its own history to meet its ideological and practical needs, and that for a "generation of competition" a history of hospitals as private-institutions-gone-awry has, obviously, much to commend it. And we could leave the matter there. Yet there are compelling reasons to reexamine both the history and the myths. This chapter begins with an overview of the historical record, to demonstrate government involvement in voluntary hospitals well before the Depression of the 1930s. It then examines more closely the different meanings of public and private that have been inherited and that haunt contemporary debate. Finally, we return to the nature and utility of myth. I shall suggest that a poor sort of memory has, in fact, only short-term benefits.

Development of Cooperative Patterns of Aid

The modern hospital, with its trained nursing staff, well-equipped laboratories, and operating room facilities, its emphasis on organization and cleanliness, and a patient clientele drawn from all social classes, dates only from the 1880s. As noted in "Sweet Charity" (chapter 1), the great growth in hospital establishment took place between the years 1880 and 1910; in the latter year there were over 4,000 hospitals in the United States, and these were catering increasingly to paying patients.[2] Nevertheless, the hospital as an institution long antedates the scientific changes in medicine of the late nineteenth century. Federal, state, and local governments had established precedents for the aid of hospitals well before the 1880s. The hospital was already a "public" institution.

In 1798 federal aid was made available to both governmental and private hospitals that served as marine hospitals under the terms of legislation for the "relief of sick and disabled seamen." Then, as now, the prospect of government funds could be a heady inducement for private groups. One of the speakers at hearings on marine hospitals in 1870 remarked that an appropriation for a hospital was "a favorite mode of starting a new town in the West, if it was anywhere on a stream or on a good sized puddle..."[3]

States were involved in subsidizing voluntary hospitals to a greater or lesser extent. Early examples are the Pennsylvania Hospital, which received 2,000 pounds from the Provincial Assembly, together with its charter, in 1751, as a matching grant contingent on an equal amount being privately subscribed; and the Massachusetts General Hospital, which was granted the Province House Estate, with authority to sell and use the proceeds, on that hospital's foundation in 1811. In 1816 Massachusetts also began to make annual grants to the Eye and Ear Infirmary, and the New England Hospital for Women and Children.[4] Such grants were not seen strictly as substitutes for government hospital provision. States were heavily involved in the provision of psychiatric hospitals, but they were not usually involved in the provision of general hospital care, although, interestingly, California did experiment with the establishment (in 1851) of short-lived state accident hospitals in the mining areas of Stockton and Sacramento.[5] Later, Pennsylvania and West Virginia were to establish state accident hospitals, and some states provided welfare medical care through the teaching hospitals of the state university system. But these were the exceptions that proved the rule. Generally, states that provided funds for voluntary general hospitals did so on a selective, ad hoc, individualized basis, responding to specific requests from influential local groups. The state of New York was unusual in having a relatively extensive subsidy scheme for hospitals and dispensaries before the Civil War, continuing to the early 1870s. After the 1870s, Pennsylvania became the outstanding example of state aid. A critical report complained that "managing officials [of voluntary hospitals] seem to develop almost a mania to get possession of and disburse public funds."[6]

Local governments established infectious disease and isolation hospitals (pest houses), necessary evils in ports and major cities, awaiting the recurring epidemics of smallpox, cholera, typhoid, and diarrhea. Counties and cities provided a substantial amount of hospital care in almshouses for those who had nowhere else to go. Some local governments participated in the founding and support of voluntary hospitals by providing land. Milwaukee, for example, donated land in the 1850s for a Roman Catholic hospital; Philadelphia, in the 1870s, for the new hospital of the University of Pennsylvania. Conversely, as the need arose, a voluntary hospital might serve a government function, acting, for example, as did Mercy Hospital, Pittsburgh, as a public pest house in major epidemics. The beginnings of today's welfare medical system were also evident. In an area where it made little sense to have two separate hospitals—a voluntary hospital for the "deserving poor," selected and admitted by volunteer trustees, and a local government hospital for the residual "indigent"—a small grant to the voluntary hospital to care for the indigent made practical sense. Similarly, in cities with large immigrant populations, such as New York City, government payments to voluntary hospitals supplemented the local governmental hospital system. Where government aid existed, its form was determined by a combination of local political conditions, commonsense, the strength of local interest groups, and the taxing structures that obtained in different states.

There are no systematic surveys of hospital financing across the United States in the nineteenth century. However, the distinguished British hospital critic Henry C. Burdett examined the income of seventeen American hospitals, mostly in the Northeast, in 1889 and 1890; his findings illustrate, at least, the range of practices with respect to government aid. Maine General Hospital received a state appropriation of $5,000 (13 percent of its income in 1890); Methodist Episcopal Hospital, New York, received both state and city money (amount unspecified); Garfield Memorial Hospital in Washington, D.C., received federal funds through congressional appropriations; Hartford Hospital, Connecticut, received $5,000 from the state (12 percent of its income), plus some additional public funds for the care of veterans; and City Hospital, Worcester, Massachusetts, received city appropriations to meet its balances. The percentage of income met by patient payments ranged from less than one percent (at the well-endowed Protestant Episcopal Hospital, Philadelphia) to over 70 percent (at the Pennsylvania Hospital and Harper Hospital, Detroit).[7] There were, in short, enormous variations. A more detailed survey of government aid in 1909, undertaken by the acknowledged "dean" of hospital administration, S. S. Goldwater, when he was superintendent of Mount Sinai Hospital, New York, listed examples of local government aid ranging, alphabetically, from Birmingham, Alabama, to Sheboygan, Wisconsin. Goldwater, presenting his findings to the annual meeting of the American Hospital Association, called his listeners' attention to the "distinctively American practice of appropriating public funds for the support of hospitals managed by private benevolent corporations."[8]

The Voluntary Hospital as a Public Institution

This "distinctively American practice" reflected, in large part, the lack of distinction between "public" and "private" functions in the development of American charitable institutions. Voluntary, not-for-profit institutions grew in the uncharted area between governmental and profit-making ventures. However, as charities they were much more akin to government than to business enterprises. For most of the nineteenth century there was little clear distinction or concern as to what fell most appropriately into the sphere of government, what into the realm of voluntary initiative. Both types of organization were assumed to serve, benevolently, the public interest. In the various programs of government subsidy, at least up to the 1890s, the good will—the "public role"—of private charitable agencies was assumed; at all levels of government, appropriations were made on a cooperative, often cozy basis. If charitable care was seen as a legitimate or necessary public function, it remained a public function whether offered in a governmental or a private facility.

As a result, for most of the nineteenth century the word "public" (as used, for example, in the phrase "public charities") meant *for* the public rather than under governmental ownership or control. The State Board of Charities in Connecticut could remark quite naturally in 1906: "There is now public hospital provision in each of the eighteen cities in the state." Assumed as "public" were many hospitals we would now call "private"; for example, the Grace and New

Haven Hospitals in New Haven, the Hartford Hospital, and St. Vincent's Roman Catholic Hospital, Bridgeport.[9] Each of these hospitals, with others, was regularly aided by the state. The term public was both independent of such aid and a rationale for its provision.

The willingness of government agencies to aid not-for-profit organizations in the nineteenth century, if only at the margin or at times of economic distress, allowed government both a responsive and a residual charitable role: responsive, that is, to claim for support from "worthy" groups, and residual in the sense of filling recognized gaps in care. Government hospitals were established where community need was self-evident and private efforts were unavailable: to safeguard the health of the merchant marine, to protect the general public from infectious diseases and contagions, to isolate and treat the mentally unfit, and to provide care and shelter to persons wanted by nobody else. Government aid to private charities, whether these were hospitals or universities, assumed a broader, if unspecified, public good, a mutual interest in charitable care, and cooperative patterns of development. In a city such as Philadelphia there were distinctions in culture, prestige, and clientele between an endowed hospital without regular government (state) aid, such as the Pennsylvania Hospital, which could pick and choose among entering patients; a voluntary hospital with state aid, such as the University of Pennsylvania Hospital, relatively free to organize itself as it saw fit but carefully attuned to the political system; and a local government hospital, such as Blockley (the Philadelphia General Hospital), which was necessarily a medical and social dumping ground for social outcasts and the morally unfit.[10] However, all were assumed to be public institutions.

Liability and Tax-Exemption

It was in this broader sense of the term "public" that not-for-profit hospitals were given legal advantages with respect to liability for injury to a patient caused by their negligence, even where much of the care given was not strictly "charitable" in the sense of being free. (Traditionally, public charities were exempt from such liability.) In the 1870s, for example, the courts held that the Massachusetts General Hospital was a public charity and thus not liable for injuries suffered by a patient—even though it required patients to pay for board according to their circumstances and type of accommodations, limited admissions so that no person individually had the right to demand admission, and let the trustees decide which patients were to be admitted.[11]

Tax-exemption also affirmed the public nature of the voluntary hospital. In Minnesota and South Carolina public hospitals were exempt from taxes on personal property under state constitutional provision.[12] Elsewhere, rulings upheld tax-exemption for nonprofit hospitals on the grounds that they were nonprofit, public charities, even where profits were made on at least some patients or services.[13] Thus, the voluntary hospital, developing an increasingly eager market of private, paying patients, was given public sanction to expand its plant, services, equipment, and endowment—not necessarily primarily, or even partly, to serve the poor. The Massachusetts General Hospital had endowments or invested property with a reported worth of $1.9 million in 1890.[14] The value of the property alone of "benevolent hospitals" (voluntary and government hospitals combined) in the United States had reached $306 million by 1910.[15]

Within the hospital the tax-exemption cases ratified the development of profit centers, allowing for what was later called cross-subsidization: the development of a surplus in some areas (in this instance, services to private patients) in order to subsidize charity care, or add to the institution's wealth through construction, purchase, or endowments. That charity, in the sense of giving services free of charge to the poor, was not the overriding public purpose of the hospital at the turn of the twentieth century is illustrated in contemporary tax-exemption cases. In one Illinois case, a hospital was upheld as tax-exempt where only 5 percent of its patients were charity patients; in another, 6 percent were county patients, but reimbursement of $7.00 a week was paid. Even the Chicago Polyclinic—where the great majority of the patients paid for at least part of their care, and where one out of seven patients paid rates at more than cost—was held by the courts to be tax-exempt: on the grounds that no one made a profit, that the hospital was open to all patients (although the nursing school was racially segregated), and that it received emergency patients from the police.[16] A pattern of mutual dependency had developed between voluntary hospitals and government agencies, on the assumption that public needs were thereby met.

Government and Hospitals at the Beginning of the Twentieth Century

Given this history, it was not surprising that a national census of benevolent (i.e., voluntary and governmental) institutions published in 1905 concluded that the hospital for the sick was becoming "more and more a public undertaking."[17] Over one million persons were admitted to government and not-for-profit general and special hospitals in 1904. Only one-fourth (24.7 percent) of these were treated in government-owned (chiefly local government) hospitals, the remainder in "ecclesiastical" (30.2 percent) and other not-for-profit institutions (45.1 percent). Outside of profit-making hospitals and almshouses, for which information is not available, the great majority of general hospital care was being given in what we now call voluntary hospitals, which were assumed to serve public ends.

Taking the hospital system as a whole, subsidies to voluntary hospitals were a relatively small part of the total picture, with total grants of $2.3 million in 1903, representing 8 percent of the total costs of hospital care in the United States. However, there were large variations. In four states (and the District of Columbia) government subsidies to private institutions represented 20 percent or more of the total cost of hospitals in the state. In contrast, in states such as Illinois, Michigan, Ohio, and Massachusetts, such aid represented less than 5 percent of the collective income of hospitals in each state. And in California,

Idaho, North Dakota, Oklahoma, Tennessee, and Utah, no government aid to hospitals was reported. While these figures should be interpreted with caution, if only because of the relatively poor state of cost-accounting in hospitals in 1903, the figures suggest a patchwork pattern of aid, more predominant in the northeastern states, and expressing decisions taken, consciously or unconsciously, about appropriate governmental and private activities.

The census takers suggested that, in some states, subsidy of voluntary hospitals was a matter of policy, an alternative to the provision of government hospitals. But the figures do not bear this out directly. Delaware, for example, with no government-owned hospitals, reported government subsidies to not-for-profit hospitals of only 1.8 percent of the total cost of hospital maintenance in 1903. In Idaho and Oklahoma, there were neither government hospitals nor government aid to voluntary hospitals.[18] It can equally well be argued that the test was not a choice of where tax money should be spent but whether it should be spent at all, irrespective of the ownership versus subsidy question. The responsive and residual roles of government meant that there was little aggressive policymaking by government agencies, although the District of Columbia may be an exception. The figures reported in 1903 are probably the result not of deliberate principle or choice but of the relative availability of tax funds, the ability of voluntary hospitals, profit-making hospitals, and almshouses to meet apparent needs without additional tax expenses, the role of lobbies and vested interests, the inertia of policymaking, and an accretion of tradition.

Some clear observations can, however, be drawn from this early census. First is the relatively important role of government funding as a whole by the early twentieth century. Besides the $2.3 million in subsidy to private hospitals, almost $6.2 million was spent on government-owned hospitals in 1903. Added together, these government funds represented 30 percent of the total hospital income of government and voluntary general and special hospitals as a group. The largest single income category was paying patients (full pay or part pay), representing 43 percent of reported income. Government funds, however, were more important than contributions and endowments. "Other income," including endowments, contributions, and loans, represented 27 percent of total hospital income.[19]

Second, the western states tended to rely more heavily on income from private patients than the eastern states. Indeed, in Utah and Oregon, reported income from private patients exceeded the total costs of hospital maintenance in 1903. In California, income from paying patients represented 56 percent of the total cost of hospital care, a much larger proportion than in New York (29 percent) or Pennsylvania (29 percent). California reported three federal hospitals and eleven city/county hospitals, including those in San Francisco and Los Angeles. However, well over 80 percent of the income of its voluntary hospitals came from paying patients in 1903. There was, in short, a striking distinction in type of income between California (and other western states) and eastern states, notably New York and Pennsylvania, with their long histories of mixed public-private hospital development. California was much more of a market system, in the terms we use today. However, in all states the idea of hospitals as public institutions remained, that is, serving the public, not liable for injuries, and tax-exempt.

A third observation is the dominant position of New York and Pennsylvania as states with the largest commitment of tax money to voluntary hospitals. In terms of dollar amounts, Pennsylvania and New York spent many times the amount of tax funds on voluntary hospitals as other states. Since their methods of appropriation were quite different, the two states provided a showcase, and to some a cautionary tale, for discussions on the pros and cons of subsidizing hospitals, as distinct from the more general questions of public versus private charitable interests.[20]

Pennsylvania and New York Compared

Pennsylvania's system of state appropriations to individual hospitals had crept into being over many years. (See supra, chapter 1.) By 1910 the state subsidized voluntary hospitals to the tune of between $2 and $3 million a year. The appropriations were lump sum subsidies, not dependent directly on how many charity patients were treated. Hospitals interested in state funding first petitioned the State Board of Charities, the formal government advisory agency (and weaker forerunner of the Department of Welfare). The applicants then lobbied members of the legislature. In turn the legislature appropriated specified amounts to different institutions, each in a separate piece of legislation. Among legislators, logrolling and back-scratching insured that most appropriations were successful. As a result, Pennsylvania's voluntary hospitals received one-third of their income from government sources in 1910. However, the lump sum or block grant nature of appropriations, earmarked individually to specific hospitals, appeared by the early 1900s to be corrupt and wasteful, and there was an increasing body of criticism.

New York City's system appeared, in contrast, a model of reform. New York City had a per diem reimbursement system for indigent patients, with standardized rates (the surgical treatment rate was $1.10 per day in 1909), implemented after a report presented to the comptroller of the City of New York, Bird S. Coler, in 1899. Coler justified the new system on grounds of efficiency; but the change from block grants to reimbursement was also a change of purpose and of power.[21] Payment on the basis of actual work done for specified indigent persons underlined the central authority of the city to contract for and to reimburse as it saw fit—and to regulate and inspect hospitals. Municipal grants to voluntary hospitals were made under the strict supervision of the City Board of Estimates and Apportionment. These regulations included accounting systems, inspections, controls on which patients would count as proper charges against the city with respect to reimbursement, and publication of amounts received in the hospitals' annual reports. New York City's subsidy system was thus accompanied by regulation to an extent unheard of in Pennsylvania.

New York City's system was also considerable. In the government hospitals of New York in 1906, Bellevue and Allied Hospitals gave 354,000 days of hospital treatment at a cost of $613,000. The second branch of the municipal service, the hospitals of the Department of Public Charities, gave 898,000 days at a cost of $798,000. But in addition, almost 998,000 days of treatment were given at the city's expense in private hospitals at a cost to the city of $699,000 (less, per capita, on average than the cost at municipal institutions). For some of the largest voluntary hospitals in New York, as in Pennsylvania, tax funds represented only a small proportion of their total budgets, but for some with large poverty populations, the city contribution was significant. The amounts received from tax funds by individual hospitals would also have been difficult, perhaps impossible, to replace by other income. In 1907, for example, Lincoln Hospital received over $62,000 from government funds, Mt. Sinai over $54,000, and Beth Israel Hospital over $27,000.[22] Pennsylvania's system of hospital appropriations might have been sloppy and corrupt. Some might have called it a "crying evil." But New York City's hospitals, too, were firmly tied to the public trough. New York's experience provided both an antidote for critics of Pennsylvania and an argument that government subsidy did not necessarily lead to graft and greed among public officials.

Whether government subsidy diminished or discouraged private contributions was, however, a matter of some debate. Critics claimed that private charities, by avoiding the stigma of poverty associated with governmental institutions, encouraged individuals to abandon their parents and their children to institutions; that indiscriminate government subsidy encouraged duplication and waste in voluntary institutions, making it impossible to unify or systematize services; and that the availability of tax funds forced charities to become lobbies with one-sided vested interests. Others believed quite simply that public services should be provided in government institutions. On the plus side of subsidy was the supposed advantage of economy. It might be less expensive to subsidize a voluntary hospital or other charity in a small town than to maintain one at public expense. The "spirit" of the private institution, including the supposed lack of the stigma of pauperism associated with government institutions, was also cited in favor of subsidies. Moreover, while the political process of subsidy might corrupt the charities, the private system was at least outside the political spoils system.[23] From the voluntary hospital's perspective, perhaps the ideal relationship was one where government guaranteed services and thus resources, but ceded further authority by recognizing the autonomy of the voluntary institution as the "moral family of dependents": in short, subsidy without regulation.

The New York City reimbursement process suggested that voluntary hospitals were no longer to be regarded as autonomous, quasi-governmental agencies, but rather as sellers of services in the medical marketplace—with government as purchaser of care for the indigent. Yet the question of whether government aid to private hospitals was justifiable recognition of these institutions as quasi-public institutions, or whether the money was to be seen as direct purchase of services for identifiable poor persons, represented potentially sharp differences in administrative relationships between government and private agencies, as well as differences in principle. It was one thing to say that tax appropriations of any sort are liable to abuse, and therefore must be carefully regulated. It was quite another to assert that government was only involved because it was, in effect, purchasing medical care for its own convenience in the private sector—and that hospitals were only involved in public services because they happened to provide such care.

Block Grants versus Reimbursement

Goldwater's study of 1909 noted government appropriations to private hospitals in thirty-five states and the District of Columbia; Canadian government agencies made similar provision in the provinces of Alberta, Manitoba, New Brunswick, Quebec, Nova Scotia, and Ontario. As superintendent of the Mount Sinai Hospital, New York, a major beneficiary of city aid, Goldwater could not be expected to recommend abolishing government aid on principle, but he did favor, with others, a more rational system of tax support. He represented a general reformist concern that abuses in the system be removed, and that regulation should encourage efficiency and the need to work towards a "useful and desirable form of social cooperation" between government and voluntary agencies.[24] Any concerns about public versus private interests were being overtaken subtly by the more general banner of "cooperation."

Even in a state like Massachusetts, with its general prohibition on direct state appropriations to private hospitals, government cooperation with private institutions could be found: in the tax-exemption granted by the state to charitable institutions; under a state law committing cities and towns to pay voluntary hospitals for public care; and in state appropriations to certain special institutions. Although often in relatively small amounts, tax funds were trickling into the voluntary hospitals, typically via local government support for a limited number of "free patients." The idea was growing that hospitals ought to be paid for charity care and that the appropriate source of this payment was government.

If hospitals were to be subsidized because their functions were public, simple block grants had some advantages. The hospitals could be seen, in effect, as acting as government's delegates or agents, and be given a budget to fulfill such purposes. But the block grant system, symbolized by the large state system in Pennsylvania, had produced a dilemma. The hospitals, scrambling for additional appropriations, were behaving competitively rather than cooperatively. As a result, Pennsylvania was criticized as a state that fostered the development of unnecessary institutions, was detrimental to private charitable work, had made the philanthropies of the state part of the political system, and was, in operational terms, "unscientific."[25] New York City's system, on the other hand, ran the risk of being over-regulated and bureaucratic.

Where amounts were relatively small, the lump sum system was clearly more efficient. Thus, the city of Birmingham, Alabama, appropriated $100 a month in 1909 for the support of five beds in St. Vincent's Hospital; Jacksonville, Florida, appropriated $5,000 per year for the support of dependent patients occupying beds in St. Luke's Hospital; Macon, Georgia, provided $6,000 to the Macon Hospital for poor city patients sent to the hospital by public officials; Wichita, Kansas, paid $600 a year to the Wichita Hospital and the St. Francis Hospital; Lexington, Kentucky, and Terre Haute and LaFayette, Indiana, also paid grants for the indigent to selected hospitals.[26] In these cases the grants represented general expectations of service to the indigent or accident victims rather than a specific amount of care. The hospital held itself in readiness as a charitable institution.

Yet the more formal reimbursement system was beginning to demonstrate its appeal, even before 1910. Other cities besides New York had developed per diem reimbursement. Detroit, for example, paid $6.00 per capita, per week, for the care of city patients receiving general medical and surgical care. (Higher rates were available for the acute care of delirium tremens and mental disease.) Portland, Oregon, paid for its poor at the rate of $1.00 per patient, per day, for city patients cared for in local private hospitals. Houston, Texas, contracted with the Sisters of Mercy to pay $0.60 per day for each patient cared for in St. Joseph's Infirmary.

Whether tax funds should be given to privately managed charities at all could be described as the "sore thumb of public administrative policy."[27] A major advantage of discussing a per diem reimbursement system was that it moved debate about government aid away from such uncomfortable questions of general principle to contractual and administrative considerations. It was one thing to discuss, in theory, the advantage of voluntary philanthropy over government institutions, in terms of the supposed superiority of voluntary effort in invention and initiative, its ability to lavish unstinted care on particular patients, and in its superior moral influence. It was entirely another question to assume that government agencies had a duty to pay for at least minimal care for the poor in private institutions and merely talk about how this should be accomplished. A per diem reimbursement system had the apparent advantage of equity, in that each institution might receive the same payment for each individual, and of accountability, since standard procedures would be worked out. In addition, abuse and fraud by patients might be more readily avoided through stringent public investigations as to who was eligible for medical assistance. Such issues were under discussion well before the 1920s.

Contemporary critics saw some advantages for hospital autonomy in a reimbursement system over grant-in-aid. In Pennsylvania, for example, the state grants system could theoretically have been used to force hospitals to close, merge, or change. Legislative hearings in Pennsylvania between 1910 and 1912, and sweeping proposals from the Municipal Charities Association of Philadelphia in 1913, suggested that such thoughts were by no means unknown. One speaker at hearings in Philadelphia in 1910—the same year the Flexner Report recommended major consolidation of medical schools—suggested that the five medical school hospitals in Philadelphia should be merged into one. Consolidation of hospitals was a recurring theme of the hearings.[28] The Municipal Charities Association suggested a planned system for hospitals in Philadelphia under which each hospital would act as the receiving hospital for a 50,000-population area. The system would be enforced where necessary through the withholding of state grants; hospitals would be controlled as a "proper governmental function."[29] One-fourth of the income of Philadelphia's hospitals was then flowing from the state. Government could thus have taken an effective proprietary interest, and voluntary hospitals become, formally, quasi-governmental. There was little danger of such radical change in Pennsylvania (or elsewhere) at the time. Nevertheless, the possibility of a per diem reimbursement system offered a possibly useful alternative for the future, because it reduced the potential threat to hospitals of government aid being used as a consolidated weapon for reform (i.e., by forcing multi-institutional hospital planning). More critically, per diem payment redefined the relationship between government and hospitals from one of principal and agent to one of buyer and seller.

At the most fundamental level, a shift in payment systems, coupled with careful decisions over who was and was not an appropriate government beneficiary (i.e., a medical assistance recipient), changed the notion of charity in the hospitals themselves. If a "free" patient could be charged to the state or (more usually outside of Pennsylvania) to local government, the patient was no longer "free" as far as the hospital was concerned. If the state or local government reimbursed on a per diem basis, what rationale was to be given for a particular per diem rate? If "free care" were regarded as something that government should reimburse, why should hospitals offer it without such reimbursement? By making the government system more efficient through a per diem reimbursement system, a wedge was to be driven between government and nongovernmental agencies. Block grants had assumed, at least, that voluntary hospitals were socially responsible and administratively capable. Decades before the implementation of Medicare and Medicaid, contractual reimbursement pushed voluntary hospitals toward the "private" end of the public-private spectrum.

Re-Definition of "Publicness"

The growing expectation by hospitals that funding ought to be available for the hospital care (but not necessarily for physician bills) of poverty patients modified the voluntary ideal. The successful community hospital of the 1920s had ceased, in many respects, to be a charity and become much more like a business. Hospital incomes rose rapidly between 1910 and the early 1920s under the impact of increasing specialization, expansion of services and equipment, and the lure of the market for private patients. Neither tax appropriations nor donations could keep up with the continuing increases in the cost of care. Baltimore was but one city where, despite increases in state and city appropriations, all the private hospitals that had provided a significant volume of free care in 1912-1913 had reduced the number of free days by 1929-1930.[30] As the percentage of private patients rose rapidly in hospitals everywhere in the United States, the poor became the residual beneficiaries of care in voluntary hospitals. Instead of being seen as the primary purposes of charities, the poor increasingly became a nuisance. Students of the hospital scene no longer described voluntary hospitals as "public" because they gave away care to the needy, but because of the source of their capital investment drawn, as it was, from a combination of "public" sources, such as donations, gifts, bequests, and taxation.[31] Concurrently, in the 1930s, "public medical services" tended to be defined as those provided under government auspices.[32]

Workers' compensation plans and contributory hospital funds added to the notion of reimbursement for hospital care. The fact that New York City's payments to voluntary hospitals for public charges represented only a fraction of the total costs of such patients was regarded by the hospitals as a serious problem, even in 1910. Workmen's compensation began in 1908 for civil employees of the federal government; by 1920 all but six states had some such legislation. While these laws had relatively little impact on hospital income, their existence, coupled with the pervasive discussions of state health insurance between 1915 and 1920, buttressed the idea that the care of unexpected, accidental sickness ought to be funded by an agency other than the hospital. Before 1900 hospitals could argue, plausibly, that they were public service institutions and thus entitled to some level of subsidy or aid. After 1900, increasingly, the more persuasive economic argument was that hospitals were private community agencies with which government might contract for services. The shift was, however, gradual, and for years there continued to be debates about the proper relationships between government and private agencies.

A national census of hospitals and dispensaries conducted in 1923 found that about 50 percent of the total patient days reported for general hospitals in the United States were attributable to paying patients, 19 percent to part-paying patients and 31 percent to "free" patients.[33] Increasingly, however, the notion of a free patient meant that the service to the individual was provided without an out-of-pocket charge, not that the hospital was expected to pay for such care out of its own endowments or donations.

Meanwhile, voluntary hospitals continued to be the focus for charitable aid by physicians, who were expected to render services free to those who could not afford to pay. The odd situation was reached that a local or state government might reimburse a hospital for care given to indigent patients only where the physician did not charge a fee. Where patients were charged a fee for their hospital care, the hospital usually had first call over the physician on collection. The voluntary hospital thus remained the locus of public service by physicians, even as the institution itself became more business-minded. The notion of the "public" hospital was thus becoming more complex.

The Sectarian Hospital as a Special Case

Sectarian institutions provide a good illustration of both the nature and the slowness of the shifts in perception and the continuing ambiguity in the term "public" institution. Government aid to sectarian institutions—whether schools, homes, or hospitals—had been a heated issue in the years immediately following the Civil War, but even then the meaning of "sectarian" was often not clear. In Pennsylvania, for example, the state constitution of 1873 denied aid to all sectarian institutions. Nevertheless, in 1919, sixty-six hospitals that could be termed denominational or sectarian were receiving aid from the state. The fuzzy terms "sectarian" and "public" were bound eventually to be called into question.

Following specific complaints, the Pennsylvania courts finally ruled, in 1921, that institutions with religious affiliations were, indeed, sectarian or denominational and thus *not* eligible for state aid—even where local boards that were largely independent of religious organizations had been established to conduct the hospital, and even though the hospital was open to all alike, without distinction to creed, color, or race, and was thus "public" in terms of accessibility to patients.[35] The legal test was whether the hospital in some way promoted the interests of a sect, whether this was the Institution of Protestant Deaconesses (Passavant Hospital, Pittsburgh), Duquesne University (renamed from Pittsburgh Catholic College of the Holy Ghost in 1911), the Jewish Hospital of Philadelphia, St. Timothy's Hospital, or the Sisters of Mercy of Crawford and Erie Counties (Dubois Hospital), all five of which were involved in related legal cases. In effect, the courts ruled that these were not "public" (or quasi-public) but "private" institutions in a limited sense. Thus the definitions of "public" and "private" became further confused.

Illustrative of the ambiguities was the resurrection of the sectarian issue in Pennsylvania only two years later, in 1923, when the state shifted its method of funding hospitals from a negotiated lump-sum grant to an amount based on the number of days of free care given. If the state was to purchase services, it seemed reasonable to suggest that it should be free to purchase that service in any hospital, sectarian or nonsectarian.[35]

The Pennsylvania courts were to disagree, in 1927: "The supervision of the distribution of the state's money to the hospitals selected, and the manner of ascertaining the amount due, effect a change of method only; there is no change in the character of payment; it is still designed to go to a sectarian institution for charitable purposes." Paying for services for the poor in voluntary hospitals was not, in short, to be compared—at least not yet—with buying a bag of flour or any other commodity from a store. State purchase arrangements were still "aid," and thus "an act of charity moving from the state, though it may be called 'hospital service,' treatment and maintenance, so many pills or so many meals."[36] Thus the prohibition against aid to sectarian hospitals remained—until the commodity approach gained general acceptance. State reimbursement of sectarian hospitals was reinstituted in Pennsylvania in the 1950s, by which time public purchase of care was seen more clearly as a method of doing business, as buying or contracting, rather than of delegating public functions to nongovernmental agencies.

Charity as a Government Responsibility

In the long run, the shift in view from charity to purchase was an inevitable accompaniment of a per diem system of government aid. Reimbursement systems linked aid directly to the recipients and the number of services given, involving government agencies in questions of eligibility and utilization, while block grants had allowed hospitals flexibility in these areas and the privilege of charging the state their deficits, including days unpaid by private patients or otherwise uncollected. Per diem methods encouraged hospitals to distinguish more sharply between private patients (private accommodations and private physicians), semi-private patients (patients in small wards, often with private physicians), and ward patients (whose physician services were usually provided free), and to charge for costs at least, wherever possible, if not to make a profit. The Pennsylvania Department of Public Welfare was not alone in encouraging hospitals in the 1920s to increase their charges to all who could pay. Between 1921 and 1924, the total income of 125 hospitals in Pennsylvania rose more than 16 percent; state appropriations dropped by 30 percent; but earnings from patients rose by 21 percent, endowment interest and income rose by 20 percent, and local grants and gifts by 176 percent.[37] Then, as later, government fostered the changing image of hospitals from agents of the state to independent contractors.

Yet despite the talk of economic self-sufficiency in the mid-1920s, the burden of the cost of care for the poor was evident, particularly in major cities. In Philadelphia and Pittsburgh, one-third of all hospital days were approved for reimbursement by the state Department of Welfare in 1924; and even in cities of under 25,000 population in Pennsylvania, almost one-fourth of all hospital days were attributable to charity patients.[38] National figures for 1922 show that 18 percent of the combined budgets of governmental and private general hospitals came from tax funds, compared with 65 percent from private patients, and the remainder from philanthropy and other sources (Table 1). Despite the rhetoric of the 1920s, and despite efforts by hospitals to reduce the number of free days, commitment of tax funds remained embedded in the system. State, county, and city appropriations to 2,570 general hospitals reporting in 1922 (three-fourths of all general hospitals) exceeded $34.5 million. There was, indeed, an increased expectation that government, local government in particular, would pay for the poor, either in government hospitals or by reimbursing voluntary hospitals.

At the same time the relative role of philanthropy had declined. The 1903 and 1922 figures are not strictly comparable; nevertheless, it is instructive to note that the census of "benevolent hospitals" in 1903 found that philanthropy represented 27 percent of hospital income for maintenance. In 1922, philanthropy represented 17 percent of the income of general hospitals. The size of the hospital industry had grown rapidly from an estimated $28 million in 1903 (for benevolent hospitals only) to almost $199 million in 1922 (for general hospitals). This increase predominantly represented an increasing number of paying patients. Hospitals were becoming financially more independent in the sense of not having to rely to a great extent on charitable or tax contributions, and more "private" in the sense of gaining most of their income from the sale of services. But tax-exemption and liability-exemption provisions of "public charities" remained.

By the early 1930s, hospitals were thus receiving conflicting messages. Perhaps it is more accurate to say that voluntary hospitals could present themselves, as circumstances arose, in guises that were essentially contradictory: that is, as institutions that were, at one and the same time, both public and private, but that were no longer to be regarded as government's agents.

The Voluntary Hospital as a Private Institution

On some occasions the term "public" hospital continued to be appealing. In 1930 (after the stock market crash) a report of an American Hospital Association (AHA) committee objected to the alleged misuse of the designation "private hospital" to cover both privately owned (i.e., proprietary, for-profit) hospitals and hospitals with general endowment. Voluntary hospitals were organizing to stake out social and political territory through clear organizational differentiation. At the other end of the scale, use of the term "public hospital" was objectionable when it was limited in meaning to government hospitals. The AHA committee was categorically firm: A "general hospital with endowments is a public institution, if it is open to the medical profession and the public."[39] This report suggested classifying nongovernmental hospitals into one class of private (i.e., for-profit) hospitals and another class of general, public, incorporated, or endowed institutions (i.e., voluntary hospitals). The three divisions became the norm: for-profit (now more commonly called investor-owned), voluntary (now not-for-profit), and governmental.

Where reimbursement was at stake, voluntary hospitals also strove to differentiate themselves from government agencies. Studies for the Committee on the Costs of Medical Care (1927-1933) reported government subsidy of voluntary health care institutions as particularly widespread in medium-sized cities such as Duluth, Phoenix, and Sioux City.[40] Newark, New Jersey, had voted to reim-

Table 1

Hospital Income by Sources, Selected Years, 1903-1958 (in Millions of Dollars)

	Source		Percentage				
			Private Payment	Tax Funds	Philanthropy and Other	Total	Total Revenue
1903	(Benevolent hospitals)[a]		43	30	27	100	28
1922	(All hospitals)[b]		59	23	18	100	259
	(General hospitals)[b]		65	18	17	100	199
1935	(All hospitals)[c]		43	47	9	100	707
	(Short-term, non-federal hospitals)[d]		62	24	14	100	430
1950	(	"	74	20	6	100	2,220
		"					
		"					
	)[d]						
1958	(	"	81	15	4	100	4,782
		"					
		"					
	)[d]						

[a] U.S. Bureau of the Census 1905. *Benevolent Institutions* 1904, Table XI, 23. Washington, D.C.: U.S. Government Printing Office.

[b] U.S. Department of Commerce, Bureau of the Census 1925. *Hospitals and Dispensaries: 1923*, 18-19. Washington, D.C.: U.S. Government Printing Office. Percentage figures are calculated form the returns of 3,470 hospitals (74 percent response rate for all hospitals) and 2,570 general hospitals (74 percent). Total income figures are for 3,524 and 2,627 hospitals, respectively.

[c] Pennell, E., Mountin, J. W., and Pearson, K. 1939. *Business Census of Hospitals*. Supplement No. 154 to *Public Health Reports*, Table 9, 22. Washington, D.C.: U.S. Government Printing Office.

[d] Klarman, H. E. 1962. "The Role of Philanthropy in Hospitals." *American Journal of Public Health* 52: 1228. The 1935 data are drawn from E. Pennell, J. W. Mountin, and K. Pearson, *Business Census of Hospitals* (Supplement No. 154 to Public Health Reports 1939).

burse local hospitals at a rate of $4.00 per day for services to charity patients, upon approval of the Municipal Department of Welfare. In the hard economic environment of 1932, the American Hospital Association recommended at its annual convention that municipal subsidies to voluntary hospitals be encouraged as a permanent source of financial support. Such developments could be conveniently seen as official recognition of the value of voluntary hospitals as private entities.

The creation of local Blue Cross hospital insurance plans during the 1930s reinforced both the idea of the "privateness" of hospitals and the idea of third-party reimbursement: Four to six million persons were enrolled in such plans by 1940.[41] The plans reinforced the spirit of voluntarism that had been bruited since at least the early 1920s—of self-help, community orientation, and nonprofit organization. With the increasing acceptance of reimbursement for the care of middle-class and indigent patients, voluntary hospitals could be presented as private institutions that had contractual relations with government—as they did with Blue Cross plans—rather than as quasi-governmental institutions. During the Depression years, the terms public and private became more distinct, although the process was by no means completed in the 1930s.

With new perceptions, new terms became accepted. The terms "voluntary hospital" and "community hospital" were widely used in the 1930s, subtly evoking 1920s distance from government, in terms of responsibility and social meaning; that is, they were not "compulsory," and they ratified and built the community spirit. Fears that voluntary hospitals might not survive the Depression fueled interest in hospital insurance and in defining the role of voluntary hospitals as distinct from, and superior to, government institutions, and thus worthy of special support. Some would even have attempted to bring back the old unquestioned lump-sum subsidy system to hospitals, with government "making up the deficits."[42] Nevertheless, the voluntary hospital survived, shored up after World War II by government aid for construction (under the Hill-Burton Act of 1946), by rapidly expanding private hospital insurance (spurred on by tax incentives to employers), and by expanded government aid for the poor through per diem arrangements. Federally assisted vendor payments became available after 1950, extended by the Kerr-Mills Act (1960) and, subsequently, Medicare and Medicaid (1965).

This more recent history has to be seen as a continuity of themes and processes inherited from the 1920s. As the older nineteenth-century spirit of delegatory charity (from government to private charities) was overtaken by a stronger stance for government in the Progressive years, so this in turn was replaced by the more market-oriented environment of the 1920s. The disasters of the Depression provided another set of actors and ideas, but the general directions were inherited. Government aid to hospitals was already, in the 1920s, an important residual element of hospital financing: Tax funds to voluntary hospitals to pay for the indigent were regarded by hospitals of the late 1920s as a reasonable expectation. The Depression may have consolidated these expectations, but it did not establish radical new directions.

History, Memory, and Myth

If, indeed, there was considerable (if scattered) government involvement in hospital care before the Depression, why do contradictory impressions now exist [in 1982]? Tunnel vision is one possible explanation. Federal programs have been so important to hospitals since 1965 that the word "government" has often been used in the limited sense of federal government. In turn, state and local government roles outside of federal programs have sometimes been dismissed as relatively trivial. Only in the 1980s, with serious discussions of state and local government responsibilities and other aspects of the "New Federalism," does the word government reassume its full meaning. Nevertheless, this explanation seems contrived and incomplete.

The simplest response to the question is lack of information. Studies of the role of government, both in terms of developing government hospitals and with respect to government aid to voluntary hospitals, are still largely nonexistent—with some notable exceptions.[43] Reliable or comparable national, historical data sources for hospitals do not exist. Studies of hospital income and expenditures usually start with 1935, when Elliott H. Pennell, Joseph W. Mountin, and Kay Pearson conducted a "business census of hospitals" for the U.S. Public Health Service. Statistics can be powerful persuaders, and this census may well suggest 1935 as a natural baseline for policymaking. If comparable figures went back to 1922, or 1903, our perspectives on historical trends in hospital financing might indeed be subtly changed. All of which is to say that perceptions are imprisoned by limited data.

But this cannot be the entire explanation. The relatively heavy commitment of tax funds to voluntary hospitals in Pennsylvania and New York City was well publicized in the contemporary hospital and social service literature. Direct expenditures on hospitals by local governments were known at the time to have increased steadily, relative to the population, between 1902 and 1927. More likely, the rhetoric of voluntarism that distinguished the 1920s spilled over into perceptions of hospitals as the embodiment of benevolent, quasi-public "privateness," assuming, in President Hoover's phrase, the "probity and devotion in service which no government can ever attain."[44] From here it is easy to assume that government had never been in the picture at all. Hence, myth conforms to the rhetoric of the day.

The Ahistorical Appeal

There is undoubtedly a reluctance, identified among historians of other sectors of the economy, to accept a large role for government in the history of the United States. Hartz, for example, has described the emergence of negative views towards the role of government in nineteenth-century business development in Pennsylvania as a pragmatic creation of the 1840s and later—after a long period of mixed public and private economic development, including the building of canals, railroads, and banking systems. Antigovernment theory rationalized the appearance and strengthening of corporate enterprise. It "mobilized democratic individualism in behalf of the corporation, it contrasted corporate operators favorably with politicians, and it cherished the judiciary as a barrier against legislative power."[45] In short, what had been a legitimate role for the state in the past had become a historical encumbrance to be jettisoned. Whitehead, describing the development of Harvard, Columbia, Dartmouth, and Yale as quasi-public institutions until the late nineteenth century—when the "private" university was largely invented—concludes that Americans try to free themselves from their own past by developing interpretations of history with which to defy that same history—and, thus, untrammeled, move ahead. "Once the visible legal connection between college and state disappeared, some men announced that the colleges and states had never been allied at all…"[46] Such arguments suggest a vigorous utility for historical myths and underline the observation that myths are obviously more than misunderstandings of fact, based on insufficient information. They also act as wish fulfillment and as functional, crafted self-portrayals of institutions and their ideologies, adapted to particular times and circumstances. The charismatic politician builds on the emotions and wishes inherent in myths. Indeed, a commonly held language—signifying apparently common beliefs—in "free enterprise," a "right to health," "competition," or whatever—is an important element in American coalition-building. Since a commonly accepted history may also serve the interests of consensus builders, it follows that views of history may be periodically readjusted to meet contemporary perspectives and/or needs.

The meaning of words, of course, changes too—like names for children, popular in one generation, old-fashioned in another, only to be rediscovered later. Once-threatening "un-American" words, such as rationing, take on a new acceptability. Other traditionally "good" words, such as "competition" or "quality," acquire new meanings. In the history of voluntary hospitals the mutations of the phrase "public" attest to the usefulness of this process to the changing scene. Voluntary hospitals have been described as public institutions at various times for many different reasons: because they were open to all; because they were not profit-making; because they were charities; because they were not liable for negligence; because they were open to scrutiny; because they were tax-exempt; because they were essential public utilities; because they relied on the general public for capital investment. Each time develops its own meanings. Present times (the early 1980s) define the phrase public hospital as virtually synonymous with a government-owned institution, thus pushing voluntary hospitals firmly into the private sector. But, of course, this meaning may change again. There is charm, as well as considerable political utility, in the lack of a single meaning. With words like public (or, for that matter, private, voluntary, or community) subject to a potentially wide range of meaning, consensus can be built and change take place under the umbrella of apparent semantic consistency.

Myths about history can also be unconsciously reinforced through accepting a restricted view of events as if it represented wider conditions. Two recent articles in leading law journals on nonprofit enterprise provide a good example of this phenomenon.[47] Both assume that the term "nonprofit" describes an institution's tax status, and that alone—thus suggesting, by omission, that tax-exemption has nothing to do with public duties or expectations. Hansmann, for example, sees private hospitals as maintaining nonprofit tax status in part as a matter of inertia and tradition, and tax-exemption as giving a potentially important competitive edge over investor-owned institutions. Clark concludes that the "legal favoritism for the non-profit form is based not on sound reasoning and hard data but on intuition." Such arguments reinforce prevailing dicta that not-for-profit hospitals are part of a private sector ranged with profit-making organizations as an alternative to, or distinct from, government intervention; and that the differences between profit and not-for-profit organizations are technical rather than substantive, matters of fiscal management rather than any difference in the purposes of the organization. Such views do not take into account the social assumptions—the values—behind not-for-profit institutions as they have developed: that is, that voluntary hospitals have strong roots as public institutions, and, indeed, that the early tax-exemption cases assumed that hospitals fulfilled public roles.

Voluntary Hospitals as Adaptive Institutions

Acceptance of the meanings and mythology of the present may channel discussion within too narrow a range of possibilities and inhibit thinking about long-term causes and effects. Voluntary hospitals of the 1980s may have more to gain from alliances with investor-owned hospitals than with asserting quasi-public functions. But what of a longer-term perspective? History has shown that the ambiguous status of voluntary hospitals as simultaneously both (and neither) public and private institutions has been useful and selectively advantageous in the past, as financial and ideological conditions have changed. There is a danger of a self-fulfilling prophecy in overeager identification with the private sector. The more "private" the institutional posture, the greater the chances in the future of private sector-government confrontations. Will we continue to have three different types of organizational form in medicine: investor-owned, not-for-profit, and government institutions? Or shall we be content with two: a basic structural dichotomy between a public (governmental) and a private (nongovernmental) sector linked through regulation and contractual obligations? Although for very different reasons, the idea of the voluntary hospital is threatened in the 1980s, just as it was in the 1930s. It seems sensible to keep all options open.

In the past, voluntary hospitals have shown remarkable survival and adaptive skills. The lack of any overarching philosophy for care of persons deemed unable to pay—and the resulting ambiguity as to the appropriate role for government intervention—has provided some political advantages for hospitals over the years. As medical care has been transformed from charitable relief to the purchase of a commodity, the voluntary hospitals have been able to present themselves, as political and economic exigencies arose, as private or public charities, as public utilities, and as businesses. How long this willingness and ability to take on public and private roles continues, in an industry whose rapid expansion appears to have stabilized (if not ended), may depend on a continued acceptance of change and uncertainty and a propensity for redefinition.

In the long term it may be advantageous for voluntary hospitals to differentiate themselves from investor-owned institutions. Competition for limited

Medicare and Medicaid reimbursements may encourage the not-for-profits of the future to rediscover or invent the image of the voluntary hospital as an altruistic, quasi-public institution, distinguished in kind from profit-making. We may see calls for block grants and other forms of government aid to replace present reimbursement systems.[48] Thus, the swings of history may continue.

This chapter was originally published as "'A Poor Sort of Memory': Voluntary Hospitals and Government before the Depression," *Milbank Memorial Fund Quarterly/Health and Society*, 1982, 60 (4): 551-584.

Notes

1. See Franklin 1754.
2. Rosen 1964; Rosenberg 1977, 1979; Vogel 1980; Kingsdale 1981; Lynaugh 1981; Rosner 1980, 1982.
3. Cited by Mustard 1945: 43.
4. Massachusetts Board of State Charities 1872: lxviii.
5. Cahn and Barry 1936: 139-141.
6. Pennsylvania Special Committee on Charities and Corrections 1891: 32. For Pennsylvania, see "Sweet Charity," supra, chapter 1.
7. Burdett 1893: 719.
8. Goldwater 1909: 243.
9. Connecticut Board of Charities 1907: 101.
10. See Rosenberg 1982.
11. *McDonald v. Massachusetts General Hospital* (1876).
12. Ely 1888: 396.
13. *Philadelphia v. Pennsylvania Hospital for the Insane* (1893); *Pennsylvania Hospital v. County of Delaware* (1895).
14. Burdett 1893: 719.
15. U.S. Department of Commerce, Bureau of the Census 1913: 22.
16. *Sisters of Third Order of St. Francis v. Board of Review of Peoria County* (1907); *Cook County Board of Review v. Provident Hospital & Training School Ass'n* (1908); *Cook County Board of Review v. Chicago Polyclinic* (1908); *German Hospital of Chicago v. Board of Review of Cook County* (1908).
17. U.S. Department of Commerce, Bureau of the Census 1905: 16-17.
18. Ibid.: 34-35.
19. Ibid.: Table XI.
20. See, for example, Fetter 1901-1902; Warner 1908; Fleisher 1914; Dripps 1915.
21. Rosner 1980.
22. Goldwater 1909: 267-273.
23. Warner 1908: 399-419.
24. Goldwater 1909: 243.
25. Fleisher 1914: 111-112.
26. Goldwater 1909.
27. Fleisher 1914: 110.
28. Pennsylvania Joint Legislative Committee 1910.
29. Philadelphia Committee on Municipal Charities 1913: 83-84.
30. Kingsdale 1981: 368.
31. Rorem 1982.
32. Davis 1937.

33. U.S. Department of Commerce, Bureau of the Census 1925: 3.
34. *Collins v. Kephart* (1921).
35. Hunt 1923: 105.
36. *Collins v. Martin* (1927): 389, 402.
37. Frankel 1925: 9.
38. Ibid.: 69.
39. Babcock 1930: 3.
40. Falk et al. 1933: 495.
41. Anderson 1975: 41, 45.
42. American Foundation 1937: 1273.
43. For example, Stern 1946; Rosner 1982.
44. Cited by Abbott 1940: 660.
45. Hartz 1948: 316.
46. Whitehead 1973: 192, 240.
47. Hansmann 1980; Clark 1980.
48. Sigmond 1982.

References

Abbott, E. 1940. *Public Assistance: American Principles and Politics.* Chicago: University of Chicago Press.

American Foundation. 1937. *American Medicine: Expert Testimony Out of Court.* New York.

Anderson, O. W. 1975. *Blue Cross since 1929: Accountability and the Public Trust.* Cambridge, Mass.: Ballinger.

Babcock, W. L. 1930. *Report of the Committee on Hospital Organization and Management.* Bulletin No. 76. Chicago: American Hospital Association.

Burdett, H. C. 1893. *Hospitals and Asylums of the World.* Vol. 3. London: Churchill.

Cahn, F., and Barry, V. 1936. *Welfare Activities of Federal, Sate, and Local Governments in California, 1850-1934.* Berkeley: University of California Press.

Clark, R. C. 1980. "Does the Nonprofit Form Fit the Hospital Industry?" *Harvard Law Journal* 93: 1417-1489.

Collins v. Kephart, 271 Pa. 428 (1921).

Collins v. Martin, 290 Pa. 388 (1927).

Connecticut Board of Charities. 1907. *Report, 1905-1906.* Public Document No. 28. New Haven: Tuttle, Moorehouse and Taylor.

Cook County Board of Review v. Provident Hospital & Training School Ass'n, 233 Il. 243 (1908).

Cook County Board of Review v. Chicago Polyclinic, 233 Il. 268 (1908).

Davis, M. M. 1937. *Public Medical Services: A Survey of Tax-Supported Medical Care in the United States.* Chicago: University of Chicago Press.

Dripps, R. D. 1915. "The Policy of State Aid to Private Charities." *Proceedings of the National Conference of Charities and Corrections* 42: 458-473.

Ely, R. T. 1888. *Taxation of the American States and Cities.* New York: Thomas Y. Crowell.

Falk, I. S., Rorem, C. R., and Ring, M. D. 1933. *The Costs of Medical Care.* Publications of the Committee on the Costs of Medical Care, No. 27. Chicago: University of Chicago Press.

Fetter, F. A. 1901-1902. "The Subsidizing of Private Charities." *American Journal of Sociology* 7: 359-385.

Fleischer, A. 1914. "State Money and Privately Managed Charities." *The Survey* 33: 110-112.

Frankel, E. 1925. *State-Aided Hospitals in Pennsylvania*. Bulletin No. 25. Harrisburg: Pennsylvania Department of Welfare.

Franklin, B. 1754. *Some Account of the Pennsylvania Hospital; from Its First Rise, to the Beginning of the Fifth Month*. Philadelphia: B. Franklin and D. Hall. (Reprinted by the Johns Hopkins Press, 1954).

German Hospital of Chicago v. Board of Review of Cook County, 233 Il. 246 (1908).

Goldwater, S. S. 1909. "The Appropriation of Public Funds for the Partial Support of Voluntary Hospitals in the United States and Canada." *Transactions of the American Hospital Association* 11: 242-294.

Hansmann, H. B. 1980. "The Role of Nonprofit Enterprise." *Yale Law Journal* 89: 835-901.

Hartz, L. 1948. *Economic Policy and Democratic Thought: Pennsylvania, 1776-1860*. Chicago: Quadrangle Books. (Reprinted 1968).

Hunt, C. W. 1923. "The Department of Public Welfare in Pennsylvania." *Annals of the American Academy of Political and Social Science*, Special Issue, *Public Welfare in the United States*. January, 105: 104-112.

Kingsdale, J. M. 1981. "The Growth of Hospitals: An Economic History in Baltimore." Unpublished Ph.D. dissertation, University of Michigan.

Lynaugh, J. E. 1981. "The Community Hospitals of Kansas City, Missouri, 1875 to 1915." Unpublished Ph.D. dissertation, University of Kansas.

Massachusetts Board of State Charities. 1872. *Eighth Annual Report*. Boston: State Printer.

McDonald v. Massachusetts General Hospital, 120 Mass. 432 (1876).

Mustard, H. S. 1945. *Government in Public Health*. New York: Commonwealth Fund.

Pennsylvania Hospital v. County of Delaware, 169 Pa. 305 (1895).

Pennsylvania Joint Legislative Committee. 1910. *Report upon a Revision of the Corporation and Revenue Laws of the Commonwealth*. Pursuant to Joint Resolution of May 13, 1909.

Pennsylvania Special Committee on Charities and Corrections. 1891. *Report*. Harrisburg: State Printer.

Philadelphia Committee on Municipal Charities. 1913. *Report*. Philadelphia.

Philadelphia v. Pennsylvania Hospital for the Insane, 154 Pa. 9 (1893).

Rorem, C. R. 1982. *A Quest for Certainty: Essays on Health Care Economics, 1930-1970*. Ann Arbor, Michigan: Health Administration Press.

Rosen, G. 1964. "The Impact of the Hospital on the Physician, the Patient and the Community." *Hospital Administration* 9: 15-33.

Rosenberg, C. E. 1977. "And Heal the Sick: The Hospital and Patient in 19th Century America." *Journal of Social History* 10: 428-447.

———. 1979. "Inward Vision and Outward Glance: The Shaping of the American Hospital, 1880-1914." *Bulletin of the History of Medicine* 53: 346-391.

———. 1982. "From Almshouse to Hospital: The Shaping of Philadelphia General Hospital." *Milbank Memorial Fund Quarterly/ Health and Society* 60 (Winter): 108-154.

Rosner, D. 1980. "Gaining Control: Reform, Reimbursement and Politics in New York's Community Hospitals, 1890-1915." *American Journal of Public Health* 7: 533-542.

———. 1982. *A Once Charitable Enterprise: Hospitals and Health Care in Brooklyn and New York, 1885-1915*. Cambridge, Mass.: Cambridge University Press.

Sigmond, R. M. 1982. "Paying for Hospital Services: Alternatives and Prospects; An Historical Perspective and Overview." Presented to the Hospital Financial Management Association, May 13-14, Washington, D.C. Unpublished.

Sisters of Third Order of St. Francis v. Board of Review of Peoria County, 231 Il. 317 (1907).

Stern, B. J. 1946. *Medical Services by Government: Local, State, and Federal.* New York: Commonwealth Fund.

Stevens, Rosemary. 1982. "Sweet Charity: Pennsylvania's Aid to Private Hospitals, 1870-1910." Unpublished at the time this article was published. See supra, chapter 1.

U.S. Department of Commerce, Bureau of the Census. 1905. *Benevolent Institutions*, 1904. Washington, D.C.: Government Printing Office.

————. 1913. *Benevolent Institutions*, 1910. Washington, D.C.: Government Printing Office.

————. 1925. *Hospitals and Dispensaries*, 1923. Washington, D.C.: Government Printing Office.

Vogel, M. J. 1980. *The Invention of the Modern Hospital: Boston, 1870-1930.* Chicago: University of Chicago Press.

Warner, A. G. 1908. *American Charities.* Second edition. New York: Thomas Crowell and Company.

Whitehead, J. S. 1973. *The Separation of College and State: Columbia, Dartmouth, Harvard, and Yale, 1776-1876.* New Haven: Yale University Press.

II. Negotiating a National Governmental Role

Introduction to Section II

The challenge for much of the twentieth century and into the twenty-first was whether a unified—that is, a national—policy for health care was desirable in the United States, and if so on what terms. Whether it was achievable was quite another question. From the progressive reformers who sought unsuccessfully to rationalize and extend payment for health care through government sponsored health insurance, state by state, between 1915 and 1920, through the failed (national) Clinton health reforms of 1993-94, that history is one of intermittent enthusiasm followed by resignation and defeat. "Dead on Arrival" is the apt title of Colin Gordon's analysis of attempts to achieve universal health insurance for the American population.

Nevertheless, the national health presence in health care grew steadily in the twentieth century. The chapters in this section come at this apparent paradox from different points of view. "Can the Government Govern?" (chapter 3) asks what happens when there is a national demand for health care that only the federal government can meet—in this case the provision of services for sick and wounded veterans of World War I. These men, many with tuberculosis or neuropsychiatric conditions, could not easily be served in the private, not-for-profit hospitals of the day. Civilian hospitals varied enormously in standards. Over and above that, the voluntary hospitals did not want pajama-wearing, cigarette-smoking, coughing, possibly swearing, sad and/or noisy long-term male residents walking around their quiet enclaves, which aimed in the 1920s at brief stays for children coming in for tonsillectomies and adenoidectomies, the drama (and hopefully the triumph) of surgery, and middle class women delivering healthy babies.

I finished *In Sickness and in Wealth* in 1988, and it was published in 1989. The establishment of veterans hospitals raised questions beyond the covers of the book. Veterans were promised benefits: They were not to rely on "charity" if and when they needed care, but were to receive benefits after leaving the military as an entitlement of service. Health benefits were justified as workers compensation for the damage done in dangerous industries, whether in the stateside factory or the mud of a foreign trench. The political arguments for action were thus in place. But how was a national veterans hospital program actually achieved? My search in the National Archives in Washington, D.C. turned up illuminating materials in the form of minutes of the consultants on hospitalization, who were the experts who designed the first national veterans hospital network, and the federal board of hospitalization, which continued the effort. In parallel, I followed the colorful story of the first director of the Veterans Bureau, Charles R. Forbes, whose demonstrable malfeasance in that role—he went to jail—engendered reams of additional materials. Recently (in 2006) I have gone back to look at different aspects of that story. Here it is part of a broader discussion of whether the federal government can function or "govern."

"Can the Government Govern?" concludes that when circumstances called for it, government could (and by extension, can) produce. This question was of particular interest in 1990, when I spoke on this topic, and 1991, when this chapter was originally published. A decade of pro-market rhetoric (this was the beginning of the managed care movement), and the sheer complexity and busy-ness of organizational maneuverings to achieve hoped-for advantage in terms of market power and money, made the government seem at times curiously irrelevant. The essentially pragmatic character of national policymaking in the United States was, however, worth remembering. Only two years later, in 1993, President Bill Clinton was to launch a massive campaign for national health insurance, though this foundered and failed the following year on the rocks of dispute and lack of consensus. There was no overwhelming agreement about the rhetoric or need for change, in contrast to the much earlier veterans' case.

In the early 1920s, when proposals for compulsory health insurance were recognizably dead, the establishment of a national network of hospitals for veterans run by the federal government might have been labeled "socialistic," and certainly as backdoor government health insurance. This case illustrates, as do many other cases of successful American policymaking, that multiple ideologies are available to justify (or reject) a specific proposal—one reason it is so difficult to predict future legislative change. When there is strong consensus for programmatic change, as shown in this case, plausible, "pro-American" arguments for change can be made that override competing ideological positions. Implementation was made possible by the use of outside experts, thus removing decisions from the apparent realm of politics by suggesting a management or technological solution to the highly contested question of where the new hospitals should be placed. Veterans hospitals are an American anomaly to this day.

"Letter from America, 1961" (chapter 4) was my first published piece, published the year I came to the United States. I have it included it here, though, not for sentimental reasons (well, perhaps a little), but to give a contemporary, outsider view—and a rather opinionated one at that—of the debates leading up to the Medicare and Medicaid legislation in 1965, when the federal role in paying for health care was phenomenally increased. Great Britain and the United States were at that time, as before and perhaps still, two nations divided by a common language, notably in the realm of political rhetoric. The chapter shows how much I myself, a twenty-five-year-old immigrant, was a product of British positions, including more than a whiff of displeasure that U.S. commentators of the time were ignoring, if not vilifying, the British experience, with its top-down, governmental National Health Service, then thirteen years old. Tutored as I had been by Richard Titmuss and Brian Abel-Smith, I was well aware that "socialism" carried very different meanings each side of the Atlantic, but was nevertheless surprised by the unexamined animus it generated in my new country. In perhaps crude and naïve terms, I sought to depict American values for the British hospital administrators for whom this piece was written. To them as well as me, in those days before global television, America was a mystifying place. The result is a snapshot of a particular time and set of events.

The basic theme of "Letter from America" is that there was a serious move to bring the federal government into health care through insuring members of the population aged sixty-five and over for the costs of hospital care. As with veterans, the private health sector could not provide services at a cost they could pay, either through insurance premiums or out-of-pocket costs. The government's role would thus be to address market failure, protect the private sector so that insurers could provide insurance to those who could afford to pay premiums, typically through employers (the working population), and in the process provide financial relief to capital-strapped hospitals. The unsuccessful King-Anderson bill, discussed here, was a direct forerunner to Medicare Part A (hospital insurance), and offered a theater for opposing views. My interest was in the apparent recognition, even in America, that only the national government can organize massive payments for an entire social group. Suddenly the American system had greater relevance for outside observers. I make comparisons between the two countries explicit (for the 1970s) in chapter 6. Meanwhile, here is my British take on America's debates almost fifty years ago about "free care" and "old age pensions," using British terms. The language of "Letter" also illustrates how far concepts of aging have changed for the better in both countries since the 1960s, when I accepted without openly questioning them the terms "old," "elderly," and "aged" to describe the entire population at or over the age of sixty-five—a group of which I am now a member.

In what has become a well-known political tale, legislators from different political perspectives crafted Medicare, Parts A and B and Medicaid into one piece of legislation in 1965, though each of the three parts had a separate history and created different programs. "Anatomy of a Dilemma: Creating and Implementing Medicaid, 1965-1970" (chapter 5) is an analysis of how Medicaid was implemented. In the late 1960s, when Robert Stevens was teaching law and I was teaching public health at Yale, we collaborated on an evaluation of Medicaid, including parallel research seminars on Medicaid in each school in the fall of 1969. Very little research was being done (or has been done since) on Medicaid's implementation. Our published work includes a long law journal article, replete with detailed footnotes, from which I have distilled the much shorter chapter here, and a book also authored by us both, *Welfare Medicine in*

America: A Case Study of Medicaid. I greatly appreciate Robert's willingness
for me to play with the prose, ignore most of the footnotes, and draw from the
article in the way I have done here.

Medicaid was, and is, a program of federal matching grants to states, distinguishing it from Medicare, which is a wholly federal program (administered
through private intermediaries). Each state had to develop its own Medicaid
program, building on its own resources, interests, and initiative. Not surprisingly,
as we show here, implementation was done differently in different states. There
were federal guidelines, but there was little or no national policing or national
managerial direction in the critical early years. While many initially heralded
Medicaid, like Medicare, as a national program (for good or ill, depending on
point of view), it was always dependent on state budgets, state politics, and state
expectations. As a national program Medicaid could be defined in two major
ways: first, as a policy of national responsibility for many, though not all, of
the needy, through extending the resources available for this purpose to states
across the nation (at least all states that wished to participate); and second, as
a huge new economic obligation, which almost immediately sparked runaway
federal, as well state, costs. Medicaid has been a political football ever since.

Looking back to the late 1960s it may seem odd that many at the time saw
Medicaid as a vehicle that might lead to national health insurance; but such was
indeed the case. Medicare was largely hospital-based, and was implemented in
1966 on the pattern of existing private hospital and medical insurance policies.
Medicaid, initially open-ended in terms of federal funding, expressed demonstrable willingness to commit federal resources to states. The states served, in
turn, as a collection of demonstration projects. In any event, both high hopes
and dire predictions that Medicaid might lead to more general population coverage were quickly dashed. Raw politics and the reality of tax expenditures in
the states reverberated back to Washington. This early history of Medicaid has
more in common with the earlier history of welfare in the states (as shown for
Pennsylvania in chapter 1) than with any progressive model of national responsibility for health care. The idea of "medical indigence" built into Medicaid
suggested that an American could be poor because of medical bills, rather than
just poor to begin with (such as those already on cash assistance under state
welfare programs), but this was quickly accommodated to link eligibility to
means test provisions under welfare in the states.

The notable exception turned out to be nursing home provision for the sixty-
five-and-over population. Medicaid provided the financial incentive to establish
new, largely for-profit nursing homes, and many of the new residents were not
(and are not) on Medicaid when initially admitted. As a result, Medicaid joined
Medicare in signifying massive government aid that was targeted at older rather
than younger members of the population. In turn, this generated concern about
intergenerational equity—too much to the elderly, too little to children—as well
as to the combined fiscal impacts of the programs as a whole. Instead, then, of

symbolizing greater social opportunity in the receipt of medical care, Medicaid became, oddly, the symbol of unfairness in the social use of federal funds.

But that is looking ahead. In 1970 Medicaid, though an administrative quagmire and fiscal mess, could be praised as a brave experiment. Indeed, in the original article we noted that the reluctance of American reformers to be daunted by disaster was one of the great attractions of the United States. If one solution fails, we wrote, the urge is to try another, preferably pouring in still more money, while blithely ignoring the lessons of history. This enthusiasm to try things out, irrespective of potential costs, has been a general characteristic of American health policy. Medicaid's implementation remains a cautionary tale of what happens when legislative opportunity trumps long-term policymaking.

As I write this in 2006, the Medicaid program is larger than Medicare. But while Medicare is a national force for policy change, Medicaid is still a collection of fifty programs, each with its own standards, rules, and regulations. Hard-pressed Medicaid administrators in one state often do not know what other states are doing. Federal administration is weak. Within CMS (Centers for Medicare and Medicaid Services), where federal responsibility for both programs resides, Medicaid is the stepchild of federal health encouragement and oversight. There is a running joke among the Medicaid community that the single "M" in CMS is meant to ignore Medicaid as a national program altogether. An outsider looking at both programs now would, I think, be surprised that there are not common national standards for both Medicare and Medicaid—or for that matter common statistics or data sets.

Medicaid has also hewn to its welfare roots. The New York program, discussed in chapter 5, is still relatively generous, compared with other programs, although—also like other programs—its managers, contractors and beneficiaries struggle with problems of eligibility, lack of participation among specialists, waiting lists, and horrific paperwork for all concerned. One expert commented in 2005 that New York "looks at each applicant as a potential criminal." (Elisabeth Benjamin, quoted by Richard Pérez-Peña, "At Clinic, Hurdles to Clear before Medicaid Care," *New York Times*, October 17, 2005, B5). Medicare, based on national Social Security rules, does not have Medicaid's excruciating eligibility requirements, but generates paperwork in the billing process for services rendered by largely private providers. As one patient put it, "You can't just be sick. You have to be sick and drowning in paperwork." (Patient Ellen Mayer, quoted by Katie Hafner, "Treated for Illness, Then Lost in Labyrinth of Bills," *New York Times*, October 13, 2005, A5).

Instead of creating an efficient, cost-effective national program in 1965, Congress gave birth to a three-headed hydra. Medicare Parts A and B (joined over the years by the largely unsuccessful C, to persuade beneficiaries to join managed care plans, and the new D, a torturously complex program to subsidize prescription drugs), reflected and added to the administrative complexity of health insurance; Medicaid, to the problems of running welfare programs in the states. The 1965 legislation ducked national government responsibility for the organization and provision of services (indeed, strictly forbade system change). As a result, Medicare embodied some of the worst features of the private sector, and Medicaid of the public, at least from the perspective of the patient.

Perhaps this outcome was foreordained in the 1965 legislation. One can easily argue this position. But this argues back from what happened later: If we know the ending, it is easier to explain the beginning. There was optimism in 1965. There seemed at least a remote possibility that these huge programs could, instead, reveal the best of private and public action in the United States—not just the best intentions. In retrospect, Medicare and Medicaid seem the gesture of a rich nation that was unwilling to assume a strong governmental role. There was debate about principle: for example, whether services for the elderly should be designed under the equal opportunity provisions of social insurance rather than via a means test, and whether the ultimate goal of either (or both) Medicare and Medicaid should be universal health insurance coverage. But there was little forethought about long-term economic outcomes or the political impact of the programs on the national budget. Medicare and Medicaid played a political role as a delaying or palliative tactic, putting off further discussion of national health insurance. President Jimmy Carter's administration (1977-1980) followed the same policy of segmented, incremental change, pushing (unsuccessfully) for federally supported health care for children.

"Governments and Medical Care" (chapter 6), published in 1977, was written for a Scottish-American symposium on medical education and medical care that was organized by the Nuffield Provincial Hospitals Trust, and held in Edinburgh; hence a few Scottish citations. This paper explores the distinctive histories of health services in the United States and Great Britain, in order to ask the then contemporary question, namely, Are health services converging? The underlying question, of course, was whether there was movement toward a similar national governmental role. This was a tempting theme in the 1970s, given the uncertainties and changes taking place on both sides of the Atlantic. The 1970s seemed—even at that time—a watershed between a more settled past, organizationally speaking, and an evidently more rambunctious future. Contemporary British policy was pushing toward decentralization of the National Health Service, while federal standard-setting seemed on the rise in the United States. Arguably, perhaps they would eventually settle into a similar or parallel balance in the exercise of central and local authority. I thought then as I think now: This hypothesis is far too simplistic.

The convergence question was, however, a serious one in the 1970s, if only as a device that might lead to a more robust, distinctive version of the federal role in health in the United States that could provide a vehicle for change. This thread of public discussion has since been largely lost, but is worth remembering; for it may return. The government role—or plethora of roles, illustrated in a huge number of separate programs—had expanded rapidly in terms of monetary commitment in the 1960s, and into the 1970s, as government-sponsored health care planning came into vogue.

What was intrinsically "American" about American health care, including its political and economic rationale and its diffuse, segmented management? It was easy to observe, as I did in another comparative presentation in 1977, at an NIH conference on priorities for the use of resources in medicine, that American medicine was demonstrably more entrepreneurial than its British counterpart, and that American organizational solutions promised to be most successful when most justifiable commercially, in terms of economics and efficiency. Besides differences in purpose and philosophy, the two health systems had very different cultural strengths. Britain's tradition of primary care and state responsibility for providing services universally to the population resonated with American concerns in the 1970s about access to care, coordination, and continuity. On the American side were commitment to technological excellence, apparently at any cost; the organizational fluidity of the health care system; the very fact that it was neither a unified nor a centralized system; and its seeming ability to mobilize for change. Surely American management technology and entrepreneurial energy would be applied to health care in order to create more efficient, effective health care organizations, whatever the public or private drivers for change might be.

My own transition in view over time reveals general and contextual shifts in thinking about government responsibility in the 1970s and 1980s. By the time I published a third comparative paper in 1983 ("Comparisons in Health Care: Britain as Contrast to the United States," in *Handbook of Health, Health Care, and the Health Professions* [1983], edited by sociologist David Mechanic) there seemed to be multiple conceptions of what a health service might be, but also some cross-Atlantic agreement about control. In (Conservative Prime Minister) Margaret Thatcher's Britain of the early 1980s, management terms pervaded discussion of (and hopes for) the future of the NHS. In the United States, likewise, in the Reagan years management and the market became fashionable terms. Paul Starr's well-regarded book, *The Social Transformation of American Medicine*, published in 1982, described the rise of the private corporation as the coming major force for American medicine and health care organizations—a scenario borne out by subsequent experience. While U.S. goals could be described as a private system operating with public subsidy and regulation, and the UK as one of public management, there were clear messages about reducing the role of central government in both nations.

By the late 1980s, health care management (whether of public or private organizations) had become the central critical dimension for international comparison. When I went back to specifically comparative U.S./UK themes in the 1990s, during the fifty-year celebrations and appraisals of the NHS in 1998, and in contributing to a festschrift for the extraordinary, indomitable economist Eli Ginzberg on the occasion of his ninetieth birthday, my approach to the health systems in the two countries was from the perspective of the organizational experimentation each had engaged in over the past fifty or so years. Parallel concerns had indeed been expressed in both countries over the years, about such organizational themes as the role of the hospital and the place of primary care.

These papers may tell the reader as much about the time in which they were written—and the national audience each was written for—as about the issues themselves. That is the purpose of my choices for this section. Underlying each chapter is the concept that the American view of government constantly shifts. Justifications for one stance or another may seem constant—for example, positions for or against social insurance, state versus federal control, or a deregulated market rather than strong national regulation. But talk is cheap. It is the politics of the hour that produce or decline to produce legislation. Public and private players implement laws in a specific socioeconomic, state and local context, transforming what was into a new state of play. The government role in the United States is heavily context dependent. Not surprisingly, that role is constantly questioned, and continuously reinvented.

3

Can the Government Govern?
The Establishment of Veterans Hospitals

The United States is a democracy whose citizens regard government with distrust and government intervention with suspicion. Nevertheless, there was a strong and pervasive federal presence in medical care in the twentieth century whose growth accelerated from mid-century. Federally prescribed rules and regulations not only drove the system at the local level but also set its moral tone: in espousing competition, for example, or endorsing disparities in access, or rewarding a rampant managerialism. Yet at the end of the century Congress appeared no more enthusiastic about accepting responsibility for the health care system than it had been in earlier decades.

What are we to make of this? One set of hypotheses focuses on the nature and structure of America's democratic institutions as adequate vehicles for national policy in the late twentieth century. "Can the government govern?" asked a Brookings Institution publication in 1989. This question was clearly designed to shed doubt, if not to suggest major restructuring; at issue was the "problem of governance."[1] Alternatively, the problem was one of consensus. In the American system, the argument goes, consensus has to be built across chasms of conflict and indecision and managed across competing interests. Since agreements may be fragile and temporary, there is no necessary consistency of view between one decision and the next, and the policy process is inherently unstable.[2] We may be prisoners of rhetoric (or masters of denial), clinging to unexamined tenets about the superiority of private medicine over an undefined "welfare state." Or we may lack the political "will" (whatever this is) to develop policies long-range. Or perhaps we suffer from a dearth of imaginative experts.

It is difficult to study such questions in the moving target that is the present, both because it is moving and because it is difficult to sort out what themes are new and what are permanent aspects of the policymaking system as it has developed in past decades. There is no point in reinventing the wheel. What I want to do here, instead, is to draw on an important, largely unexamined case study: how the federal government became involved in a massive program of government hospital services to veterans.

The federal hospital system for veterans, established in the aftermath of World War I in a context of decentralization, privatization, and rejection of compulsory health insurance, seems an anomaly in health care policymaking. It is actually a good case of how the federal government achieves results in an area fraught with conflict: via normalization of crisis, containment of political decision-making, and the association of the program with previously accepted goals (in this instance, workers' compensation). In the veterans' case, political judgments were transformed into scientific and bureaucratic decisions via the pragmatic use of experts. The system worked; the federal government governed.

This case has particular advantages both as a comparative and as an historical study. First, I want to show that the debates over how hospital services should be provided to the four million U.S. veterans of World War I illustrate enduring characteristics of national medical policymaking in the United States. Second, the creation of a national, government-run hospital service for veterans, a prime case of "socialized medicine" that exists to this day, is a good example of the way in which the federal government has become involved in medical care in a big way within a culture that assumes, nevertheless, that minimal government intervention is the desired form of social organization.

Political philosophy has actually had little to do with how specific federal policies have been made in the United States, as this case illustrates. In the past as in the present, federal policy has typically been a response to sectional or immediate needs, the crisis of the moment, rather than to any long-term, integrated social agenda. One result is that it is possible to speak of a congeries of separate medical policies (in the plural), each with its own internal rationale and lobbying groups: for example, biomedical research policy, medical care of the elderly, or, as in this case, hospitalization of veterans.

This observation leads to a second: that health policy in the United States is often the secondary result of other more pressing policies, designed primarily for something else. Hospitalization of veterans was a byproduct of larger issues of veterans' benefits, rather than a subset of health care decisions. Similarly, medical care for the poor can still be understood as a subset of American welfare policy rather than as a health policy; and biomedical research is better seen in terms of national commitments to science and technology, or even to the linked cultural power of university, government, and corporate networks. This characteristic is so deep-seated that we need to give much more consideration than we do to whether it makes sense to talk about national health policy at all, even today, in terms of any a single, overarching concept or mobilizing vehicle.

A third prevailing theme, evident in the case of veterans' hospitals but with many more general ramifications, is the role played by national debates. I want to show here that the congressional and administrative discussions surrounding the veterans' hospital issue provided a forum not only for the negotiation of views but also for conflict avoidance. Decisions were displaced in two directions: to experts (whose views were supposedly apolitical) and to administrative agencies. The results of this displacement were, and are, instructive. This is a tale of national medical leadership and the limitations of medical (private) power in the U.S. political system; of national hospital policy made by experts; of congressional reluctance, logrolling, and conflict; and of administrative confusion and chicanery.

Setting Hospital Policy for Veterans

When the United States entered World War I in April 1917 there was a patchwork of private and public hospitals across the country, most of them established in the previous thirty years. Hospitals were beginning to be seen as a national enterprise. The U.S. Census Bureau had singled them out for major national surveys in 1904 and 1910. Prominent members of the American Hospital Association had also lobbied Congress unsuccessfully for a federal bureau of hospital information within the U.S. Public Health Service.[3] The United States Public Health Service ran a string of federal hospitals at major ports of call along the coasts and major rivers and thus had some claim to national hospital expertise; there were twenty marine hospitals, with 7,200 beds in September 1918.[4] But their role was largely that of quarantine and the care of sick and injured sailors. Hospitals were overwhelmingly local affairs, far more attuned to local power structures, than to what went on in regional, state, and national arenas. It was the "business of every community to look after its own wear and tear in human life," wrote the ubiquitous Abraham Flexner.[5]

However, in striking contrast to this decentralized responsibility and rhetoric of "community" for hospitals, the medical profession was rapidly consolidating and extending its influence as a *national* force, through reform of medical schools, clinical education, and pressures for medical licensing. National health associations were also forming around specific health problems, notably tuberculosis and mental hygiene. Whatever the rhetoric of local or even institutional autonomy for hospitals, the interests of organized medicine were already turning toward a national system of hospital regulation. The profession was centralizing, then, while the major medical institutions—the hospitals—were diffused. In 1914 the American Medical Association began to survey hospital internships throughout the United States. Leading surgeons organized themselves into an American College of Surgeons. In 1917 the college was establishing national standards for surgeons and moving toward the inspection and certification of hospitals in order to upgrade the practice of surgery, which was the mainstay of general hospitals across the country. In short, there were national medical interests and the beginnings of national policymaking for hospitals in the United States before World War I, but through private (professional or voluntary) organizations rather than through national government or the political system. So strong, relatively, was private medical influence and expertise at the national level that the army and navy delegated the organization of U.S. military hospitals for the European front to U.S. medical schools and teaching hospitals. Eighteen medical schools and forty-two major hospitals across the United States organized huge mobile "base hospitals" for the U.S. government in the war, sending members of their own medical and nursing staff, with others, to the front.[6]

In contrast to the effective centralization of the medical profession, the federal government's role in health before the war was fragmented and weak; responsibility for public health resided largely in the states. Unlike most western European countries, friend and foe alike, the United States had no national health insurance program. Several states were considering compulsory health insurance during the wartime period, but none of them passed the necessary legislation, and after the war interest waned. There was thus no obvious framework of public policy—national or state-based health insurance—for the medical needs of sick and injured veterans. In the case of veterans' hospitalization, as in many other cases since, national policy toward a "worthy" or particularly needy target group within the population had to be invented. How, in particular, were ex-soldiers, who were receiving state-of-the-art medical care in base hospitals run by the nation's top medical schools and teaching hospitals, to be fitted into the fee-paying, disorganized patchwork of voluntary and local government hospitals within the United States? Looking after the normal "wear and tear of life" at the local level for civilians was one thing; but soldiers were a national responsibility.

How does a country without a national health program for all justify national health benefits for the few? In the United States, programs for the few tend to have been generated by a sense of urgency, and developed in blinkered isolation. Their success rests, first, on the ability to define the group clearly as a distinct and limited class of beneficiaries, through employment, age, or means test, and second, on an economic or contractual justification that is not seen to apply to the whole population. The federal government's early foray into health insurance, insuring merchant seamen (under legislation originally passed in 1798), remained self-limiting. Similarly, the veterans were a clearly definable group of people whose attitudes in battle, as well as their prospects for recovery if they were wounded, might well affect the well-being of the republic.

The entitlement of veterans to health benefits was framed by the War Risk Insurance Act of 1914 (P.L. 63-193), as modified in 1917 and 1919. Hospital and medical services for veterans were dealt with in a single paragraph in a section of the legislation that dealt with disability compensation. By definition this was not *health* policy but *disability* policy. There was no necessary connection between the provision of care to veterans and other federal health programs, notably the hospital program of the U.S. Public Health Service for the merchant marine, as there might have been in a piece of legislation designed for hospitalization per se. Section 302 of the war insurance law, as framed in October 1917, simply stated that the United States would provide the individual with medical, surgical, and hospital service, supplies, and appliances, as determined to be useful and reasonably necessary by the director of the War Risk Bureau, a section of the U.S. Treasury Department.[7]

As with the underlying rationale for protecting the merchant marine, this legislation was originally designed to protect American shipping. Commerce, rather than individual safety, was the driving interest. The War Risk Act of 1914 insured vessels and their cargoes from the risk of German submarine attacks before U.S. entry into the war, because insurance in the private sector had become prohibitively expensive. Thus, in a way, the act buttressed the role of private insurance companies as well; its intention was commercial insurance, pure and simple. Insurance was extended to the lives of officers and crews in mid-1917, after the United States had entered the war. But by this time there was general military conscription, requiring every male between the ages of twenty-one and thirty, inclusive, to register for the draft. It certainly seemed reasonable that they, too, should have life insurance, at least. Indeed, insurance had become a national preoccupation; there were 49 million private life insurance policies in effect in 1917, up from 25 million in 1907.[8]

Before World War I veterans had only received pensions, although a few disabled veterans were also living in soldiers' and sailors' homes. But quite apart from shifts in benefit policy away from charity toward entitlement, the Great War raised new issues of scale. In August 1914 there were only 785,000 living veterans, about half of whom had served in the Spanish-American War.[9] Conscription promised to create more than 4 million new potential veterans overnight. Progressive social policy suggested the same kind of deliberation that was being given, concurrently, to workers' compensation laws and to proposals for compulsory (state) health insurance and mothers' pensions.

The new veterans package of benefits was in fact written for the Council of National Defense by a small group of experts on insurance, the family, and dependency, chaired by federal appeals court judge Julian W. Mack. This group, drawn from the private and public sectors, worked hard through the summer of 1917, with staff provided by Columbia University through its legislative drafting research fund. Mack was a member of the Council of National Defense's Committee on Labor, chaired by union leader Samuel Gompers. In the wartime spirit of public-private cooperation, Mack's subcommittee included Assistant Secretary of the Treasury Leo S. Rowe, well-known accountant S. H. Wolfe, Children's Bureau representative Julia Lathrop, President of the National Civic Foundation V. Everit Macy, and Professors Henry R. Seager and Thomas I. Parkinson of Columbia University.[10] True to prevailing progressive ideas, the focus was on readjustment, rehabilitation, and family protection. The committee framed the problem of veterans' benefits in large part as one of absent or incapacitated fathers and sons. Enlisted men with dependents were subject to specified, compulsory family contributions, and besides compensation entitlements for death and disability, life insurance was provided on a voluntary basis.

The main task of the War Risk Bureau became the marketing and processing of individual insurance forms, with agents even signing up soldiers in the trenches.

In the absence of government health insurance programs, workers' compensation legislation provided the most direct prototype for the provision of medical benefits for veterans. Suddenly, in 1917 the federal government became a major employer of workers—in a dangerous and unhealthy occupation. Occupational health and industrial medicine were obvious civilian models for translation to the wartime theater. There were appalling casualties in factory or railroad work or grubbing in a mine; according to a member of the Industrial Accident Committee of California, Will J. French, on average, one American worker was killed every fifteen minutes, and one injured every sixteen seconds.[11] Fighting was also a dangerous occupation. Workmen's compensation laws had been established in virtually all major industrial states by 1917, in a flurry of legislative activity. Compensation was also available to civilian federal employees.

Politically, compensation for injury was non-controversial by 1917, though there was considerable debate about ways and means for implementation in different states. At a major conference on social insurance called by the U.S. Department of Labor in December 1916, speakers from a wide variety of interests—business, labor, politics, state officials, progressive reformers, even President Woodrow Wilson—had agreed on the importance of investing in human capital as part of the "new industrialism."[12] It made no sense, said one speaker, that America "throws on the scrap heap its human machines, while tending machines made of wood and iron."[13] A speaker from the B.F. Goodrich Company of Akron, Ohio, called workers' health insurance, life insurance, and pensions, too, "just a plain horse-sense business proposition"; his firm, he said, happened to have "seen the vision a little before the mass has seen the vision."[14] This vision was readily transferable to veterans by analogy to private industry.

There was far less consensus in favor of health insurance than there was for workers' compensation among the same groups. Where workers' compensation seemed a logical extension of the costs of employment (and could thus be justified as "practical economics" rather than "sociology" or "politics"), closely tied to accident prevention, health insurance addressed a much larger set of social needs. Thus a representative from General Electric, West Lynn, Massachusetts, could dissociate workmen's compensation entirely from other progressive social policies. Workmen's compensation was not "social insurance," he said, because it dealt with the obligation of industry to workers, rather than the duty of society to the citizen.[15] Although such remarks were clearly designed to stop other forms of government-sponsored social insurance (notably health insurance) dead in their tracks, they also implicitly imposed a duty on the federal government, as an employer, to prevent its conscripts from ending up on the "scrap heap."

Secretary of the Treasury William Gibbs McAdoo voiced the new philosophy of veterans' benefits in stark terms in transmitting the administration's bill for the extension of war risk insurance for servicemen to President Wilson on 31 July 1917:

> The minds of our soldiers and sailors should be put at rest, so far as their loved ones are concerned, by the knowledge that they will be amply provided for by their government as a part of the compensation for the service they are rendering to their country. In like manner they should know in advance that if they are killed in battle, definite and just provision has been made for their dependents, and that if they are disabled, totally or partially—if they come back armless, legless, sightless or otherwise permanently injured—definite provision is made for them, and that they are not going to be left to the uncertain chances of future legislation or to the scandals of our old pension system. Every man should know that the moment he is enlisted in the military service of the government these definite guarantees and assurances are given to him not as charity but as a part of his deserved compensation for the extra-hazardous occupation into which his government has forced him.[16]

As with other forms of workers' compensation, there was the difficult question of how best to provide medical benefits. The inclusion of medical service benefits in the 1917 legislation made the program more than just a matter of setting rules for entitlement and managing money, efforts appropriate to the Department of the Treasury. However, it was expected that, for the duration of the war at least, injured and sick men would remain in the service until they had reached maximum improvement, so this was largely an academic question in 1917. Meanwhile the mixed experience of civilian workers' compensation offered a confused maze of practices that made it only a partial and unsatisfactory guide. Connecticut and the federal employees' program were unusual in providing medical and surgical services to those eligible for workmen's compensation that were unlimited with respect both to time and to amount. The typical pattern was to specify a number of days of care and/or a low ceiling on the dollars available to hospitals and doctors per case.[17] There was growing concern among physicians about methods of payment, particularly the "certain inherent evils" of capitation payments under contract practice (notably overworked doctors and poor quality service)[18] and widespread criticism of the general standards of hospital care. A review of industry done by state officials in Missouri after the war concluded that there were few adequate facilities for industrial accident cases in hospitals anywhere in the United States; and that hospitals had "never desired this sort of work particularly."[19]

With the signing of the armistice agreement in November 1918, the question of medical benefits to veterans suddenly became of acute, practical concern. Rather than stay in the service until maximum functioning was reached depending on their condition, thousands of disabled men and women decided to return to civilian life, carrying their guaranteed benefits with them, and more would follow behind them. The War Risk Bureau was caught unprepared; there was as yet no general hospitalization program, nor even any plan for the medical screening and rating of veterans. The bureau rapidly began to implement its responsibility for determining individual eligibility for medical benefits through designating a string of medical examiners. Compensation and medical care were to be provided to those who could show disability of ten percent or more from disease or injury "incurred in or aggravated by military or naval service in the World War."[20] However, hospitalization remained a problem. By mid-1919, over 3,200 veterans were receiving hospital care in overcrowded U.S. Public Health Service hospitals on contract to the War Risk Bureau, in the army and navy hospitals attached to cantonments in the United States (which were often unsuitable for rehabilitation and long-term care and far from patients' homes), and from civilian hospitals ranging from excellent to terrible. There was a huge backlog of pending cases. A congressional study estimated that 204,000 U.S. soldiers had been "wounded not mortally," and uncounted legions suffered from tuberculosis and neuropsychiatric conditions.[21] Perhaps 300,000 or more veterans would need further hospital care.[22]

Neither Congress nor the administration had been blind to the problem of hospitalization. The question was one of ways and means. In a country lacking a defined or generally agreed-on national health policy, it was tricky to establish a national health policy for veterans. Structural characteristics of American federalism and of the major political parties militated against the development of unified postwar social welfare policies based on a consistent political ideology. American political parties were (and are) essentially un-programmatic. Each major political party included members with very diverse political views. All else being equal, federal influence promised to grow weaker as centralized wartime coalitions disbanded and the nation relaxed into the promised "normalcy" of the 1920s, with a strong reliance on private institutions.

In a federal system, too, the role for the states was a matter of importance. Public health and safety were functions that fell primarily to the states rather than the federal government. Hence the discussion of health insurance by state legislatures and commissions rather than by Congress, and the establishment of state workmen's compensation programs. "What is best for one state or section," the U.S. Commissioner of Labor Statistics remarked, in reminding the conference on social insurance of its purpose in 1916, "may not be the best for another state or section."[23] For veterans, the tension between national policies and state or regional variation would have a particularly poignant relevance for racial politics, north and south, with powerful southern interests standing out for racial segregation of veterans hospitals in the South. (This political stance ultimately led to the establishment of a national hospital for black veterans at Tuskegee, Alabama.) But veterans hospital policy also hinged on the inability and/or unwillingness of states to define health and hospital policies of their own. Ultimately the federal government would become a service agency for veterans hospitals because no one else was doing it.

Quite apart from ideological divisions and structural constraints, there were major differences of opinion about whether new hospitals were needed for veterans at all. One of the problems was that the first group of claimants were not really "veterans" at all, but unhealthy and unfit young men who had passed the cursory medical screening of their local draft boards but had then been discharged from the service after reporting to base camp: over 70,000 men in all. These individuals, most of whom were suffering from tuberculosis, were entitled to compensation and medical benefits under the War Risk Act, which hardly seemed fair to other civilians. The War Risk Bureau asked the U.S. Public Service to admit those needing hospitalization to their hospitals. Not surprisingly, by mid-1918 the Public Health Service was overwhelmed with patients and was looking for funds for expansion of its own string of hospitals. Meanwhile the huge sum of $99 million was being poured into military hospitals located in and around thirty or so army cantonments in the United States.[24] However veterans, as civilians, could not use these. The system appeared inherently illogical, with no clear policy directions.

Congressional debates on veterans hospitals in 1918 illustrated only too clearly the problems of designing a national program in a federal system—and a federal system, moreover, that lacked strong state administration in the health and welfare area. Elected representatives engaged in an unseemly free-for-all. Squabblings over the location of new hospitals for veterans began during hearings in the House of Representatives in October 1918. An enterprising group of private citizens in Dawson Springs, Kentucky, had offered the federal government a piece of land provided that a veterans hospital was constructed there, bringing with it of course federal tax money to Dawson Springs. Kentucky Democrats supported this proposal. Republicans in the House rallied against it. If federal money was available as a potential plum, why not put a hospital in the salubrious Republican stronghold of Amarillo, Texas, instead? (Amarillo did get a veterans hospital, constructed on a donated site, but not until 1940.) Or French Lick, Indiana? Or somewhere else? It was obvious to all concerned that a national veterans hospital system could not be planned in Congress without an out-and-out contest for federal funds, with vote trading, logrolling, and the general "odor of pork."[25]

The political rifts over Dawson Springs (which was built) suggested that the only fair way to design a national hospital program for veterans was to remove it from the political process altogether. A prime ingredient of the eventual veterans hospital program, then, was the inability of Congress to design a national program itself. Consensus was to be achieved by agreement in principle that a hospital program was needed, by the appropriation of funds, and by the displacement of political decision-making to the realm of experts, who were to be drawn from the national organizations of health and medicine.

By the spring of 1919 veterans had become a political force. Two organizations, the American Legion and Veterans of Foreign Wars, were proving effective lobbyists, and cries of "equity" and "national obligation" were focusing political interest. In 1919 alone, fifty-five bills were introduced in Congress to "adjust" the rates of pay servicemen had received during the war up to the levels they might have received had they stayed at home and profited from the boom in wartime industry.[26] There was growing consensus in Congress that something should be done about hospitals, but there was no agreement about what should be done or by whom. The Public Health Service's estimates that over 30,000 hospital beds would be needed for veterans within the next two years, predominantly for psychiatry and tuberculosis, were criticized in Congress as unnecessary. Expertise from within the federal bureaucracy was not to be readily accepted; indeed it was tainted by being part of government at all, for almost everyone agreed that government bureaucracies were inherently grasping and inefficient, especially where construction and supplies were involved.[27]

Limited funds were made available for the adaptation of existing army hospitals, but the system was getting worse rather than better. Field investigations made by the American Legion reported stories of shell-shocked veterans sent to hospitals for feeble-minded children, where they were forced to sit on infants' chairs, and of tuberculosis patients sent to marshy districts detrimental to their health.[28] By the beginning of 1921, more than two years after the war had ended, the hospital program for veterans was a nightmare of red tape, inefficiency, confusion, and neglect.

Congress finally appropriated $18.6 million for veterans hospitals in March 1921. President Woodrow Wilson, weakened by illness, signed the law (P.L. 66-384) on his last day of office.[29] He thus left a major new domestic program to a new administration, that of President Warren G. Harding. The Secretary of the Treasury, not the now-discredited Public Health Service, was made directly responsible for organizing the new facilities. The way was now clear, it seemed, for hiring the outside experts who would decide how the money would be spent. In charge was the new Secretary of the Treasury, millionaire banker Andrew W. Mellon.

In recognition of the role of national medical expertise, Secretary Mellon sent for a well-known tuberculosis specialist, Dr. William C. White. White was a prominent member of the National Tuberculosis Association and had directed the wartime hospital program for tuberculosis for the Red Cross in France and Italy. Mellon and White then selected three other national experts. Dr. Pearce Bailey, a New York psychiatrist, had served as chief of the U.S. Division of Neurology, Psychiatry, and Psychology during the war and also represented the National Mental Hygiene Association; Dr. Frank Billings, professor of surgery and medical school dean, had chaired the American Red Cross mission to Russia in 1917, was ex-president of the Association of American Physicians, and was twice elected president of the American Medical Association; and Dr. John G. Bowman, then chancellor of the University of Pittsburgh, had formerly run the hospital standardization program of the American College of Surgeons.[30]

These experts served without pay as "consultants in hospitalization." They reported directly to Secretary Mellon and were served by staff in the Treasury Department. This delegation of public power to a coalition of private interests was not unlike other cooperative public-private arrangements for organizing national resources during the war.

In the two years that they served, 1921-23, the consultants on hospitalization conducted their own hearings with over one hundred groups, from senators to local chambers of commerce, each of whom wanted a veterans hospital in their own area. The consultants made visits to hospitals across the country, sought advice from major hospital groups and philanthropic foundations, and produced copious, detailed maps of where all hospitals were across the United States. They published standards for construction, equipment, and personnel, and rated hospitals in different areas as satisfactory or unsatisfactory. Holding fast to the general principle that they had observed in wartime, that veterans should be served in federal rather than local hospitals as far as possible on grounds of quality of care, the consultants approved the building of over 6,000 beds in new hospitals, strategically placed across the country. The consultants also acted as broker and decision-maker for the building of the segregated hospital for black veterans at Tuskegee, over the opposition of black veterans' groups, but with the support of the national philanthropic foundations and powerful southern politicians. The consultants were, in short, extremely influential. They even attempted to set up machinery for federal oversight and federal standards for *all* hospitals in the United States, so that "uniform care of the citizens of the United States" could be achieved, rather than relying on the "influence of individual or local interests."[31] But this was going too far, even for their own constituencies.

In a period of diminishing federal influence over American institutions, then, a coterie of private citizens drawn from national medical and health associations established the veterans hospital program, a huge new federal service commitment. There was a remarkable dichotomy between the high-handed, bureaucratic idealism of these experts, used to wielding power through private associations, the Red Cross, and the military, and the muddling-through, deal-making politics of Congress.

It would be misleading, though, to interpret the role of the consultants merely as an example of the public power of private interests. Equally, the experts were Congress's servants, hired guns with a limited mission. The use of the experts served to break congressional deadlock and to create a design for hospitals that could be justified as "scientific." In essence, they were technocrats. They engaged in the practical politics of policymaking under the umbrella of rhetorical agreement that was made by Congress—that "we need to do something about hospitals for veterans." Private experts are typically also used in the United States to create regulations for the implementation of federal programs, and to design programs that may then be legislated; their role, past and present, needs to be emphasized much more in health policy research than it has been.

A further strong and major implication in the use of experts in creating the veterans program, as in other cases of health policy that might be cited, was the assumption that the federal bureaucracy itself could not, or should not, create policies for implementation. One question here, of course, was, Which department? A collection of departments was involved in veterans hospital affairs: the army, the navy, the U.S. Public Health Service, the War Risk Bureau. The creation of a Federal Board of Hospitalization in 1921 was supposed to bring them all together, but there were problems of policy and jurisdiction here, too. The chairman of the new board was Dr. Charles E. Sawyer, President Harding's personal physician (actually Mrs. Harding's physician) and an old crony of his from Ohio. Sawyer was well-known for his view that it was a waste of money to establish new hospitals when empty beds were available in hospitals on military bases. But he became, more generally, a thorn in the flesh of the director of the new Veterans Bureau, which was also established in 1921 to take responsibility for the entire veterans benefits program. According to Director Forbes' self-justifying and pugnacious recollection, written after both Harding and Sawyer had died, Sawyer "carried falsehoods to the president and sought to locate hospitals in a way that would be advantageous to his own interests." The description continues:

> A homeopath himself, he sought to have homeopaths replace allopaths. He established a stool-pigeon system within the bureau and in other departments of government as well. He was a vain, strutting little creature and fancied that he had a great attraction for women. He held himself out to be the personal representative of the president and he spoke with a great show of authority when asserting his position.[32]

Dr. Sawyer's feelings toward Forbes, while perhaps less colorfully expressed, were also strongly negative. But whatever the two men's personal views, there were clear problems of where power resided, in the agencies or in the White House.

Charles R. Forbes, the first director of the Veterans Bureau, was another of the president's cronies, and he soon became the focus of a major scandal. Forbes had actually been hoping for a place on the Shipping Board, according to his account. He reportedly accepted the directorship of the bureau after some discussion as to whether he should become governor of Alaska. But whatever Forbes' character and capabilities, there was a marked difference in style between the military efficiency of the consultants and their staff, responsible directly to Andrew Mellon, and the sprawling muddle of the Veterans Bureau, successor to the trouble-ridden and over-extended War Risk Bureau. The veterans hospital program fell through the cracks. As part of the compensation package for veterans, the hospital program was appropriately housed in the Veterans Bureau. However, just as staff in the Department of the Interior were regarding oil leases as likely plums for personal enrichment, the Teapot Dome lease being the spectacular example, so the leaders of the new Veterans Bureau had greedy agendas of their own, with little apparent commitment to the medical needs of veterans, and little or no knowledge of operating hospitals.

In the glare of titillating national publicity in the years 1923 through 1925—for the story included, among other things, a flood of Prohibition-era whisky drinking, crap games, actresses, divorce, and shady deals—Charles R. Forbes was indicted for bribery and fraud in the administration of the hospital program of the Veterans Bureau, and sent to prison at Leavenworth, Kansas. Coincidentally, he resigned his position the same month that the consultants gave Secretary Mellon their extensive report on hospitalization, in February 1923. The Veterans Bureau had sold millions of dollars' worth of new materials, including mattresses, sheets, towels, and floor wax, stored at Perryville, Maryland, for twenty cents to the dollar to a private firm in Boston. Some of the new sheets arriving at one Veterans Bureau depot were, it was claimed, "*run through and out the other side*, to the waiting cars of the contractor who carried them off as part of the booty."[33] [Emphasis in original.] The transaction resembled "more the work of buccaneers in the looting and scuttling of a ship than the mere negligence of trusted government officials."[34]

The limited sympathy for Forbes that appeared in the press damned the system as well as his peculations. The *American Legion Weekly* emphasized the tensions that existed between Forbes and Sawyer and the system of patronage that had pitchforked an inadequate individual into a formidable administrative position. The bureau's total budget in 1924 was over $400 million, "or about what it took to run the whole United States Government in 1895."[35] Clearly the temptation was too much. Justifiable criticism of federal program administration in the Forbes case seemed in turn to justify public distrust of government as a system. The Forbes case, like the Teapot Dome, could be seen as a self-fulfilling prophecy that government did not—could not—work.

By the mid-1920s, too, there were shifts in the views of those who initially supported veterans' benefits. The coalitions of interest were breaking down. Most notably, the widening scope of medical benefits was troubling the medical establishment. Consultant Frank Billings' elite efforts to control all hospitals on grounds of science and technique hardly squared at all with the interests of the average practicing physician. Indeed, the rapid rise in hospital beds for veterans soon had unexpected practical consequences for private practitioners, threatening out-and-out competition as veterans' organizations joined with federal officials, who wanted to see the new beds filled, and pressed Congress to expand veterans' benefits. The initial requirement had tied eligibility to conditions acquired or exacerbated in military service. In June 1924 veterans became eligible (under P.L. 68-243) for care for *any* condition, whether connected with their service or not, provided hospital space was available; preference was to be given to those unable to pay for hospitalization and traveling expenses. With one stroke of the pen, then, the original hospital and medical program, which had been designed as workers' compensation, was translated into comprehensive hospital insurance for veterans.

In the late 1920s and early 1930s over 60 percent of all veterans hospital admissions were for conditions unrelated to period of service.[36] Far from being pleased, the American Medical Association rose in aggressive opposition to this new competition with private medical and hospital practice. The new benefits were deemed, not unreasonably, "very much like 'state medicine' pure and simple"—and this was not meant as a compliment.[37] In 1928 the association officially declared that any further extension of veterans hospitals would be "socialized medical practice"; in 1930 the word was "communistic."[38] From the mid-1920s on, the association viewed the veterans program with watchful apprehension. Note how quickly the politics of veterans had changed. Within four years the medical establishment had shifted in role from being the domain of expertise on veterans hospitals to being the reactionary opposition. The program had acquired a life of its own, independent of its creators.

Within the veterans hospital system, too, the power structures shifted from structures for implementation to those for maintenance. Forbes, the operator (in more than one sense), had taken the reins from the planning experts, whose role appeared one of temporary expedience. After the consultants on hospitalization made their report in 1923, accounting for the expenditure of the $18.6 million designated to them, they disbanded. Their job was done. Their individual futures lay in the private sector. Decisions on the location of new veterans hospitals passed to a group of federal officials, the Federal Board of Hospitalization, chaired by General Frank T. Hines, who had been chief of the army's Embarkation Service in World War I. Hines brought probity, continuity, and expertise to the bureau (which became the Veterans Administration, or VA in 1930), directing it from March 1923 through August 1945. Veterans' affairs were thus also shielded in these years from the grosser elements of political patronage as one administration followed the last. In a sense the bureau was "professionalized." The hospital program settled into a bureaucratic routine. Even the more political elements of the program—where new hospitals should be sited—now fell to the Federal Board of Hospitalization, with its members drawn from across federal agencies, including the U.S. Public Health Service. The board's minutes[39] depict a stream of members of Congress and representatives of private groups making their pitch for a hospital to these federal officials.

One nice example in the 1930s involved Congressman Lister Hill (later Senator Hill, sponsor of the federal Hill-Burton hospital construction program for civilians in 1946) in lobbying for a VA hospital in Montgomery, Alabama. The tussle over whether to site a new (white) veterans hospital in Birmingham or Montgomery pitted Congressman Luther Patrick against the already powerful Lister Hill, chairman of the Military Affairs Committee, in 1937. Hill won the decision for Montgomery. The *Montgomery Advertiser* remarked, "Just what

Lister Hill said to General Hines to get him to select it, we don't know, but it must have been good." Patrick called the chairman of the Alabama Hospital Committee to complain and received a laconic reply: "Maybe Lister Hill had the longest pole and he got the persimmons away from you." Birmingham did not have long to wait, however. Approval for a new hospital there was given in 1946. The system of decision, although intensely political, was contained in such cases through (1) placing it in the federal bureaucracy, not Congress, although local congressmen remained powerful players; (2) confining decisions to locations within states, where existing power structures came into play; and (3) openly recognizing federal funding as a "delightful plum" to quote the *Montgomery Advertiser* again, no matter whether it fell into local hands to build a hospital or for something else—an airport, for example, such as Maxwell Field, which was cited in this case.[40]

Once implemented, the idea of a federal hospital program became remarkably entrenched; federal hospitals for veterans were "just the way things were." (Medicare was to have a similar acceptance in the 1960s). There was surprisingly little talk of turning over veterans' care to civilian hospitals after World War II, despite concerns elsewhere in policymaking about "socialized medicine," states' rights, and the primary importance of local communities, and despite widespread criticisms of the quality of the VA system as it had evolved in the 1930s. Under another massive new construction program after World War II, veterans hospitals were virtually reinvented, rebuilt, and affiliated with medical schools. The new watchwords were teaching and research.[41]

By the 1980s, when I wrote this account, the veterans' system, with an aging, poverty-stricken population, was struggling to define its future. It was far less important as an instrument of federal policy than Medicare and Medicaid, even though neither of these owned or operated health care institutions. With its clientele arbitrarily defined by war and its basic purpose still in large part that of workers' compensation, the VA hospital system lay uneasily outside the realm of the most powerful private interests. Nevertheless the veterans' health system still exists as a large federal enterprise, in direct line from the early 1920s.

Past and Present: Generic Themes

What does this study tell us, if anything, about federal policy for health in general? I have six observations to offer. The first is that crises offer opportunities: To policy analysts, they offer the opportunity to study policy in the making, and to practitioners who want to see change, the chance to achieve it. Nothing was done to give veterans the hospitalization to which Congress itself had entitled them until the sense of frustration on all sides made it possible to act. Indeed, an overwhelming sense of the need to act may be required before Congress will take action on domestic social welfare policies. Without the sense of crisis, diverse, pluralistic interests, inside and outside Congress, are unlikely to rally together to support any one proposal; hence the stalemate of veterans hospitals until 1921.

At least up until 1990, policy analysts in the health care field tended, as a group, to seek an overarching rationality as an appropriate goal for health policy in the United States; at heart, I remarked in the original conclusion, "we tend to be old-style Progressives." One conclusion to be drawn from this study was the need for a serious reappraisal of the underlying assumptions of policy-relevant health services research. Rather than deplore the practice of policymaking by crisis, I suggested, it probably made more sense to accept it as normal practice. It still does. It follows that policy analysts and practitioners who wish to achieve change would be more fruitfully employed in identifying, establishing, or nurturing a shared sense of crisis across potential members of powerful coalitions, rather than writing elegant plans that attempt an overall policy synthesis.

My second observation was (and is) that in the American system major policies are often defined not by philosophical intention (e.g., "We should set up a federally operated hospital system"), but by the pragmatic effects of implementing vague agreements. Major programs can arise out of decisions that make sense of the exigencies of the moment; for example, delegating the design of a program that turned out to be a new federal hospital system, to the consultants on hospitalization. The veterans hospital system was a feasible approach to the national medical care of veterans after World War I in a country without national health insurance. Only later was it attacked as "socialized medicine."

This observation raises a connected issue. Political philosophies attached to programs are contingent, and can shift as the program matures and/or the social context changes. The veterans program was designed to provide workers' compensation of the type that, in industry, would thrive as a form of "welfare capitalism" in the 1920s, with major employers providing services directly to their workers. Compensation was implemented with respect to veterans hospitals as an exercise of military or wartime public-private cooperative strategy that was carried over into peacetime. And it could also be seen as an extension of the national, private regulatory program for "standardizing" hospitals that was then engaging the American College of Surgeons (and is now hospital accreditation) and of the national data gathering for hospitals that was established by the American Medical Association in 1921. But finally, as that association made clear, the veterans program could be branded as a socialist proposition. Ideologically, the program was the empty shell for others' views.

The lack of a fundamental philosophical position as a basis for social legislation in the United States makes such legislation the subject of never-ending dialectic as to what in fact it is; so that any powerful group can attach any label it thinks fit. Thus President Harry Truman had to decide whether to defend proposals for health insurance, which could have been labeled business protection, against charges of socialized medicine after World War II. The symbolic importance of labeling—of rhetoric as a means of establishing consensus and marking out political positions—is a fundamental attribute of the U.S. system. The fact that veterans' health benefits were labeled workers' compensation gave them a legitimacy that they would not otherwise have had. They were part of an established language of employer responsibility and employee protection, removing the debates from any hint that this was compulsory health insurance. Thus, for example, Samuel Gompers, who was president of the American Federation of Labor in 1917 and a strong antagonist of "social insurance," could support the veterans program as written; indeed he probably helped to write it.[42] In contrast, social insurance, as he defined it, was bondage, "gyves upon the wrists." Government power, he maintained, "grows upon that which it feeds," sapping the strength of a "virile people."[43]

A later example of the symbolic power of labeling was the transmutation of prepaid group practices into health maintenance organizations in the early 1970s. Health maintenance was linked, symbolically, with income maintenance, local autonomy, and corporate innovation, removing group medicine from political views on the left, and allowing for coalition building for new legislation. Out of words come agreements.

My first observations from this case, then, are the opportunity to achieve policy change under a perceived crisis situation, joined by consensus-building rhetoric. A second set of opportunities arises after legislation is achieved. In other words, policy is made through a continuing process of implementation. Much of what is interesting about U.S. policy is the politics of implementation, with subsequent adjustments to an ongoing program (here, for example, the backhanded inclusion for veterans of hospital benefits for all conditions in 1924, at a time when compulsory health insurance had been abandoned as a policy of choice for other members of the population). As a basic research hypothesis, political and social analysts should expect to find more policy-relevant research findings *after* a piece of legislation than in the battles and compromises that led up to it.

A third observation is the role and utility of experts as instruments in the process of implementation—more specifically, as a way to break deadlock in the political arena. The importance of expertise may seem as self-evident today as it did in informing policy in the late 1980s: days of diagnosis-related groups, outcomes research, and physician payment mechanisms. But the veterans case further demonstrates how experts (in this case, from medical and health associations) can be brought in to break the deadlock on policy in Congress. The decisions of the consultants on hospitalization over where to put hospitals and why, decisions that were administrative, political, and judgmental, were accepted because they were thought to be disinterested; that is, as technical and scientific, drawing on the best hospital planning expertise that then existed. Hence congressional votes were mobilized and consensus achieved at a general level, with the critical decisions displaced to experts.

In one sense major medical interests "captured" the decision-making process, at least temporarily.[44] However, it is equally true that the experts were used by it, and were discarded when no longer necessary. The experts made some logical proposals for planning for all hospitals in the country that went much further in terms of federal control than either Congress or the national medical associations would accept. Those proposals were simply jettisoned. After they had produced their report the consultants' utility was finished. One way to interpret this is to remark on the efficiency of this particular system of implementation. The experts came and the experts went. Ultimately, they were expendable. They left behind no continued power base. Their authority was exercised for only two years. They shored up rather than threatened the power of continuing democratic institutions.

A fourth set of observations centers on the role of U.S. federal agencies as administrators of service systems, particularly where construction and supplies are in play. Forget whether the federal government ought to run major service systems on grounds of principle. Practical doubts have also been expressed, beginning with the Marine Hospital system in the nineteenth century, as to whether the U.S. government is competent to run major health service systems on grounds of administrative capacity. This country may just be too big for the central administration of peacetime service systems (I'll leave the military out of this discussion). But even if the federal government can administer such systems, there remains a long history of administrative irresponsibility within at least some federal agencies.

Could a national health service system ever be well run by a federal agency? The veterans case gives two unpromising scenarios up to World War II. The first (the Forbes administration) is a story of graft and greed, including the nicely symbolic though probably apocryphal tale of President Harding choking Forbes in rage in the Red Room of the White House. "You yellow rat!" the president reportedly cried. "You double-crossing bastard!"[45] The second is the story of the far tamer Hines administration; during this period the veterans hospital system was criticized for failing to develop its scientific and technical capability. It became, in a nutshell, third rate. Are we condemned to the prospect of federal administration as essentially corruptible, lackadaisical, and/or inefficient? Or have we not found the model yet, at least as far as health services are concerned?

When I wrote this article, I thought the jury was still out on these questions. Veterans health services were reinvented (and linked with medical schools) after World War II, but were in the doldrums again by the late 1980s. I am now (in 2006) more negative than I was then about prospects for efficient federal service systems, at least with respect to health services. However, the VA became a leader in hospital and health care quality evaluation in the early 2000s—something that could not have been predicted fifteen or twenty years ago. For other programs, the familiar federal model is now standard-setting and rule-making. Medicare administration, predicated on provision and administration of service in non-federal institutions, carries the weight of detailed federal audit and regulation. By avoiding the appearance of a federally dictated health care system, the United States has created an intensely regulated health care system.

A fifth observation from the veterans case concerns the role played by organized medicine. The American Medical Association has often been criticized for its powerful, reactionary role in the history of American health policy. However, one essential point has often not been made and deserves far more attention than it has been given. Namely, what is, can, and should be the role of a national profession in a federal political system? Organized medicine has been extremely visible in American medicine because it has often been much more effectively "organized" in its political views than the very diverse group of individuals and interests in Congress. American medicine had an effective, centralized power structure by 1918 (actually more than one, for both the American Medical Association and the American College of Surgeons should be mentioned) but little or no parallel national political structure (or even national party platforms) with which to work. And there was no permanent senior civil service to provide continuity across administrations. Arguably the medical profession was more consistent in its policy views than Congress in the twentieth century, and more willing, too, to couch policies in terms of ideology and political philosophies. Be that as it may, it would be helpful to have a series of studies of the role of national professional associations in national policymaking in federal systems, not just in the United States, but also in Canada, Germany, and Australia, at least.

Sixth and finally, there are the questions of piecemeal rather than global policymaking for health care in the United States. On one level, it made no sense having separate federal hospital systems for the Public Health Service and for veterans, even in the 1920s. But in terms of their legislative history, it did. Veterans hospitals served veterans and were subsidiary to the primary legislative purpose of veterans' compensation. In the absence of a larger national health system, all parties were probably best served this way, rather than through administrative attempts to cobble together federal programs that, however logically they were joined through professional expertise (hospital administration), were not joined through congressional intent. Those of us who are Machiavellian might also deduce from this history that the best way to get health legislation passed is to disguise it as something else.

The result of federal policymaking in the United States has been (and is) a constantly negotiated health care system or, more accurately, a series of systems, filled with discoveries and surprises, temporary coalitions, changing rhetoric, new experts, new solutions. Federal policy lurches from one perceived crisis to the next, and consensus, is narrow and ever-shifting. Resistance to government in principle is matched by pressures from specific interests for more government intervention, for limited purposes or specific populations. Each case is "special."

This process tends to lead, overall, to an increased federal role by a process of accretion. It seems highly unlikely that federal responsibility for health care will become a unified whole in the near future, as the consultants suggested (for hospitals, at least) in the early 1920s. The United States will probably continue to lurch along with separate programs for the elderly, the poor, the disabled, children, the unemployed, veterans, Indians, and other worthy groups, wherever consensus is achieved. Perhaps, as Rashi Fein argued years ago, a future band of pragmatists, responding to a sense of administrative chaos, will argue successfully for a national health service. However, there is a strong political rationale for continuing the present system of policy by accretion. So long as decisions are fragmented across numerous different programs, conflicts over a single national health policy can be sidestepped.

There was never a single or simple "capitalist" medicine to set in opposition to "socialized" medicine or to offer as the basis for considering the new "post-welfare state." If there is any consistent theme it is, as Gerald Holton (1989) put it, the theme of improvised arrangements and entrepreneurial experimentalism.[46] What, I asked in 1991, were experts in health care to do in the 1990s and beyond? Much health services research had focused on short-term quantitative analyses, sometimes for designing detailed federal regulations. Given the highly political nature of health care, the United States was appallingly short of good political, anthropological, and social analysis. While much has been done since then, this remains a major task for the future.

Equally important is how experts in health services research actually see the system as it functions in the present. The veterans case is a good example of American flexibility in policymaking, maddening though this process may be. The system worked! There was no national health insurance; nevertheless, a health care system was designed for veterans once their entitlement to such benefits had been agreed upon. There was no consensus about how to establish hospitals; nevertheless, hospitals were established, through the useful device of an expert committee. True, the hospital system was late, wasteful, and initially corrupt. But it was present. There was—and is—no necessary flaw in the institutions of government itself. Could the government govern? The answer was yes: despite the lack of party discipline, the sectional interests of Congress, distrust of government, and very varied performance by federal agencies. Today, as yesterday, the critical questions revolve on the creation of sufficient consensus to pass enabling legislation and an effective machinery for implementation.

This chapter was originally published as "Can the Government Govern? Lessons from the Formation of the Veterans Administration," *Journal of Health Politics, Policy and Law*, 1991, 16 (2): 281-305.

Notes

1.   Chubb and Peterson 1989: 3.

2. See Fox 1986; Morone and Dunham 1985.
3. See Stevens 1989: 378, passim.
4. Adkins 1967: 102.
5. Flexner 1911: 363.
6. Medical Department 1923: 92-93.
7. See Glasson 1918: 291.
8. U.S. Bureau of the Census 1919: 645.
9. Adkins 1967: 87.
10. Ibid.: 92, 95-96.
11. French 1917: 267.
12. U.S. Bureau of Labor Statistics 1917.
13. Holman 1917: 249.
14. B.F. Goodrich, with four hospitals or dispensaries in the plant, reportedly employed nine full-time physicians and twenty-two full-time nurses for its workers, and its district nurses were "each equipped with a Ford coupelet and a driver." About half the population of Akron was dependent on wages earned at B.F. Goodrich (Dudley R. Kennedy, director, Labor Department, B.F. Goodrich Company, cited in U.S. Bureau of Labor Statistics 1917: 345-46). On the broader picture of corporate responsibility for social services in this period, see Brandes 1970; on working conditions, Rosner and Markowitz 1989; and on health insurance, Numbers 1978.
15. "Workmen's compensation is not social insurance. Morally and legally it is based, not upon the duty of society, but upon the duty of industry to the worker.... Underlying the whole theory of workmen's compensation is the recognition that when the worker devotes his services to a particular industry, he subjects himself to the peculiar hazards of its environment and that the injuries incurred during the course of his service are in the general nature of things part of the accepted incidents of production and therefore part of the ultimate cost of the product.... The employer has not discharged a social duty; he has merely done justice as between himself and his employees" (Magnus W. Alexander, General Electric Company, cited in U.S. Bureau of Labor Statistics 1917: 765-66).
16. Cited in Adkins 1967: 94.
17. See, for instance, Williams 1917: 292-304. F.M. William was chairman of the Workmen's Compensation Commission of Connecticut.
18. According to Alexander Lambert (1917: 656), chairman of the Social Insurance Committee of the American Medical Association. "Capitation has certain inherent evils.... The evils of it are that it produces overcrowding of work on the part of the physicians, forcing hurried and inadequate service, and worst of all, under such circumstances that the really sick patients who need the greatest amount of attention are the least adequately cared for. It produces the kind of contract practice against which the profession has protested for years."
19. Missouri Bureau of Labor Statistics 1920: 249, passim.
20. Rogers 1921: 1081. J. B. Rogers was assistant medical adviser at the Bureau of War Risk Insurance.
21. Ibid.; Adkins 1967: 102.
22. Adkins 1967: 104; Cumming 1921.
23. Meeker 1917: 14.
24. Adkins 1967: 92, 102.
25. See Leigh 1927: 177-178.
26. Ibid.: 150.
27. A nice example is from the Conference on Social Insurance, from Edson S. Lott, president of the United States Casualty Company: "Service! My friends, have any

one of you been so unfortunate as to have a contract, for construction or what not, with the government? How long did it take you to get your money, and did the man in charge show judgment or fairness in settling disputed matters? Delays, red tape, indifference—these are the often everyday diet of the citizen who contracts with his government. The insurance company is a corporation, but in its dealings with its patrons it is at least polite, prompt, and fair. It has to be. Competition compels it" (U.S. Bureau of Labor Statistics 1917: 100). The problem of corruption was also not unknown in the letting and administration of federal contracts. A notable example, disclosed at congressional hearings on military hospitals in 1919, was the Speedway Hospital, a huge $3 million hospital to be built by private contractors, ostensibly for the military, on an automobile racetrack in Chicago. Charges of bribes and special deals surrounded this project, including an alleged bribe of $100,000 to a senior War Department official (U.S. Senate 1919: 5). The army eventually accepted the hospital, but it was an embarrassing white elephant. In 1921, for example, it reportedly had one thousand beds and only five patients (Consultants on Hospitalization 1921).

28. Leigh 1927: 192-193.
29. Wilson's incapacity, joined with tussles over power between Congress and the executive, probably contributed to the delay in veterans policy. His Secretary of the Treasury described him in the spring of 1920 as old, worn, and haggard, one of his arms useless, his jaw dropped on one side, his voice weak (Houston 1926: 70-72).
30. Pearce Bailey resigned after three months and died soon after. He was replaced by Dr. George H. Kirby, director of the New York Psychiatric Institute at Ward's Island and former medical inspector of the New York State Hospital Commission.
31. U.S. Department of the Treasury 1923.
32. Forbes 1970: 27-43.
33. U.S. Senate 1924: 68.
34. John F. O'Ryan, cited in Mertz 1924: 440. General O'Ryan was counsel to the Select Committee on Investigation of the United States Veterans Bureau. The latter quote appears verbatim in the body of the Senate committee report, where Forbes' conduct is described as criminal (U.S. Senate 1924: 40).
35. James 1923: 18.
36. Veterans Administration 1933: 11.
37. Haggard 1925: 1664.
38. American Medical Association 1959.
39. In the National Archives.
40. Quotes are from Federal Board of Hospitalization 1921: 48.
41. See Gronvall 1989.
42. See Adkins 1967: 92.
43. Gompers 1917: 845, 847.
44. I am indebted to Lawrence D. Brown for the point about the need to rethink the "capture" theory.
45. Adams 1939: 297.
46. Holton 1989.

References

Adams, Samuel Hopkins. 1939. *Incredible Era: The Life and Times of Warren Gamaliel Harding*. Boston: Houghton Mifflin.
Adkins, Robinson E. 1967. *Medical Care of Veterans*. Report prepared for the House Committee on Veterans Affairs. 90th Cong., 1st sess. Committee Print 4.

American Medical Association. 1959. *Digest of Official Actions, 1846-1958.* Chicago: American Medical Association.

Brandes, Stuart D. 1970. *American Welfare Capitalism, 1880-1940.* Chicago: University of Chicago Press.

Chubb, John E., and Peterson, Paul E., eds. 1989. *Can the Government Govern?* Washington, D.C.: Brookings Institution.

Consultants on Hospitalization. 1921. Minutes, 14 September. Record Group 121, Box 233. National Archives, Washington, D.C.

Cumming, Hugh S. 1921. "The Work of the Public Health Service in the Care of Disabled Veterans of the World War." *Public Health Reports* 36: 1893-1902.

Federal Board of Hospitalization. 1921-48. Records of the Federal Board of Hospitalization (1921-1948), Site Files, 1921-1948, Box 1. Record Group 51 NA 21.5. National Archives, Washington, D.C.

Flexner, Abraham. 1911. "Hospitals, Medical Education, and Research." *Transactions of the American Hospital Association* 13: 363.

Forbes, Charles R. 1970 [1927]. "Inside the Harding Administration". In *Politics in the Nineteen Twenties*, ed. John L. Shover. Waltham, MA: Ginn-Blaisdell.

Fox, Daniel M. 1986. "The Consequences of Consensus: American Health Policy in the Twentieth Century." *Milbank Memorial Fund Quarterly* 64: 76-99.

French, Will J. 1917. "Accident Prevention in California." In *Proceedings of the Conference on Social Insurance.* Bulletin of the United States Bureau of Labor Statistics No. 212. Washington, D.C.: U.S. Government Printing Office.

Glasson, William H. 1918. *Federal Military Pensions in the United States.* New York: Oxford University Press.

Gompers, Samuel. 1917. Address. In *Proceedings of the Conference on Social Insurance.* Bulletin of the United States Bureau of Labor Statistics No. 212. Washington, D.C.: U.S. Government Printing Office.

Gronvall, John A. 1989. "The V.A.'s Affiliation with Academic Medicine: An Emergency Post-War Strategy Becomes a Permanent Partnership." *Academic Medicine* 64: 61-66.

Haggard, William D. 1925. "Address of the President-Elect." *Journal of the American Medical Association* 84: 1664.

Holman, Dudley M. 1917. "The Problem of the Handicapped Man." In *Proceedings of the Conference on Social Insurance.* Bulletin of the United States Bureau of Labor Statistics No. 212. Washington, D.C.: U.S. Government Printing Office.

Holton, Gerald. 1989. "From Colony to Developed Nation." Paper presented at the Eighteenth Congress of History of Science, Hamburg, August.

Houston, David F. 1926. *Eight Years with Wilson's Cabinet, with a Personal Estimate of the President.* Vol. 2. Garden City, NY: Doubleday, Page and Company.

James, Marquis. 1923. "What's Wrong in Washington: The Latest Muddle in the United States Veterans Bureau." *American Legion Weekly*, 9 March, p. 18.

Lambert, Alexander. 1917. "Organization of Medical Benefits under the Proposed Sickness (Health) Insurance System." In *Proceedings of the Conference on Social Insurance.* Bulletin of the United States Bureau of Labor Statistics No. 212. Washington, D.C.: U.S. Government Printing Office.

Leigh, Robert D. 1927. *Federal Health Administration in the United States.* New York: Harper and Brothers.

Medical Department of the U.S. Army in the World War, The. 1923. Vol. 1. Prepared under the direction of Surgeon General M.W. Ireland. Washington, D.C.: U.S. Government Printing Office.

Meeker, Royal. 1917. "Introduction." In *Proceedings of the Conference on Social Insurance*. Bulletin of the United States Bureau of Labor Statistics No. 212. Washington, D.C.: U.S. Government Printing Office.

Mertz, Charles. 1924. "The Betrayal of Our War Veterans: The Forbes Story as a Factor in the Campaign." *Century Magazine* 108: 440.

Missouri Bureau of Labor Statistics. 1920. *Missouri: Red Book 1920, 1919, 1918*. Pt. 2, Wartime Industrial History of a Progressive Commonwealth. Jefferson City: Missouri Bureau of Labor Statistics.

Morone, J. A., and Dunham, A. B. 1985. "Slouching Towards National Health Insurance: The New Health Care Politics." *Yale Journal on Regulation* 2: 263-91.

Numbers, Ronald. 1978. *Almost Persuaded: American Physicians and Compulsory Health Insurance, 1912-1920*. Baltimore, MD: Johns Hopkins University Press.

Rogers, L. B. 1921. "The War Risk Act and the Medical Services Created under It." *Journal of the American Medical Association* 76: 1081.

Rosner, David, and Markowitz, Gerald, eds. 1989. *Dying for Work: Workers' Safety and Health in Twentieth-Century America*. Bloomington: Indiana University Press.

Stevens, Rosemary. 1989. *In Sickness and in Wealth: American Hospitals in the Twentieth Century*. New York: Basic Books.

U.S. Bureau of Labor Statistics. 1917. *Proceedings of the Conference on Social Insurance*. Bulletin No. 212. Washington, D.C.: U.S. Government Printing Office.

U.S. Bureau of the Census. 1919. *Statistical Abstract of the United States, 1919*. Washington, D.C.: U.S. Government Printing Office.

U.S. Department of the Treasury. 1923. *Report of the Consultants on Hospitalization Appointed by the Secretary of the Treasury to Provide Additional Hospital Facilities under Public Act 384*. Washington, D.C.: U.S. Government Printing Office.

U.S. Senate, Committee on Public Buildings and Grounds. 1919. *Military Hospitals: Hearings Pursuant to S. Res. 386*. 65th Cong., 1st sess.

U.S. Senate, Select Committee on Investigation of the Veterans Bureau. 1924. *Report Pursuant to S. Res. 466*. 67th Cong., 2d sess.

Veterans Administration. 1933. *Annual Report for 1933*. Washington, D.C.: U.S. Government Printing Office.

Williams, F. M. 1917. "Medical and Hospital Fees under Workmen's Compensation." In *Proceedings of the Conference on Social Insurance*. Bulletin of the United States Bureau of Labor Statistics No. 212. Washington, D.C.: U.S. Government Printing Office.

4

Letter from America, 1961

It is not often that debates in the Congress of the United States are of interest and importance to students of the British National Health Service. The controversial King-Anderson bill to provide medical care for the aged does, however, fall into this category. Strongly supported by President Kennedy, it raises the fundamental question of free medical care. This bill proposes to extend the social security system, which already provides the old age pension and disability and certain survivor benefits, to include the provision of some free medical care for persons receiving the old age pension (Social Security insurance benefits). The extra cost would be met by an increase in social security contributions, which are collected as a percentage tax on incomes up to a certain income level.

Under the provisions of the bill old age pensioners would be entitled to ninety days of continuous hospital inpatient care in any one year (with a deduction for the first nine days), 180 days of skilled nursing home services where they immediately follow inpatient care, the cost of outpatient treatment over and above $20 (four pounds sterling in buying power), and visiting nurse and related home health services for a limited, unspecified period. There would be no financial help toward drug bills, inpatient or outpatient doctors' fees, or preventive medical care.

A Crying Need

In spite of its limitations and deficiencies the bill is a positive attempt to remedy a crying social need. At present old people pay for the cost of medical care in the same way as others: through their income, savings, or through private insurance. Unfortunately, in America as elsewhere, the income of the elderly tends to be small and many have little or no insurance coverage: for it is not always possible to pay medical insurance that will cover costs incurred beyond the age of sixty-five. Since the elderly require more medical care than any other group, life savings may be quickly drained, insurance benefits (where they exist) exhausted, and the old people left to struggle on as best they can or become destitute and/or eligible for public assistance. Less than half of those sixty-five years of age and over who receive social security pensions (and only 60 percent do) own health insurance of any type; 57 percent have no insurance against hospital costs; and 71 percent have no insurance against surgical costs. Moreover, in equivalent buying power more than half of the elderly in America have a money income of less than 200 pounds annually. Yet the medical cost to married couples in this group with one or both members in the hospital averages 140 pounds and many have to find a great deal more than this.

Something has to be done; there is no disagreement on this point. Dissidence only arises as to what should be done. The bill raises two controversial issues: first, whether medical care should be provided free of charge to individuals other than on the basis of financial need (via a means test); and second, whether medical care, even to this limited degree, should be allowed to fall under the control of the federal government. Since the bill's proposals do incorporate the idea that medical benefits would be given to all contributors as a right irrespective of their ability to pay, critics have seized on the term "socialization" to suggest that the scheme would undermine the American way of life—a sentiment that almost invariably ensures popular sympathy. Four clergymen of different denominations recently testified before the House of Representatives Ways and Means Committee that free medical care through social security would interfere with individual responsibilities and the responsibilities of those caring for those in need of assistance. The supreme importance of self-reliance and self-help is at the root of the traditional image of the "American way of life." The hero of the myth is the individual who, by his own unaided efforts, makes his own life a success. Traditionally, America is a society whose economic vision is perfect competition, its social vision equal opportunity, and its psychological vision individual autonomy. In theory, everyone should find his or her rightful place. These ideas are so deeply embedded in the American subconscious that they are sometimes accepted as independent moral ideals.

In spite of the fact that the King-Anderson bill provides medical care through an insurance system, there is a widespread feeling that people would be getting something for nothing. The first major objection is that no effort would have to be made by the individual to provide for his or her own health care needs through savings, private health insurance, or group prepayment plans. The lazy or negligent individual would receive the same benefits as a farsighted one. Nor would the individual have a choice as to whether or not to participate in the scheme: Free benefits would be available to everyone covered. Moreover, those not wishing to benefit would still have to contribute during their working life the same way as everyone else. Both these concepts of individual effort and individual choice are part of the American myth. To disregard them is deliberately to weaken the moral fiber of the nation, say the critics, particularly medical associations that see in the bill the loss of the doctor-patient relationship, the loss of a right to choose one's own physician, and, perhaps most of all, a threat to the inflated incomes of American doctors.

The second main objection is to federal rather than state or local control, and that is for some a more serious cause of apprehension. Increasing centralization, they feel, will lead eventually to a vast, impersonal organization, wielding immense power, wasteful and inefficient. State control would be weakened and local initiative disregarded. Thus medicine would be become prey to the bureaucratic machine.

Charity or Social Insurance

There has never been any question about helping the indigent. Those who need financial help outside social security may get it from public assistance, from voluntary organizations, or by the waiving of physicians' fees. Outpatient charity clinics are held in public hospitals. Voluntary bodies such as Goodwill Industries provide employment for the disabled. Donations and bequests keep the private hospitals alive. All these, however, embody the precept of giving to the poor, the needy, or the unemployable by the rich, the more comfortable, the employed. They discriminate in fact between the "haves" and "have-nots."

The Eisenhower administration secured legislation last autumn (1960) that perpetuated and strengthened this attitude. The Kerr-Mills Act was designed to placate those who feared government intervention and those loath to relinquish the charity principle, at the same time leaving the details of providing assistance to the individual state legislatures. Under the Act, the states are each entitled to legislate to give free medical care to persons already on public assistance and to those who, although they are not on public assistance, are pronounced "medically indigent" according to means test provisions determined by the states themselves. The federal government provides matching funds to enable the states to do this. So far less than half the states are participating in the plan; and the compromise has largely failed.

The King-Anderson bill attempts to remove this discrimination. "We do not want charity—we want care with dignity," proclaimed leaflets distributed by the old age pensioners who picketed the American Medical Association's annual meeting in the summer of 1960. They were echoing Kennedy's statements a year before, when he testified on his previous health bill before the Senate Finance Committee: "They should be eligible for retirement benefits—as a right they have earned."

Thus the American people are being presented with the choice between two principles: charity or social insurance. Charity as at present organized (both private charity and public assistance) is insufficient to meet the need. Old people who cannot pay their medical bills are not necessarily otherwise indigent. Yet charity, an integral part of the free enterprise system and the American myth, is not easily relinquished. There is a great reluctance to help those not actually in need or to encourage dependence on a state welfare program. Even many of those who favor medical care for the aged through social insurance are suspicious of how it would work in practice.

Comparisons with the British National Health Service

In these circumstances it is not surprising that there should be great interest on this side of the Atlantic in the working of the British National Health Service (NHS). The principles of free enterprise in the economics of the two countries are sufficiently close for direct comparisons to be drawn. Compulsory contributions toward the service, free benefits regardless of ability to pay, and control by the central government are all incorporated in the British system. Does the British experience foreshadow the pattern of future health care organization in the United States, or is it an example to be avoided? The AMA takes the latter view, frequently with great vehemence, pointing to the NHS as a miserable failure. Their self-interest in this matter is obvious, as is that of the private insurers and pharmaceutical firms, who also strongly oppose the King-Anderson bill.

The views of critics of the NHS (particularly those from the United Kingdom) are widely publicized; but more and more thinking Americans are trying to find more objective reports. It is not easy for them to make intelligent comparisons from the reports available. They read of the increased cost of the service from year to year, of the waste of materials provided free (one lady from Whitstable was recently quoted in the *Wall Street Journal* as claiming her husband used bandages supplied free on prescription for cleaning the car), and of the introduction and steady increase of direct charges to patients. They also read of a reported increase in British United Provident Association membership (private insurance) from 65,000 to 850,000 since the beginning of the service. To such persons it appears not only that the British system is financially unsound, but that two of the strongly-held American principles—fee for service and voluntary insurance—are gradually creeping in. Whereas it appears that America is heading toward some sort of blanket coverage, it appears that at the same time Britain is not entirely happy with it, and indeed is slowly withdrawing to a system of individual payment.

By the time this article is published the fate of the King-Anderson bill will be known. It appears unlikely that it will be passed in this session of Congress. But even if it fails, President Kennedy has said that it, or a similar bill, will be brought up again next year. When the problem is reexamined, one thing is certain: The spotlight will again be turned on the NHS as a basis of comparison. Let us hope that by this time more accurate and detailed information on the NHS will have been made available to the American public. When the facts have been properly presented, Americans will have much to learn from the British system; and if America draws closer to the principles embodied in the NHS, Britain in its turn may receive useful ideas for the future development of its services.

"Letter from America, 1961" was originally published in the British journal, *The Hospital*, October 1961: 623-25. It is edited here for clarification.

5

Anatomy of a Dilemma: Creating and Implementing Medicaid, 1965-1970

Rosemary Stevens and Robert Stevens

The Medicaid program—title XIX of the Social Security Act—was passed amid great hope on the part of liberals as the so-called "sleeper" of the Social Security Act of 1965. The optimistic saw Medicare (title XVIII) as a step towards a Swedish form of social insurance and title XIX as a step towards something like the British National Health Service. They could not have been more wrong. While title XVIII was to achieve general acceptance, title XIX lived up to almost none of the expectations of its proponents. By the early 1970s, when the paper from which this chapter was drawn was published, Medicaid had served only to confirm many of the doubts about government programs of medical care on the part of professional critics and fiscal conservatives.

How did it come to pass that, in five brief years between 1965 and 1970, title XIX grew astronomically in its financial demands (it was originally projected to cost the federal government $0.7 billion annually and by 1970 was in fact costing Washington $2.8 billion, with a total estimated annual cost from all governmental sources of some $5.5 billion) and yet failed to satisfy the persons it was supposed to serve as well as the hopes of its supporters? The answers, vital to policy evaluation, include these: Medicaid was built on a program—Kerr-Mills—which was itself a failure; the structure of the program ensured that it would never be able to escape the debilitating effect of its welfare parentage; the concept of "medical indigency" was (and is) meaningless; and the administration of the program was a failure at every level.

The inappropriateness of a welfare-means-test approach was not only particularly noticeable in a program of services but also economically unrealistic as a means of providing medical services. "Medical indigence" proved a less rigorous concept than "poverty" itself, if only because the breakthroughs and potential of modern medicine made it possible for virtually any American to be "medically indigent" by the late 1960s—a heart transplant could be paid for by very few Americans out of their own assets. What a significant percentage of the American population was suffering from was "health insurance indigency."

Medicaid also failed to achieve its initial expectations because of inadequate administration. Supervision was assigned to a division of the federal bureaucracy with insufficient prestige and resources to administer, make policy for, or police the program. Administration was equally unsatisfactory in the states. Both these administrative weaknesses, coupled with congressional unwillingness to come face to face with the powerful medical lobbies, meant that the traditional medical monopolies, privileges, and forms of practice were left untouched—as they were in the simultaneous implementation of Medicare. The economic advantage of the providers over the purchasers in these early years, coupled with inadequate administrative safeguards, virtually assured that the Medicaid program would be plagued by a series of financial crises between 1966 and 1974.

Predecessors of Medicaid

Provision of medical care to the poor has long been a recognized part of the American system of public relief. Early arrangements were made on an ad hoc, decentralized, local, and often erratic basis, following the patterns of cash relief in the towns, counties, and states. With the introduction of federal grants-in-aid under the Social Security Act of 1935 for population groups (or "categories") who were at that time most urgently in financial need, came old-age assistance (OAA), aid to the blind (AB), and aid to dependent children (later, aid to families with dependent children, AFDC). A fourth categorical cash assistance program, aid to the permanently and totally disabled (APTD), was added in 1950. These joined the earlier programs of general assistance by the states or local government units, and in large part supplanted them as states recognized the benefits of Medicaid's federal matching funds. Between 1940 and 1966 the number of individuals receiving cash payments under general assistance declined from four million to less than 600,000, while the number receiving categorical assistance rose from three million to over seven million persons.[1]

Federal-state grants for certain medical services were made available as separate programs under the 1935 legislation, most notably for maternal and child health services and for services to crippled children; but these were service programs provided by the states and not directly related to welfare programs. No separate provisions for paying health providers were made in the federal matching grants for categorical assistance programs. In some areas, notably California and the City of New York, health services at low cost for the indigent were provided in public hospitals and clinics. But in general the provision of health services for the poor remained, at best, a subsidiary part of cash benefit programs and a neglected area of state and local welfare responsibilities, until the establishment of a federally-supported program of vendor payments for medical care under the Social Security Act Amendments of 1950.

The new vendor payments were designed to reverse, at least partly, the formal federal unconcern with medical care for the poor. "Vendors" were providers of health services—the model was state government as buyer (buttressed by federal subsidy) and the largely private providers as sellers. Under the 1950 amendments the federal government agreed to share with the states the cost of direct payments to physicians, hospitals, and others who provided medical care to persons on public assistance. States responded to the availability of the new federal grants-in-aid. By 1960, vendor payments under all public assistance programs had reached a total of $514 million, well over half of which was for hospital and nursing home care.[2] These payments were still, however, limited to persons on the existing welfare rolls. For almost all of these recipients, the states were also recovering part of their cash benefits from the federal government through one of the categorical cash assistance programs.

Concern over the plight of the elderly in the 1950s was also focusing congressional attention on the medical needs of that increasingly articulate, numerous, and medically needy group, over and above the meager provisions, means test requirements, and welfare stigma of OAA. In 1960, there were 16.5 million people sixty-five years of age and over, representing 15.4 percent of the population twenty-one years and over. This sizeable proportion of "aged" potential voters could not be ignored politically. Proposals for Health Insurance for the Aged, the forerunner of hospital benefits under Medicare, appeared forcefully in 1957 under the sponsorship of Senator Aimé Forand. By 1960 health insurance for the aged had become a political hot potato. In that year, as a countermeasure to proposals for a federal program of hospital insurance for all of the aged (what would eventually become Medicare), the Eisenhower administration proposed a new federal-state program to protect low-income elderly persons against the cost of long-term illness; Vice President Richard Nixon was a strong supporter. This proposal would have established a national means test eligibility level for assistance, with specified medical, hospital, and nursing benefits. The House Ways and Means Committee rejected this too. Instead, proposals sponsored by the committee chairman, Representative Wilbur Mills of Arkansas, and by Senator Robert Kerr of Oklahoma, were added to the omnibus social security bill (H.R. 12580) and enacted into law as the Kerr-Mills Act of 1960 (P.L. 86-778). For the time being, health insurance for the aged was defeated.

The Kerr-Mills Act provided more generous federal matching grants for vendor medical payments under old-age assistance. But it also included a new category of assistance in a separate program of federal grants to the states: medical assistance to the aged (MAA). This applied to "medically needy" aged persons who were needy because of their health care bills but were *not* cash assistance recipients; after 1962 the blind and disabled were included under a similar category (title XVI). The new beneficiaries were defined as elderly or blind persons (or totally disabled persons over twenty-one) not on public assistance, whose income might be above state eligibility levels but not high enough to meet their medical bills. Kerr-Mills provided matching grants to participating states of 50 to 80 percent of the cost of vendor payments, depending on the state. The structure, later to be followed by Medicaid, was one of open-ended federal cost sharing, without limitations on individual payments or total state expenditures; cost control was left to the states. The matching formula favored lower-income states, including those of Representative Mills and Senator Kerr. State participation was optional, as with other assistance titles.

The act suggested a broad range of hospital, nursing home, physician, and other services, and required each plan to include both institutional (hospital and nursing home) and non-institutional care as a condition of federal sharing. Thus while the new program was left in the hands of state administrators, it included as an important precedent the concept of federal standard-setting of benefits. There were provisions that a recipient could not receive medical care under both OAA and MAA, that states were not to set up enrollment fees for participation, and that (as with other categorical public assistance programs) the program had to be in effect in all administrative subdivisions of a state. Two innovations set the new MAA apart from other public assistance programs: States were not to impose long-term residency requirements for eligibility, nor were they to impose liens on the recipient's property during his lifetime or that of a surviving spouse. The Department of Health, Education, and Welfare was responsible for approving state plans, issuing guidelines, and receiving reports on their operation. The program began on October 1, 1960.

In theory the Kerr-Mills program could have provided extensive services to a substantial proportion of the elderly population and to the other two adult groups included in at least some of its provisions. But—prefiguring the experience of Medicaid five years later—the nature of Kerr-Mills was predetermined by its heritage as a defensive political compromise in Congress. This was not a health insurance program but a supplement to existing forms of poor relief. Kerr-Mills was also, importantly, a means of increasing federal grants for vendor payments in the states. Counties in the United States that were subsidizing medical relief welcomed Kerr-Mills as a source of additional state support; hospitals and doctors as a means of reducing their own private contributions to medical care to the indigent, by the introduction of more realistic fees for welfare patients who were elderly; while the states had the pleasant prospect of expanded federal funding. California defined its new MAA program quite clearly as being designed "to supplement the financial ability of counties to meet the health needs of aged persons."[3]

At the federal level, the program was administered by the Bureau of Public Assistance, not by the Public Health Service. Not surprisingly, the states in implementing their programs designed means tests for the medically indigent under MAA, which, though more liberal than the means test for both cash and health programs under OAA, were similar in administration and intent. The atmosphere of "welfare" was all-pervasive. Under MAA, the elderly were forced to spend down to the relatively low-income eligibility limits of the program before receiving any benefits. As Secretary Celebrezze pointed out in the 1963 hearings on hospital insurance for the aged, Kerr-Mills did not prevent dependency but only dealt with it after it had happened.[4]

The implementation of Kerr-Mills in the states was similar in flavor to the later implementation of Medicaid. The federal Bureau of Public Assistance, renamed the Bureau of Family Services of the Welfare Administration, issued a series of State Letters summarizing the provisions of the legislation and reflecting the department's view that both the extended OAA vendor payment provisions and the new MAA program would result in the improvement of programs of health care for the elderly. The bureau prepared information leaflets, met with state directors of public assistance, appointed a group of consultants on medical matters, prepared a guide and a handbook of regulations, published statistics, and assisted the states through technical medical consultation. As a voluntary program of grants-in-aid, however, MAA imposed little responsibility on the Department of Health, Education, and Welfare. Apart from exhortation, the federal role was minor.

The states embraced Kerr-Mills as an extension of existing welfare programs and a new source of federal budgetary assistance. Because of the higher federal sharing provisions under MAA there was an immediate incentive, particularly in the richer states with large vendor payment programs, to shift part of their existing programs into the new category. Indeed, one report in 1963 found that the combined percentage of old people who were covered for medical care under OAA and MAA had actually declined after the adoption of the new program, from fourteen to thirteen percent.[5]

An important byproduct of the funding arrangements was that, instead of encouraging services where they were most needed through higher federal matching grants to the low-income states, Kerr-Mills proved more attractive to states that already had substantial vendor programs. In 1965, the five states of New York, California, Massachusetts, Minnesota, and Pennsylvania, which together included about 31 percent of the nation's sixty-five-plus population, received about 62 percent of federal MAA funds.[6] By then forty-four of the fifty-four jurisdictions had some program in effect, but in many cases programs were minimal and there were wide and confusing variations. Only five jurisdictions were judged to provide comprehensive medical services (Indiana, Massachusetts, Minnesota, New York, and North Dakota). Eligibility levels varied widely; indeed, in fourteen of the states the MAA income levels were found in 1963 to be more rigidly interpreted and often lower than those for OAA. The continuation of family responsibility for the medical care of elderly relatives, the custom of attaching property after death (although forbidden during the recipient's lifetime), and the pauperization provisions of the means test all added to the political failure of Kerr-Mills to provide even a minimal alternative to a general program of health care benefits for the elderly.

One major difficulty, which was to be transported lock, stock, and barrel into Medicaid, was the financial inability and thus unwillingness of low-income states to afford a medical assistance program even when the federal matching grant was up to 80 percent of the total cost. Georgia, for example, authorized MAA in 1961 and Mississippi in 1964, but no state funds were ever appropriated. Even the richer states were already aware of state funding problems. Governor Brown of California stated in 1963 that the cost of making MAA a comprehensive medical care program in that state "would bankrupt the State and county governments."[7]

Kerr-Mills was built on the dilemma that foreshadowed Medicaid. Benefits for the medically indigent were, arguably, a program of health services, or even a form of private health supplement. But if so, there was no particular virtue in attaching them administratively to a program of public assistance cash benefits whose primary capability lay in determining individual eligibility through means tests—not in providing services. The states universally defined "medical indigence" in terms of standard means test provisions, even though the "medically indigent" were emphatically not "indigent" in the sense of being on cash relief. Kerr-Mills thus fell between two stools. It was both a reflection of inadequate medical services to those with low and middle incomes and an extension of traditional notions of assistance.

More Radical Changes?

While the states—and potential beneficiaries—struggled with the administrative complexities of Kerr-Mills, pressures built up in Congress for hospital insurance for the aged through Social Security for persons at *all* income levels. Specific medical services would be added as a covered benefit (or entitlement) under the Social Security program, free of state variations and of the administration of a means test. The two movements—the growing failure of Kerr-Mills and pressures for health insurance for the aged—gathered momentum in the years after 1960, culminating in the Social Security Amendments of 1965, which established both Medicare and Medicaid.

With the Democratic landslide in the elections of November 1964, the composition of the House of Representatives (and of the Ways and Means Committee) changed in favor of adding hospital insurance as a benefit for the elderly under Social Security. Other proposals for financing health care were, however, by no means dead. Indeed, it was the eventual combination of several major proposals that was to give the 1965 legislation its peculiar and distinctive character. In 1961 Senator Jacob Javits had revived the Eisenhower proposal for federal support of extensive state programs for those over sixty-five whose individual incomes did not exceed $3000, or whose joint incomes did not exceed $4500. The AMA developed its own "Eldercare" proposal, sponsored in the

Congress by Representatives Curtis and Herlong and by Senator Tower, which called for a federal-state program to subsidize private health insurance policies for the elderly. A similar bill, sponsored by Representative John W. Byrnes and endorsed by the House Republican leadership, "Bettercare," suggested a federal (rather than a state) program whereby the elderly would be encouraged to contribute part of the premiums of a voluntary health insurance program with public subsidy of the remainder. There were also continuing proposals for tax credits and deductions for health insurance premiums, and for expanding the struggling Kerr-Mills program.

Representatives Mills, King, Herlong, Byrnes, and Curtis were members of the House Ways and Means Committee, and the outcome of the debate over Medicare was by no means predictable. In the end, the bill reported out of the Committee was not one bill but (as by now is well known) a compendium of three originally separate, and in some respects competing, proposals. The administration's proposals for hospital insurance for the aged, financed through the Social Security system, became Part A of Medicare for all those eligible for Social Security retirement benefits. Medicare Part B, as a second layer, offered federal subsidies to enable individuals age sixty-five and over to buy into a voluntary program of insurance for their doctors' bills (the Byrnes proposal). Medicaid was the third proposal, to liberalize and extend the program of federal grants to states for the indigent and medically needy. President Johnson signed Public Law 89-97, amid some flourish and in the presence of former President Truman, on July 30, 1965. Thus Medicare became a new title XVIII, and Medicaid title XIX of the Social Security legislation. Medicaid was, in fact, Kerr-Mills applied to a much wider audience than before: an extension of state welfare provisions rather than a new health service program.

The Medicaid Provisions of Public Law 89-97

The somewhat vague, or at least poorly drafted, provisions of title XIX took up only nine pages in the official version of the act—a relatively small space for what was to become one of the more expensive and most controversial pieces of federal legislation of the 1960s. Such brevity was not always matched by clarity of expression.

Title XIX extended medical assistance to all those in the categorical public assistance programs, thus applying across-the-board the principle that had been introduced for the aged by MAA and extended to other groups by title XVI. In addition it combined the separate public assistance medical vendor programs for cash recipients into a single program. The act did not require the states to establish such a program, but it put very considerable pressure on them to do so by providing that after December 31, 1969, there would be no further federal funds for medical vendor payments under the categorical titles for OAA, AFDC, AB, APTD, and Kerr-Mills. Perhaps even more important as an inducement—especially to the larger states, which had "suffered," in their own view, under the earlier variable formula—was the provision in title XI (section 1118) allowing states establishing title XIX programs to use the more favorable title XIX reimbursement formula for their other categorical assistance programs. The pressures were effective. Although some states barely made the deadline—Alabama, Arkansas, and Mississippi did not begin their programs until January 1, 1970—only two, Alaska and Arizona, had failed to implement it by that date, pleading extenuating circumstances in that virtually all Eskimos and Indians would be eligible, and the potential costs would be unbearable.

The 1965 law, as interpreted by the regulations, required the states to provide five basic services for those covered by Medicaid: physician's services, skilled nursing home services, inpatient hospital services, outpatient hospital services, and other laboratory or X-ray services. The states also had the option of providing a number of other services, such as those furnished by other licensed practitioners within the scope of their practices as defined by state law, home health care, private duty nursing services, dental services, and other services; the potential range was broad. Eligibility was also potentially generous. A state might choose to cover all those who were under twenty-one and "medically indigent" even if they were not eligible for a categorical program—that is, were not blind, disabled, or in a family eligible for AFDC; in the jargon of the time, this group was called the "noncategorically related medically needy."

The 1965 law normally required payments directly to the providers of services. In the case of hospitals the test for reimbursement was "reasonable cost." This phrase was also applied to hospital reimbursement under Medicare. There was no requirement that Medicaid and Medicare regulations be combined (or even similar), but it was agreed after debate in HEW that hospital reimbursement under Medicaid would follow the same broad test as in Medicare—a double bonanza to hospitals in these relatively generous early years. States were free to apply their own standards with respect to other medical services, though there was a hope that other medical providers would be paid according to locally prevailing (private) fees—again suggesting there would be rapid expansion in expenditures for physicians and other health practitioners. The 1965 law prohibited deductions and cost sharing for individuals seeking services under Medicaid, at least for those recipients also receiving money payments. For those sixty-five and over and covered by Medicaid, the states were also required to meet the cost of any deductibles under Medicare. Relatives of a beneficiary were not to be held financially responsible for his or her Medicaid bills; the prohibition of liens on the later income of recipients was carried over from Kerr-Mills; and states were free to determine their own notions of who, indeed, was "medically needy." Here was an open invitation to expand the population to be served, as well as the amount to be paid per treatment, with the assistance of federal funds.

Federal contribution to the states' eligible Medicaid programs ranged from 50 percent through 83 percent, based on a variable-grant, federal-state matching formula, which paid most to the state with the lowest per capita income. The federal government covered 75 percent of professional administrative costs and 50 percent of other administrative costs. The law also sought to prevent the states from using the new federal medical care dollars to replace existing state expenditures; in other words, Medicaid programs had to be incremental. As with other federal-state programs, certain administrative standards had to be met, in terms of designating a single state agency for administration and providing uniformity throughout the state, equal medical care benefits in the different categories, fair hearing procedures, confidentiality, and similar requirements. The importance of these changes should not be underestimated. The requirement of equal medical treatment in all categories was an important step forward, while the end of relatives' financial responsibility was to have an important effect on the utilization of nursing homes.

Convoluted as the wording was, the main thrust of title XIX was expansionist. Section 1903(e), for instance, set the long-term goal:

> The Secretary shall not make payments under the preceding provisions of this section to any State unless the State makes a satisfactory showing that it is making efforts in the direction of broadening the scope of the care and services made available under the plan and in the direction of liberalizing the eligibility requirements for medical assistance, with a view toward furnishing by July 1, 1975, comprehensive care and services to substantially all individuals who meet the plan's eligibility standards with respect to income and resources, including services to enable such individuals to attain or retain independence or self-care.

At least some states took the encouragement seriously.

Implementation 1965-67

It was not surprising that many saw title XIX as the "sleeper" of the 1965 legislation; even as more important than title XVIII (Medicare), because it was more open-ended, while others saw it as the national health program of the future.[8] For both supporters and critics, the months of implementation early in 1966 were a cause of excitement, though for different reasons. Initially, most states moved to implement Medicaid at fairly modest levels; Pennsylvania set $4000 as a limit of "medical dependency" for a family of four (under "Pennsycare"), while Illinois set it at $3600. Two states, however, New York and California, established programs that were shortly the center of violent controversies. The effects of the disputes in Albany and Sacramento were soon felt in Washington, D.C.

New York—and especially New York City—had a relatively generous program of medical care for those on public assistance and Kerr-Mills, and so it was not surprising that, when the time came to prepare state legislation early in 1966, Governor Rockefeller should propose a base of $5700 for a family of four, and Speaker Travia, the Democratic leader, $6700, or that ultimately a compromise of $6000 was agreed upon. Only one day's hearings were held on the bill. The Travia bill passed the Democratic-controlled Assembly and the Rockefeller bill the Republican-controlled Senate, both almost without debate, during March 1966. In April, after a warning by Rockefeller that New York stood in danger of losing possible new federal funds, the speaker and the governor met, worked out the $6000 compromise with reasonably generous provisions for excluding essential property and savings, and the bill shot through both chambers with remarkably little dissent. In signing the bill, Governor Rockefeller called it "the most significant social legislation in three decades."[9]

After the bill passed the fireworks began. The eligibility standards came under vigorous attack, as it was appreciated, by many for the first time, that about eight million people, or 45 percent of the population of the state, would now be eligible for Medicaid. Governor Rockefeller, in a statement that tells much about medical care in America, vainly protested that experience showed that only 25 percent of potential participants signed up for public assistance medical programs. He also argued that, despite the increase in eligibility, the new program would actually save money for the state and local authorities. The governor appeared on television in a vain effort to quell the rising hostility, most of it from upper New York State, where average incomes were lower than in and around New York City. It was claimed that in some up-state counties 70 percent of the population would be eligible for Medicaid. This prospect offended local authorities, who at that time were required to provide a quarter of the cost, and local physician groups, who saw the possible evisceration of their practices. Farmers' groups, employers' lobbies, and medical groups (although not the state medical society) lobbied for repeal. In an unusual move, the legislature held post-passage joint hearings to allow hostility to be aired, but the only important legislative change to come out of the hearings was a deductible of one percent of earnings for those families earning more than $4500. The governor was heckled about Medicaid in his campaigning for reelection upstate, but by then the program was ready to be implemented.[10]

First, however, HEW had to approve the New York plan, and so opponents had further opportunity to intervene. Litigation, alleging abuse of administrative power by establishing unreasonable standards, failed in the New York courts. By then various New York groups were attempting to persuade HEW not to approve the plan, including the Citizens Committee for Responsible Government and the Association of New York State Physicians and Dentists. Eight state legislators from Erie and Niagara Counties formally asked HEW to disapprove the plan, and soon Congressman Stratton from Rochester was organizing the opposition in Washington.

At the same time, the governor and his advisers were communing with HEW, although the Department was by then showing some reluctance to move since Congress had become increasingly concerned about the federal cost of

Medicaid. On Capitol Hill, Senator Saltonstall took the same line that some of the New York legislators had espoused:

> There was little discussion of title 19; which certainly has proved to be the "sleeper" in the bill. I am certain no one dreamed that within the next five years, "medicaid" as the program established by that title is called, could come to dwarf medicare.[11]

Meanwhile, the architect of title XIX, Chairman Wilbur Mills of the House Ways and Means Committee, was holding closed hearings. Bureaucrats at HEW were in a difficult position. There was no legal reason why they should not approve the New York plan, yet that plan alone would use up almost all the money that, one year earlier, had been estimated as the total federal cost of title XIX. Before the Committee, Robert Myers, chief actuary of the Social Security Administration, was blunt about the potential fiscal situation:

> It seems quite likely that under "mature" conditions, with full utilization of the provisions by those eligible to do so, and with expansion of the provisions of many of the State plans...so that they become much more like the New York plan, the Federal cost for title XIX as it now exists would be as much as $3 billion per year (or even more).[12]

The committee report noted that "while most of the State plans raise no question at this time, a few go well beyond what your committee believes to have been the intent of the Congress."[13] The mood was set for continuing congressional watchfulness of Medicaid in the states. Increasingly Medicaid was to be regarded not as one component of state welfare programs but as a substantial national commitment of funds for medical care.

While consideration of the New York plan continued in the executive branch, the legislature sought ways to tame the financial ogre with which it now saw itself faced. Senator Javits suggested more flexibility in deductions for services under Medicaid, variations in the type of services offered to different groups within Medicaid, and variations in eligibility standards in different parts of a state. While Javits was essentially seeking to save the New York legislation, the Ways and Means Committee was working on long-term solutions to control the federal costs of Medicaid. After considering abolishing the "open-ended" funding of title XIX by putting a ceiling on the federal contribution, fixing a maximum percentage of the population to be covered in any one state, and fixing a standard for "medical indigency" beyond which states could not go, the committee finally came down in favor of cutting back certain groups that might be covered—in particular, those relatives with whom children were living who were not already receiving cash payments under AFDC. Ultimately, in the shadow of impending elections, it was decided to delay changes in title XIX until the Ninetieth Congress; and on November 15, 1966, HEW formally approved the New York program, with the expectation that the federal government would meet the first $217 million out of a total annual cost of $532 million (including services not covered by federal matching provisions).

Approval was only the beginning of other types of problems. The New York program ran into criticisms from a variety of sources as implementation proceeded. The health professions were dissatisfied with their conditions. Dentists, who were paid on a fee schedule, protested that (in the words of the Eighth District Dental Society), "Fee schedules will be determined by men who sit behind desks who have not been in practice and have no clinical experience."[14] Physicians in New York City opposed a recommendation by the state that there should be a penalty clause for physicians who abused the plan as being "unduly punitive and arbitrary."[15] Pharmacists refused to comply with a New York City order that they substitute cheaper generic drugs for brand names.[16] A citizen's committee accused the New York City Welfare Department of "gross negligence" in its administration of the program, and cited its "incomprehensible forms, unnecessary red tape and confused administration."[17] Meanwhile, especially in upstate New York, there was growing pressure to curb the spiraling costs of the program, by limiting the number of non-welfare recipients. Medicaid was vulnerable to criticisms that it gave services to the poor at vast and uncontrollable cost and made doctors rich at taxpayer expense.

The same month that HEW approved the New York program (November 1966) a Medicaid political crisis broke in the state with the second largest program, California—but for different reasons. Where New York was viewing Medicaid as a means to expand the covered population, state administration in California was more interested in liberalizing the type of care available to recipients. An act to implement title XIX as "Medi-Cal" had been approved late in 1965, and the program began in March 1966. There were the usual complications involved in the implementation of any federal-state program, but the first few months of the program did not cause the storm provoked in New York. Though the range of services was wide, the eligibility levels were relatively low in California; this was still a program for the destitute, not for low-income workers.[18]

California's initial concerns related more closely to establishing better care and paying providers more quickly than to the overall cost of the program. Medi-Cal offered a comprehensive group of services to public assistance recipients, replacing previously fragmented and incomplete programs. In addition, efforts were made to abolish the stigma of second-class poor relief in medicine by dropping previous requirements that the poor (including Kerr-Mills recipients) could only be cared for in public institutions, that is, in county hospitals and clinics.

California epitomized the views of contemporaries who wished to bring medical care for the poor into the "mainstream"—that is, to treat the poor as well as the rich in private hospitals and through private medical practice. To advance this aim Medi-Cal introduced a system of payment to physicians according to their usual and customary fees, instead of through the fixed fee schedules of earlier assistance programs. Administration was shifted from county social welfare departments to an office of Health Care Services within the state Health and Welfare Agency, thus emphasizing the health rather than welfare attributes of the program. At the same time Blue Cross and Blue Shield were designated as state fiscal agents of Medi-Cal for processing and reviewing claims. Taken together, these moves represented a significant shift in emphasis, away from a minimal, direct-service welfare system to a system more like private health insurance.

It was expected in the debates over Medi-Cal in the legislature that the substantial additional costs of the program—the amount of vendor payments per capita nearly tripled between 1965 and 1967[19]—would be largely absorbed through additional federal matching funds. But in November 1966, after the election of Governor Reagan but before his inauguration, the administrator of the Health and Welfare Agency announced that Medi-Cal was running out of money, and that either the legislature would have to vote more funds or benefits would have to be reduced before the end of the fiscal year. By the spring of 1967, with bills for services coming in slowly, it was estimated that in the first sixteen months of the program the state would be "in the red" to the amount of $130 million, with a further deficit of $80 million for the following fiscal year. It was in this atmosphere that Governor Reagan delivered a televised "Report to the People" on July 10, 1967, arguing that the program was likely to increase in cost fifty percent each year, and that "something must be done before this ill-conceived program bankrupts the state."[20]

The premature release of this information caught the program administrators by surprise and had the effect of legitimating the amount of the projected budget deficit, and of providing ammunition for the governor's office to castigate the profligacy of the previous Democratic administration. Although both the estimate and the multiplier proved to be inaccurate, they had become political facts of life.

In California, staff work on possible cutbacks in the still-new Medicaid program began in the summer of 1967. More than 40 percent of the estimated program expenditures were on behalf of 200,000 persons classified as medically needy, but a substantial minority of these were old and disabled persons in nursing homes whose benefits could not be cut off without a resulting public outcry. Instead of reducing the number of beneficiaries, the staff recommended the reduction of available services, from the relatively comprehensive benefits then available to the five basic services then required under the federal legislation (inpatient care, nursing home care, physician services, laboratory services, and outpatient clinic services). In addition, other savings were suggested, including a rollback in physician fees to the level of "usual and customary fees" prevailing as of January 1, 1967. These cutbacks were announced in August 1967 and received widespread public attention. They were immediately deplored by an effective alliance between professional organizations in the health field and representatives of poverty groups in the state.

This opposition was crystallized in a restraining order obtained the same month by California Rural Legal Assistance (a legal services program funded by the federal Office of Economic Opportunity) temporarily blocking the cutbacks. Attorneys representing medical, dental, and pharmaceutical groups appeared as amici curiae. Despite claims from the state that it would lose $5 million a day if reduction in service were not made, the Superior Court in Sacramento made the order permanent. The state appealed the case, but lost its appeal in November 1967. The California Supreme Court ruled that the Health and Welfare Agency had authority to reduce the program but that the manner in which the reductions were made was ultra vires (i.e., that it contravened) the 1965 and 1967 Medi-Cal laws, the latter requiring either elimination of medically needy beneficiaries or a proportional reduction of all services as opposed to elimination of particular services. Governor Reagan immediately put the question of Medi-Cal before the legislature, then meeting in special session, and warned that he would be forced to remove benefits from the medically needy unless the projected cutbacks could be made; the supposed deficit for 1967-68 was then claimed by the Reagan administration to be $71 million. As the months went by, however, the fiscal situation changed significantly. By the spring of 1968, the deficit had not only disappeared; a surplus of $31 million was allowed for carryover into 1968-69. But that announcement coincided with the signing of the 1967 Social Security Amendments in Washington. Congress had acted.

The Social Security Amendments of 1967

Congressional hearings on the 1967 Social Security amendments began before the House Ways and Means Committee on March 1, with proposals by HEW Secretary Gardner, who was known to be anxious that title XIX be treated as a health care program, while Chairman Mills saw the legislation very much as part of welfare. The Ways and Means Committee was on record as saying that it had never been intended that the federal government should subsidize the medical care "of the considerable portion of the adult working population."[21] The House hearings took their predictable directions. Proposed limitations on federal participation in title XIX (section 220 of H.R. 5710) were supported by groups including the American Life Convention and Life Insurance Association (who would have preferred dollar limits on federal participation), Blue Cross, Blue Shield, various chambers of commerce, the International Association of Health Underwriters, the National Association of Life Underwriters, various medical groups, and, once again, Representative Stratton (who thought H.R. 5710 did not go far enough). Federal cutbacks were opposed—predictably enough—by the AFL-CIO, the Community Council of Greater New York, the International Ladies' Garment Workers Union, the National Association of Social Workers, the National Urban League, the Physicians Forum, and the United Auto Workers.

But when all the rhetoric was done, the Committee decided to produce its own "clean," more restrictive bill (H.R. 12080). This bill limited federal participation in medical indigence categories to payments on behalf of individuals and families whose income was no more than 133 1/3 percent of the highest amount of cash assistance ordinarily paid to a family of the same size on AFDC. Among other proposed changes, instead of having to provide five basic services under the program, states were given the choice either of including those five, or any seven out of the fourteen that the 1965 legislation had enumerated as approved for federal matching.

To a very large extent the testimony before the Senate Finance Committee was similar to that of Ways and Means. AMA testimony was sympathetic to title XIX. Pro-Medicaid lobbyists appeared to protest section 220 in terms of its impact on "families who have managed to pull themselves up from the lower depths of poverty, who are just beginning to see daylight and learning to become productive members of society... We cannot rationalize the anguish of the medically needy with the unrealistic formula of H.R. 12080."[22] New York's commissioner of Social Services argued that all his state was doing was attempting to meet the "comprehensive services" requirement for all needy persons, a requirement to be achieved by 1975 under the Medicaid legislation—but New York was way ahead of other states.[23] As reported out, the Finance Committee restored the 150-per-cent-of-AFDC payments formula to the bill. Among other important changes, the new bill called for licensing the nursing homes in which Medicaid patients were living, and licensing nursing home administrators. The Finance Committee accepted the House proposal that states might choose any seven out of fourteen of the allowable services under section 1902(a) for the medically indigent, though it required states to continue to provide the five basic services for those receiving cash payments through public assistance. In further suggested squeezes, deductibles might also be imposed on the medical indigent. Responding to other specific concerns, home health services were added as a mandatory service for certain groups by 1970, as were "early and periodic screening and diagnosis" of those under twenty-one. Elsewhere in the bill, the Senate restored the administration's proposal for federal matching funding for "intermediate care facilities," which would handle those persons who were not able to live at home but did not need the services of a hospital or a skilled nursing home.

The Senate debates on the 1967 amendments were dramatic, but more because of proposed increases in Social Security and what many regarded as repressive changes in AFDC. Only one important change was made in the Committee bill with respect to Medicaid, the amendment by Senator Ribicoff requiring state plans to provide utilization review procedures. The bill finally passed on November 22 and went to conference. With the exception of the federal financial provision, the Senate version of the bill generally prevailed. The 1967 legislation encouraged states to roll back eligibility for the medically indigent to 150 percent of the top AFDC level by July 1, 1968; to 140 percent by January 1, 1969; and to the final 133 1/3 percent by January 1, 1970. There would be no federal subsidy above these limits. It was still possible, of course, for states to go beyond the limits, but only if financing was exclusively from state funds, generally a difficult hurdle to clear. Fiscal reality had struck. The first stage of the history of Medicaid was complete.

Public Law 90-248 was signed by the president in January 1968. Eight states felt obliged to come down to the 150 percent level by July 1, 1968, if only to protect their budgets. These included California and New York, as well as Delaware, Kentucky, Maryland, Oklahoma, Pennsylvania, and Rhode Island; though technically, Pennsylvania avoided the federal cutback by raising its AFDC levels. Iowa imposed a cutback on its new program to reach 133 1/3 percent by July 1968. Connecticut and Illinois imposed cutbacks by January 1969. Altogether, then, eleven of the twenty-three states that were then providing Medicaid services to the medical needy (as well as to cash assistance recipients) adjusted their income eligibility levels in response to the 1967 Amendments. A clear message was emerging that medical indigence as an expansionary health policy did not work. Governors of nine states whose eligibility levels were cut back, and twenty-five without cutbacks were polled in the summer of 1968. Six of the former and nineteen of the latter considered the cutbacks desirable, on grounds that the limits were realistic and reasonable, or would force states to raise public assistance (cash eligibility) levels to get more federal funds and keep the wealthier states from taking an undue share of available federal money.[24]

Tying means test levels for medical indigence to other public assistance programs in a state made the strong statement that Medicaid was "welfare." However, though attached to a system of cash assistance benefits, Medicaid was a health service program whose administrators had to deal with an army of medical care providers. While states purchased services in the private medical sector, they exerted little or no authority over the providers. The role of HEW was limited, with major management devolution of programs to the states. Instead, then, of a unified national policy toward Medicaid from the executive, the growing budgetary problems in the states ricocheted back to the Congress. Within three years fiscal realties had trumped any lingering national or state expectations that medical services could be extended on an incremental basis, with little economic or political pain. Medicaid's problems were not of any one organization's making; rather, they were inherent in the system itself. They were expressed in terms of Medicaid's spiraling and uncontrollable costs, but they were at root problems of goals, authority, and administration.

Rising Medical Care Costs

Problems of costs and expenditures were central to Medicaid politics from its beginning. The 1967 amendments attempted to provide cost brakes by tying state Medicaid eligibility requirements to AFDC income levels for the purposes of federal cost-sharing. In theory, too, the newly-invented category of intermediate care facilities was expected to remove some nursing home expenditures from Medicaid. Yet the rapidly rising costs of medical care and Medicaid's acceptance of market-based, provider-generated reimbursement levels—then thought to be an essential feature of the public-private mix—contributed to continuing increases in Medicaid expenditures. The patterns and pressures were similar to those experienced under Kerr-Mills. Legislators and their staffs at all levels of government were unprepared for Medicaid's fiscal impact. Between 1965 and 1970 federal expenditures for vendor medical payments increased fivefold, with similar increases in the states. And there was no sign of any lessening of the cost acceleration.

The difficulty of making accurate cost estimates for the federal share under Medicaid became a focus for sharp criticism (and much confusion) in congressional hearings. According to the chief actuary of the Social Security Administration, Robert J. Myers, the initial additional cost for Medicaid for non-institutionalized recipients was estimated as $238 million in the first full year of operation, calendar year 1966. This figure, however, reportedly excluded the costs of patients in institutions (who were to form an important group for Medicaid payments), as well as the new Medicaid category of medically indigent children. Altogether it was estimated that additional costs would be $353 million, added on to the previous medical vendor payments through the categorical assistance and MAA programs (an estimated $678 million); the total cost would thus be over $1 billion.[25]

These total costs were important because Medicaid involved substantial shifts of money among the previous categories. As states moved into title XIX their vendor payments under OAA, MAA, AB, APTD, and AFDC were absorbed into the states' medical assistance programs. In December 1969, for example, forty-five jurisdictions were receiving payments under title XIX, while another nine were still working through previous arrangements. It was not surprising that there was confusion as to what, then, were the costs of "Medicaid." This was reflected in questions by Senator John Williams to Undersecretary Wilbur Cohen in the Finance Committee hearings on the 1967 amendments:

> Your first estimate on the cost of Title XIX was $238 million, if I understand it correctly. Then you were going before the committee a year ago and were shocked to find it was going to cost around $2 billion.... Now, what is the estimated cost of this Title XIX as it stands, about $3 billion or more, is it not?[26]

Although Undersecretary Cohen reiterated the explanation of the partial and additional nature of the $238 million, the initial obfuscation hindered all later HEW attempts to explain the early estimates.

The total federal share of medical vendor payments was also consistently underestimated. As noted in further hearings in 1969, the estimate for fiscal 1969 made in December 1967 was $1.58 billion in federal funds; a month later the estimate was enlarged by $450 million; by January 1969 it had another $200 million added to it; and in the revised budget three months later another $40 million had appeared. This last estimate was 50 percent greater than the initial estimate.[27] Medicaid seemed tied to the tail of a ravenous financial beast.

Problems of cost estimation were not, of course, confined to Medicaid. The Medicare program was also caught in the same medical price spiral, consistently underestimating its own fiscal needs. Little more than a year after Medicare started, Congress increased Medicare taxes by some 25 percent to meet unexpected hospital cost increases under Medicare's Part A. The contributory premium paid by the elderly under Medicare Part B for physician services was also increased from the initial $3 a month to $4 a month, and later to $5.30 a month, effective July 1, 1970, each sum matched by concomitant increases in federal matching funds. Medicaid, even with the 1967 retrenchments, continued to be relatively uncontrollable, because its financing was still open-ended, fixed by whatever the states spent. Rising expenditures meant increased pressures both on federal funds and on hard-pressed tax funds in the states.

In Congress, the combined and rising expenditures of Medicare and Medicaid focused attention on the federal costs of medical care. Estimates of total public and private health expenditures in the United States for fiscal 1969 reached $60.3 billion, $18 billion more than in fiscal 1966, representing 6.7 percent of the gross national product [which in hindsight may not seem too bad, but then seemed huge]. In fiscal 1966, the public sector funded about 22 percent of total expenditures for medical care; three years later the proportion had risen to 36 percent.[28] The primary reason for rising expenditures lay in the costs of providing hospital and nursing home care—which were stimulated, in turn, by the purchasing dollars let loose by both Medicare and Medicaid. Expenditures for hospital care increased by 17 percent within one year, to a total of $22.5 billion in fiscal 1969. Only part of these increases could be attributed to expanded or better services.

These general cost trends had specific implications for Medicaid. Inpatient hospital care represented 37.5 percent of expenditures of $4.3 billion for medical assistance in fiscal 1969, and nursing home care another 29.8 percent, a combined total of 67.3 percent. The 1965 legislation specified that inpatient hospital care (though not nursing home care) under Medicaid should be reimbursed on a "reasonable cost" basis (rather than, for example, on a more limited, statewide fee schedule—as was to come much later). The Medicare interpretation of reasonable cost, defined in regulations by the Social Security Administration, was adopted for interim payments under title XIX, greatly facilitating payment for hospital services on behalf of elderly persons who were recipients of both Medicare and Medicaid. But, at the same time, reasonable cost reimbursement tied states both to Medicare policy and to the rising costs of institutional care. Total hospital expenditures for the elderly rose from $4.17 billion in fiscal year 1967 to $6.53 billion in 1969, while nursing home costs rose from $1.52 billion to $2.17 billion in the same period.[29]

There was no similar provision in the legislation for Medicaid to pay nursing homes on a reasonable cost basis. Apart from hospitals, suppliers of services were reimbursed according to state policies, which were to "provide such safeguards as may be necessary to assure that…such care and services will be provided, in a manner consistent with simplicity of administration and the best interests of the recipients."[30] State plans for medical assistance were to define the "best interests of the recipients" as receipt of medical care through services included in the plan "at least to the extent these are available to the general population." This, in a nutshell, is what "mainstream medicine" meant.

California interpreted the intent of Medicaid as providing services to the poor on the same basis that services were provided to the insured middle-class population through the private sector—a stand that argued for payment of services through Medicaid under similar arrangements to those made by private health insurance or Medicare. This interpretation appeared to be also the original federal policy. For institutions other than hospitals, states were advised that fee structures should focus on payment on a reasonable cost basis, equivalent to the reimbursement methods under Medicare Part A. Before Medicaid, state welfare departments had usually paid their "vendor payments" for skilled nursing home care on the basis of negotiated fees, per diem or monthly flat rates, which were in many cases below the institutions' operating costs. Not surprisingly, in states that shifted to reimbursement methods more nearly reflecting the costs incurred, there were immediate increases in nursing home expenditures.

A second factor in increasing nursing home expenditures under Medicaid was the immediate boom in nursing home development—largely the result of private speculation, which accelerated rapidly following the passage of Medicare and Medicaid. Nursing home care proved elastic in terms of demand: The more beds, the greater their utilization. In states such as Connecticut, where the great majority (70 percent) of nursing home beds were filled with welfare recipients, the expansion of facilities led to an unexpected increase in the number of eligible recipients cared within them, and thus to an unexpected rise in nursing home expenditures; and to a greater or lesser extent this was true of all states with relatively generous Medicaid provisions. Expenditures on nursing home care being met from public sources (chiefly Medicare and Medicaid) more than doubled between fiscal 1966 and fiscal 1968—from $604 million to $1,490 million, largely for institutional care of the elderly.[31] Medicaid thus became part of the cause of the rising costs of nursing home care as well as victim of their implications.

The initial approximation of reimbursement methods to the methods used in Medicare was not limited to institutions. Passage of Medicare and Medicaid in the same legislation coincided with a prevailing mood in Secretary John Gardner's Department of Health, Education, and Welfare that medical care for the poor should be provided with equal dignity and through similar channels as the medical care of other members of the population. This was a question not merely of political philosophy but also of encouraging professional participation in the program. Fee structures, it was emphasized in 1966, should be "realistic to assure eligible persons medical care and services in sufficient quantities."[32] The goal for minimum participation state by state, determined separately for each covered profession and for specialties within a profession, was for approximately two-thirds of practitioners to take Medicaid participants—and to treat them as if they were private patients.[33] For physicians, this was an invitation to incorporate into Medicaid (as well as Medicare) fees similar to those charged in private practice. As a result there was a movement, led by state medical societies, to establish payment of physicians on the basis of their "usual and customary fees" in the developing Medicaid programs. A review in 1967 found that fifteen title XIX programs had established payment of physicians through their usual and customary charging structure; only one of these states (Idaho) had previously paid on this basis.

The success of this policy in encouraging physician participation was universally commended by physician organizations. The president of the Illinois State Medical Society, for example, ascribed the jump in physician involvement in Medicaid in that state, from 3228 MDs in 1967 to over 6000 in 1969, to the move from the previous pattern of closed panel "welfare physicians" to one that allowed all physicians to participate.[34] In effect, states traded medical buy-in and patient accessibility for higher costs, a good part of which was subsidized from federal funds. Commitment by states that chose to pay the charges as determined by physicians, with only minimal state controls, added to the inflationary characteristics of Medicaid programs. A survey of states with programs early in 1968 found fourteen states reporting unwillingness of physicians or other suppliers to participate, chiefly because of inadequate fees; on the other hand, seventeen states reported sharp rises in fees and charges, and already there were charges of profiteering and racketeering on the part of providers.[35] For reasons both of extended services and rising fees, the amount paid to physicians under medical assistance programs increased fivefold between 1965 and 1969; by the latter year physician fees absorbed 12 percent of expenditures of assistance programs.

Though many of the additional expenditures represented extra services and possibly extra time spent with medical assistance patients (and perhaps even less tangible elements such as greater personal attention to welfare patients), there was undeniable evidence that much of the benefit of the additional expenditures was flowing into the pockets of providers—hospitals, nursing homes, physicians, laboratories, and other participating facilities and services. The providers had, after all, previously provided a substantial subsidy to welfare recipients. Cost increases in Medicaid between 1968 and 1970 were estimated to be three times as great as the increases in the number of persons served by the programs; a remarkable phenomenon even taking overall inflation into account.[36] By the late 1960s Medicaid could not be labeled as "sleeper" legislation for the coming of national health insurance (or if it was, only as a warning signal of out-of-control spending and games playing at every level); or even as a simple extension of the welfare safety net. Coupled with Medicare, Medicaid had acquired a new political soubriquet: the personification of confusion, extravagance, and waste.

Medicaid Budgets in the States

Medicaid's impact on state budgets, and thus state politics, was also quickly evident. Medical vendor payments represented less than one third of state welfare budgets in 1965. By 1969 medical vendor payments had risen to well over 40 percent of the welfare budgets. Reportedly, one out of every three states had been forced to raise its taxes, at least in part because of Medicaid. California, Michigan, and New York had run into fiscal difficulties even before the end of the 1967 fiscal year, and three other states, Maryland, Nevada, and Oklahoma, in 1968. In Maryland, Michigan, and New York, substantial proportions of the Medicaid payments were being made for non-welfare cases. The states were thus subject to a number of pressures. Welfare budgets were strained, with payments for medical care competing and in some cases threatening to overrun funds for direct cash assistance. Medicaid was also becoming unpopular politically, especially in terms of requiring additional taxes on those lower income groups whose own medical care was not always adequate. There seemed to be no alternative to an attempt to cut back coverage and tighten payments to providers. State retrenchments thus joined retrenchments by the federal government.

Some sense of the impact of the 1967 amendments in the states may be gleaned from the reactions in California and New York. Taken together, in the fall of 1967 the two states accounted for nearly half (48.5 percent) of all national payments to medical vendors, and for about 37 percent of all recipients of medical assistance. The experiences in these two states were thus of particular importance to the overall development of Medicaid.

Governor Rockefeller's situation in New York was unlike Governor Reagan's in California in that New York had established what other states felt to be abnormally high eligibility levels. The New York situation was thus one of justifying population coverage rather than services. But again there were immediate problems of costs grossly exceeding budget estimates. Although Governor Rockefeller had joined Mayor Lindsay of New York City in urging that President Johnson not sign the bill that became the 1967 amendments, once it was law the governor was faced with the need to raise an extra $150 million in connection with the required welfare changes. Twenty-eight municipalities had raised their sales tax, and nearly all sixty-two counties had raised their property tax, virtually all alleging the "Medicaid problem"—though in some cases Medicaid may have been a convenient scapegoat. Governor Rockefeller admitted he had been mistaken to be so enthusiastic about Medicaid, and called for cutbacks in the program in his budget message to the legislature. In the Assembly upstate Democrats forced the issue, fearing local taxpayers would revolt. The Republican-controlled state Senate cut back the program with little debate. Governor Rockefeller signed the bill almost as soon as it reached his desk—some said in the hope of obtaining conservative backing for his presidential campaign. The state's Medicaid contribution would, it was estimated, be cut by some $300 million (although experience did not bear this out), while the new eligibility levels—down to $5300 from $6000 for the family of four—were expected to remove roughly a million persons from the nearly three-and-a-half million enrolled. But even at $5300, New York's was still the most generous Medicaid program in the nation.

The medical care needs of the people cut off the rolls in New York City, as elsewhere, did not of course suddenly go away. Mayor Lindsay estimated that the eligibility cuts would mean a loss of about $80 million in state aid to municipal and voluntary hospitals, and could mean closing public health facilities. Some of the costs were shifted from one public pocket to another. To help those dropped from Medicaid, the New York City Department of Hospitals cut its own fees in municipal outpatient departments—thus aggravating the already perilous financial situation of the city hospital system. Moreover, with the coming of Medicaid, much of the former private subsidy of welfare cases had been replaced by public subsidy; Medicaid had in large part eliminated "charity." The voluntary and proprietary hospitals and, for that matter, private practitioners in the health fields, were not prepared simply to revert to the preexisting situation. Voluntary hospitals, in particular, could not afford it. It was also by then illegal for welfare workers to press a recipient's relatives to contribute. There was no adequate resource to pick up the services and patients that Medicaid dropped. All in all, the medical care available to the many thousands of poor in New York City who were no longer eligible for assistance was worse in 1968 than it was before Medicaid was enacted.

Yet still the budget rose; and the New York legislature took further measures to attempt to control it in 1969. Effective July 1, 1969, the eligibility level for a family of four was reduced to $5000 (eliminating another 200,000 persons from New York City's Medicaid rolls, and leaving about 650,000 low-income participants, together with the one million welfare recipients). Reimbursements to hospitals were frozen and a general cutback of 20 percent in fees was ordered effective as of June 1. For the medically indigent (but not those on cash assistance), doctors, dentists, and pharmacists were to collect 20 percent of bills directly from Medicaid recipients. Not surprisingly, such administrative shifts rippled through the system. The *New York Times* published a photo of a line of individuals outside a medical center, waiting to "clarify their status," in an article, "Medicaid Shifts Cause Bewilderment."[37] On behalf of users of the programs U.S. District Judge Constance Baker Motley in New York City issued a temporary restraining order against putting into effect the regulation for compulsory contributions from the medically indigent, although this was dissolved after a hearing before a three-judge court. Another three-judge federal court in Brooklyn struck down Medicaid reimbursement restrictions on hospitals in New York, on the ground that they violated federal law. But the eligibility levels stuck, and Albany's efforts to curb the state Medicaid budget continued.

The problems of Medicaid in California and New York were paralleled by similar budgetary increases in other states, if on a lesser scale. In Oklahoma in fiscal 1968 the Welfare Department's cash reserve became so low that the state was forced to draw federal funds in advance to make monthly welfare payments; as a result, services under the Medicaid program were cut for all persons receiving aid (predominantly for payments to hospitals and physicians), and the number of eligible recipients reduced. In Maryland, Governor Agnew cut eligibility for a family of four from $3120 to $3000 and for a single person from $1800 to $1500, in the expectation of cutting 22,000 persons out of the Medicaid program. In addition, for the "medically indigent" (who received a special card to distinguish them from other "indigents") a $40 deductible for each admission to hospital was imposed, together with a twenty-one-day maximum stay, and partial charges were imposed for use of dental services and emergency rooms, for drugs, and for visiting a physician. The state medical society resolved at its 1969 meeting that Medicaid services for hospital inpatients and outpatients should continue to be reimbursed at the usual and customary levels until the budget was depleted; physicians would then give care without charge. Even this apparently generous gesture was insufficient. By the end of 1969, hospital officials claimed the state owed Baltimore hospitals more than $6.3 million in unpaid bills.[38]

State legislatures were increasingly reflecting the hostility of Congress to the Medicaid program. New Mexico, which did not even cover the "medically indigent," was faced with a legislature that refused to allocate enough funds to pay even for the barebones program. Nevertheless medical vendor payments in that state rose from $5.4 million in 1965 to $16.9 million in fiscal year 1969. New Mexico became the first state to close down its Medicaid program (on May 1, 1969). Although the program was reinstated after nine days, it remained chronically underfunded. The state welfare department of Nebraska was forced to seek a $1 million deficit appropriation in 1969, three-fourths of which was attributed to Medicaid. In August 1968, Louisiana retrenched, cutting inpatient stays, drugs, and payment of coinsurance under Medicare's Part B; even then there were demands for further cutbacks. Cutting back was difficult in some states, if only because there were no "medically indigent" categories to cut.

Budgets and Controls: Increasing Federal Intervention

The defeat of the Democrats in the presidential election in November 1968 signaled a rethinking and reappraisal of Medicaid. In 1965, the message of Medicaid had seemed to be one of purchasing health services of a quality equal to private services for a substantial proportion of the population under basically state-controlled programs. One fallacy was, of course, that preexisting welfare recipients and a new group of uninsured individuals (the medically indigent) could be calmly absorbed into the medical marketplace without the terms of that market being changed; a second, that the additional costs would be politically acceptable to Congress and the states. Title XIX, as passed in 1965, had it been fully implemented, could have covered as many as thirty-five million Americans and cost as much as $20 billion a year (in 1960s dollars). From the time of the 1967 amendments, and especially after the beginning of the Nixon administration in 1969, the prevailing congressional view of Medicaid was quite different. A shift toward greater federal control over Medicaid (federal audits of 1969 were one indication) reflected concern over rising budgets, and at the same time a recognition that Medicaid could not and should not be regarded as providing the equivalent of middle-class medicine. This last point of view was stated succinctly by Dr. Roger Egeberg of HEW in the summer of 1969. Claiming that title XIX would never provide a single standard of services for rich and poor under the current system of distribution of health services, Egeberg said the slogan "let's get everybody into the mainstream" (that is, the private medical care system) should never have been used.[39]

In Congress, concern over medical costs kept increasing. The Senate Finance Committee held highly critical hearings on Medicaid and Medicare in both 1969 and 1970. In addition, the Finance Committee staff began a probing analysis of Medicare and Medicaid, whose results, published in 1970, provided a detailed review of management practices and cost deficiencies in these programs. And hearings on health care in America before Senator Abraham Ribicoff's Subcommittee on Executive Reorganization of the Committee on Government Operations in August 1968 focused on the costs of medical services. National health policy was in the forefront once again.

The Senate Special Committee on the Aging and its subcommittees held some thirty days of hearings during 1969 in Washington and around the country. Assisting its Subcommittee on Health of the Elderly, an advisory committee on health costs and aging came out in favor of "comprehensive compulsory health insurance for all Americans," and its testimony underlined the deficiencies in Medicaid, "a poor program with no standards, no quality controls."[40] Other Senate committees with an active or stated interest in health organization and costs by the end of 1969 included the Senate Committee on Public Welfare's Health Subcommittee, and the Antitrust and Monopoly Subcommittee, which was particularly interested in proprietary (for-profit) health institutions, especially those owned by physicians. All of this interest ultimately resulted from concern over costs and possible exploitation for private gain in publicly financed health programs. Medicaid, accounting for nearly one-fourth of all public medical expenditures, would have been a target for probing criticism even without its obvious difficulties.

In March 1969, in the wider frame of the Nixon administration's attempt to control increases in federal appropriations, HEW announced that procedures for reviewing the appropriate use of services would be required for state Medicaid programs, as well as for Medicare. Utilization review procedures were by no means the only attempted controls on Medicaid providers and services. One of the primary targets for cost controls was physicians' fees. As part of its growing investigation of Medicare and Medicaid costs, the Senate Finance Committee requested from HEW in April 1969 a list of all practitioners who received $25,000 or more under Medicaid in 1968. This was followed in June by an announcement by Senator Long that the resulting names would be turned over to the Internal Revenue Service.[41] Only a week after this announcement, HEW officials revealed that payment schedules would be set up for Medicaid and that these would be based on the lowest Blue Shield payment plans. Fees would thus be deliberately fixed on a lower scale than those for Medicare (which were actually higher than the average Blue Shield fees). This announcement came as a shock both to physicians and to those who still hoped to see Medicaid with a reimbursement program tied to full private fees. It was followed by a statement from HEW Secretary Robert Finch in June 1969 that payments to physicians would indeed be limited.

Following a series of discussions in HEW and with professional organizations, the interim regulations for physicians and other individual practitioners appeared in July 1969. The link to Blue Shield was dropped. Instead the regulations limited Medicaid fees to 75 percent of physicians' customary charges in January 1969. Subsequent increases would be tied to changes in the Consumer Price Index or in an alternative index developed by the secretary. Moreover, before increases were to be allowed there had to be evidence that the state and the profession concerned had established an effective utilization and quality control system, including provision for disqualifying practitioners found to have defrauded, overutilized, or otherwise abused the program. These regulations froze physician fees at a given level (although administratively that level was difficult to define), providing for each physician a kind of personalized fee schedule. With the new regulations two levels of payment were recognized, one for Medicare and one for Medicaid, with lower fees for the latter. For the elderly who were entitled to Medicare but part of whose medical bills were picked up under Medicaid, the situation was anomalous. On one hand they possessed recognized rights to medical care in the private sector; on the other, they were once more "welfare" patients with physicians donating to them at least one fourth of their normal fee. Physicians responded in different ways. The AMA, protesting the move, questioned whether HEW had the authority to set up nationally applicable regulations, but meanwhile urged local medical groups to establish effective controlling mechanisms to review services and fees as the necessary alternative to future fee reductions.

As cost controls were beginning to be developed through federal intervention in Medicaid, there was a movement—again from within the Senate Finance Committee—to slow the expansion of services that had been envisaged in the initial development of Medicaid. On the proposal of Senator Clinton P. Anderson of New Mexico, a rider was attached to a tax bill in May 1969 (and legislated),[42] permitting states to cut back some Medicaid services and suspending the requirement that states provide comprehensive care to all the medically needy by July 1, 1975. The prospect of comprehensive health services for a relatively large group of persons—the original apparent implication of Medicaid—was receding rapidly.

Management had also become a hot political issue—and to some extent the rationale for cuts. Announcing that the program was "badly conceived and badly organized,"[43] HEW established a Task Force on Medicaid in July 1969, chaired by health insurance expert Walter McNerney—with a staff allegedly larger than the federal agency administering the program, the object of its investigation. The Task Force issued its interim report in November 1969 and its final report in June 1970.[44] Medicaid ($2.7 billion in federal funds) was then run by the Medical Services Administration (MSA), a division of the Social and Rehabilitation Service (SRS), a descendent of the Welfare Administration. Not the most powerful empire in HEW, its purpose was to make grants to states rather than to innovate or run services; it was not loved on the Hill; and it did not have the power or prestige to deal with the powerful professional groups who were the providers of Medicaid. To these difficulties were added chronic understaffing. Not only did its leadership feel impotent and change frequently; senior posts were left unfilled, and the staff of MSA was so small that even had it had the will, power, and prestige to press states and providers, or to face other problems squarely, it would not have had the manpower to follow through. The unwillingness to staff MSA adequately was a major contributing factor in the "Medicaid Crisis" by 1970. Title XIX, as passed in 1965, was so vague that only a well staffed department could have implemented it effectively.

As it was, mandatory dates were not met (for example, Arizona and Alaska failed to meet the December 1969 deadline for producing a state plan for Medicaid), and cutoffs in state funds (which could, for instance, be imposed on those several states who had not met utilization review requirements) were not only not made, but never considered very seriously. Despite the fact that each year Medicaid took an increasingly significant share of the federal budget, the issuing of regulations—the very core of an effective federal-state grant-in-aid program—proceeded remarkably slowly. Basic regulations for administration of the program were not issued until 1969. MSA only just made the deadline provided by the 1967 legislation, which required federal standards for licensing of nursing home administrators and definitions of a skilled nursing home by July 1970. Even then, some of the regulations were provisional, with the result that regional offices and state welfare departments treated them with some suspicion lest the offices and departments commit limited resources only to find the regulations withdrawn.

Belatedly, in 1968 HEW set up standard audits in sixteen major Medicaid states; the reports were released during 1969. Among the findings were that Illinois had drawn nearly $1 million in federal funds improperly, New York City wasted $9.7 million in federal funds because of alleged procedural violations and administrative laxness, and Texas was using procedures that resulted in the loss of interest income to the federal government of $48,750 a month. The audits reported weaknesses in management controls, procedures for processing claims, eligibility, and other areas amounting to a total "questionable dollar impact" (that is, waste) of at least $318 million.[45] These audits served to emphasize two major features of Medicaid. The first was administrative inefficiency in the states, the second the lack of adequate federal guidelines, methods, and controls in a program that was substantially federally funded. Not until June 1970 was a federal regulation proposed for Medicaid to require that a state, in discharging its fiscal accountability, "maintain an accounting system and supporting fiscal records adequate to assure that claims for federal funds are in accord with applicable Federal requirements."[46]

Among other critiques, the Final Report of the Task Force on Medicaid (1970) reechoed the need for review of the whole federal apparatus in health and better integration of health programs and the health bureaucracy. But it did note that

> ...the haste with which it [the 1965 legislation] had to be implemented left little time for meaningful planning or imaginative leadership. MSA's management style has been characterized by a crisis orientation to the detriment of sound management practices and long-range planning.[47]

Across the country huge, multimillion-dollar state programs operated without the basic mechanisms of program accountability. The tradition of inadequate statistical data was carried through from the welfare programs into Medicaid. As a result, the administrators of the Medicaid programs (and other interested groups, including the recipients themselves) had little ammunition to defend their operations or to justify the rapidly increasing expenditures.

Everywhere states seemed to have basic problems of effective administration. New York's administration offered a continuing target for complaint within the federal government, and among providers and recipients. During 1968, private hospitals even evicted Medicaid patients for nonpayment, and the drug stores held a brief boycott of Medicaid. Standing disputes between the state Department of Social Welfare and New York City existed since the program began, because the city was anxious to have a rigorous audit of physicians, and saw the need to have some limits on freedom of choice for Medicaid patients. The city was also in trouble with the state because of its plan to mix payments made for Medicaid patients being treated in the municipal hospitals with general city funds. While that dispute was settled in favor of the state, the city in late 1968 refused to go along with a state rule requiring payment of doctors in teaching hospitals for general supervision of Medicaid patients. New York City also perpetuated other crises, not only as a center of alleged Medicaid fraud, but taking the lead in most disputes.

Criticism of state administration in the late 1960s was so widespread that even the Senate Finance Committee staff, working for a committee dominated by Southerners, demanded far more rigorous federal control. The second Task Force Report made it clear that their ideal would be to federalize health care almost entirely, while suggesting some improvements in state administration in the meantime. That the urge was to give more power to HEW, whose defects in this field were manifest, was a mark of the even graver defects perceived in state administration. Here, then, was a program—Medicaid—whose policy directions were unclear by 1970, and whose management was uncertain, if not grossly inefficient at both the state and federal levels. Disenchantment had set in.

Relations with Providers

During the crucial first years of the program the providers of services under title XIX (hospitals, nursing homes, doctors, and others) thus dealt with the state agencies in the absence of effective guidance or regulation from MSA. The one exception was inpatient hospital care, where the 1965 legislation laid down the test for reimbursement of "reasonable cost." Elsewhere there were battles between providers' groups and state agencies, and occasionally battles between groups of providers, as when the specialists fought the general practitioners in Kentucky over differential fees, or when internecine warfare broke out over differentials between optometrists and ophthalmologists in Rhode Island. But where the providers were united, it was generally the recipients who suffered.

A huge initial difficulty lay with the very concept of vendor payments. The state neither employed nor contracted with its providers of services, but merely paid the bills according to established criteria. When these criteria revolved around reduced fees—for example, lower fees for welfare patients than for private patients—the state (and the vendor) might well take the view that the provider of services was doing the state a favor. Hospitals, doctors, dentists et al. tended to react with surprise at any apparent limitation on their freedom of action under Medicaid. States, on the other hand, tended to accommodate themselves to the wishes of providers to ensure widespread participation in their Medicaid programs. Indeed, had the states not been pliable, the net result would have been to ensure a lower rate of participation.

The administrative and economic weaknesses of Medicaid, however, exaggerated the lopsided contest between well-organized, articulate providers and the understaffed, undervalued, and underinformed members of the welfare and health departments in different states. The most interesting of the battles were between the most prestigious and highly paid of the health professions—the physicians—and the state departments. This was not an entirely noble story.

The AMA had opposed Kerr-Mills because it claimed that physicians already provided care to the elderly poor free of charge. It opposed the medical care package in 1965 on the ground that no one in the United States went without medical care merely for being poor. Thus when physicians began to be paid for their services under Kerr-Mills in 1960 and under title XIX after 1965, they received a sudden and significant increase in their incomes, allegedly for services they were already donating. At the 1965 hearings, the immediate past president of the Pennsylvania Medical Society claimed that Pennsylvania doctors had provided almost $42 million worth of free care in 1960: 28 percent of their free care to private patients, 37 percent for hospital charity care, 24 percent in outpatient clinics, and 10 percent for everything else.[48] Medicaid (like Medicare) payments were a windfall.

In any event, the impression was created that physicians were ungrateful for this financial bonus and, at the same time, frequently insensitive to the attempts to change the psychological atmosphere of welfare medicine. Worse still, there was extensive evidence of profiteering, fraud on the Medicaid program, and, allegedly, a propensity to cheat the Internal Revenue Service on the part of some members of the medical profession. Such negative observations fed into a wider critique of the medical profession, evident by 1970.

Battles about usual or customary fees and the fee schedule marked disputes about Medicaid from the very beginning, and were to lead to intervention from the White House to curb fees in 1969. Meanwhile relations with the profession soured in many states. In New York the state medical society had in general supported Medicaid, but by mid-1966 there was trouble about fees. During May, a task force from the state Budget Bureau drew up a suggested scale of charges, while the medical society endorsed a more generous one. The governor claimed that the state fee scale was slightly above private insurance levels, while the doctors argued that the Medicaid reimbursement rates were considerably below those in most communities. In the end a compromise was worked out with a gubernatorial Interdepartmental Committee on Health Economics, which represented the state but was assisted by a five-man advisory committee of the state medical society. In the process, doctors looked like unionists, bargaining for whatever they could get.

A large state with a powerful governor was able to resist pressure from physicians. California, while providing for reasonable charges in the light of usual and customary fees, put ceilings on the amounts Medi-Cal's fiscal agents could in fact pay. In other states the pressure for establishing Medicaid often came from the physicians—for example, in Virginia—on condition that the physician fee arrangements were the same as in Medicare. In Pennsylvania (claims of earlier medical charity now forgotten), the state medical society organized an elaborate lobbying program to show how much they were subsidizing title XIX because they were being paid on a fee scale rather than their usual and customary fee. Each physician was asked to send statements to patients and to the state welfare department showing the degree of "subsidization" in each case. In other states—for example, Massachusetts—physicians lobbied for the appointment of Blue Shield, a physician dominated organization, as the fiscal agent.

Connecticut provides an example of a middle-of-the-road state. It established a relatively cautious program in 1967 with moderate eligibility standards and a fee schedule for physicians and other individual providers, with a Hospital Cost Commission for methods of reimbursing the hospitals. The latter had a long history in Connecticut, having been first established in 1949. Indeed its tradition was so strong that for the first few years of Medicaid it refused to apply the federal formula for reimbursement and actually paid hospitals less. More interesting, however, was the pressure put on the legislature to drop the fee schedule and pay physicians their usual and customary fees. Despite financial crisis in the state Medicaid program, the legislature passed Public Act 548 in 1967, which called for the payment of usual and customary fees for an experimental period between March 1968 and March 1969. The experiment was tried; physicians participated more readily, but costs skyrocketed. After hearings in February 1969, and the listing by name of major physician beneficiaries of Medicaid in local Connecticut newspapers, Connecticut returned to a fee schedule. The medical profession was displeased, but in the end it was the recipients who suffered, since it became much more difficult to persuade a physician to take a title XIX patient. Compared with the physicians, the other providers caused little problem.

In any event, by the summer of 1969 the idea of "usual and customary" fees was almost a dead issue in the Medicaid program, for the federal government had moved to freeze physician fees. The rather rapid change of heart had come not just because of the general rise in costs but also because a pattern of excessive payments to physicians and dentists had emerged and with them growing evidence of fraud on the part of various groups of providers.

The first rumblings were heard shortly after the beginning of title XIX. At the end of 1966, in New York State, Senator Thaler claimed misuse of funds by a Staten Island hospital. Early in 1967 the U.S. General Accounting Office reported rumors of physician misuse of drugs and nursing homes in the Cleveland area. By August 1967, as part of Senator Thaler's campaign to expose chicanery in New York City's hospitals, there were allegations of excessive Medicaid visits and prescribing in New York City—a state of affairs conceded to exist by the city's Health Services Administration. By the time the Senate held hearings on the 1967 amendments later in the fall, the Finance Committee was prepared to investigate the increasing allegations of abuses—a procedure in which the chairman of the AMA's Board of Trustees concurred. Particularly in California, the allegations of fraud by physicians, pharmacists, dentists, and others were reaching epidemic proportions. The October issue of *Parade* charged that during the first eighteen months of Medi-Cal, 1200 physicians had been paid an average of nearly $70,000 each. Although the president of the California

Medical Association denied abuse by providers, claiming that Medi-Cal had actually saved taxpayers millions because of effective utilization review, there was increasing evidence of at least excessive billing from all over the country; and this was true, on a lesser scale, for other health professions.. At hearings in Elmira, New York, in 1968, it was reported that a chiropractor had billed Medicaid unreasonably for spinal manipulation of a seven-month-old infant, and a dentist had received the then exorbitant sum of $80,000 for 1967.[49]

Inappropriate care, high costs, and fraud were not necessarily related, but they became so in the press as concern over all three mounted simultaneously. The line between inept management on the part of administrators and fraud on the part of providers is never clear. Fraud was, however, the most flagrant administrative deficiency, and egregious fraud the easiest to identify. As time passed, rumors of fraud were shown to have more than a core of truth. In November 1968, the California Department of Justice held hearings in Los Angeles, which, while giving the nonprofit hospitals a clean bill of health, found overservicing, kickbacks, and duplicate billings predominant in physician-owned hospitals. The following month the state attorney general reported that $8 million had been "drained" from Medi-Cal by unethical means. Hospitals, doctors, the fiscal agents, and almost all providers came in for attack. The attorney general of Maryland announced he was investigating frauds by physicians, dentists, and pharmacists. By the end of December, providers in Massachusetts were under attack (one dentist was said to have grossed $164,000 in 1968 from Medicaid), and the prosecution of ten physicians for fraud had begun in Maryland.

The new administration inherited accumulated evidence of fraud. On taking office as undersecretary of HEW in 1969, John Veneman announced, "We have to move toward eliminating greed in Medicare and Medicaid whether on the part of the recipients or the vendors."[50] The collapse of the Medicaid program in New Mexico was attributed by some to the greed of providers; the Associated Press reported "Medicaid Reported Bilked Out of Hundreds of Millions of Dollars," and the *Chicago Tribune*, normally more harsh on recipients than providers, claimed that "in the health programs the cheating is being done mainly by unscrupulous doctors and sticky-fingered functionaries."[51]

There was inevitably a demand for publishing the names of highly paid physicians—in the words of Senator John Williams (Delaware), "to name names and sums of money and put it on the front pages all over the country."[52] States complied. For instance, Maryland reported that one-fifth of the $4 million paid to 2470 physicians under Medicaid had gone to twenty-eight of them. By April 1969 the Senate Finance Committee was notifying states that it wanted data on all physicians paid more than $25,000 under title XIX in 1968. The California legislature introduced special legislation to punish defrauding providers. In Congress, Senator Long pressed for sending data to the IRS.

Some doctors no doubt were paid large sums under Medicaid because they chose to work in low-income areas. Nevertheless, some striking data gradually emerged. In Maryland, after a "nolo" plea, six physicians and a dental intern were put on probation and returned $68,000 to the state, representing illegal Medicaid billing. The highest payment reported to a single physician in Michigan was $169,000, but three osteopathic physicians allegedly filed over $800,000 in claims. In Kentucky, ten physicians received more than $50,000 each; the highest payment to a physician in Illinois was $110,806; and Kansas reported cases of revoking licenses and banning participation because of fraud. It finally emerged that, in 1968, at least 1329 MDs received more than $25,000 and 290 received more than $50,000 from title XIX, while over 7000 received more than $25,000 from Medicare.[53] These seemed exorbitant, if not extortionate sums. There was further agitation when, in 1970, the Treasury Department claimed that one-third of the physicians with large payments under Medicaid had cheated on their tax returns. Action appeared to have shifted to the federal government's right to police the quality of care in Medicaid and other governmental health programs.

In July 1969, the AMA passed a resolution opposing any governmental auditing of quality care in favor of professional peer review. In a biting response the New York City Department of Health refuted the AMA position, pointing out the large amount of low-quality care being provided under Medicaid, at least in New York City. This was not for lack of financial commitment. New York State in 1968 spent $63.95 per inhabitant, while twenty-one states spent less than $10 per inhabitant. In 1967 it was estimated that potential coverage ranged from 45 percent of the population in New York to seven percent in Massachusetts, although actual utilization ranged from a high of 11 percent in New York to a low of 2.5 percent in North Dakota.

Fraud on Medicaid was not limited to providers. There were well-documented frauds by recipients, ranging from the usual frauds associated with any means-test program through impersonation and excessive doctor-shopping. But it was generally held that fraud by recipients was insignificant compared with the behavior of providers, at least in terms of dollar costs. Of more concern with respect to beneficiaries were barriers to their receiving services, or at least the services they most needed. The potential recipient of Medicaid could be faced with a humiliating and complex means test and either confusing or inadequate advice. As the *New York Times* put it, the form to be filled out in New York to become a Medicaid beneficiary was "at least as difficult as the long-form tax return" and "could prove an impenetrable barrier to the least affluent who also tend to be the least educated."[55]

There was a huge variation in the services available to recipients in different states. For those receiving cash payments under federally supported public assistance, programs had to provide seven basic services by July 1970: inpatient hospital care, outpatient hospital services, other laboratory or X-ray services, skilled nursing home services for those over twenty-one, screening and treatment for those under twenty-one, physician services, and home health services. But beyond that, states had great latitude. Alabama, Arkansas, Colorado, Florida, Georgia, Indiana, Iowa, Louisiana, Maine, Mississippi, Missouri, Montana, Nevada, New Jersey, New Mexico, Ohio, Oregon, South Carolina, South Dakota, Tennessee, Texas, West Virginia, and Wyoming offered no program to the "medically indigent." Mississippi provided no services other than the required ones to the groups compulsorily covered, while Wyoming offered only transportation by way of such service. New Mexico, on the other hand, although having no program for the categorically related or the "medical indigent" category, offered welfare recipients home health services, drugs, dental services, eyeglasses, hearing aids, prosthetic devices, physical therapy, private duty nursing, optometrists' services, podiatrists' services, chiropractic services, clinic services, transportation, and other diagnostic services. At the most expansive end of the scale, California, Connecticut, Minnesota, New York, and North Dakota offered every additional service for which a federal contribution was available.

Recipients often found it difficult to obtain the services to which they were entitled. A year after Medicaid began, only 4500 of New York City's 15,000 physicians and 2400 of the city's 7500 dentists had registered for Medicaid. At different times between 1967 and 1970, pharmacists boycotted Medicaid in New York City, as did dentists in Connecticut, skilled nursing homes in Massachusetts, and hospitals in Washington, D.C. As the result of a dispute about payment for outpatient services, only two of Washington's ten hospitals agreed to cooperate. Though the program began on July 1, 1968, a compromise with all the hospitals was not finally worked out until the summer of 1969. In the process many providers of care looked bad, neglecting the needs of the impoverished or dumping them on the old charity institutions, in favor of maximum reimbursements for their own institutions.

Perhaps more frequent were situations where providers were evasive; for example, after Connecticut reverted to a fee schedule for physicians (in March 1969), following a twelve-month experiment with usual and customary fees. The AMA News announced: "Medicaid Killed in Connecticut," while *Medical Economics* described the twelve-month experiment as the "one glorious year" when Medicaid "really worked"; that is, when 3000 out of a possible 4500 physicians took part.[56] After the fee schedule was reintroduced, these reports suggested that only about 1000 doctors participated in Medicaid, a trend borne out by studies made in the New Haven area early in 1970. To the geographical and social problems involved in reaching a physician was thus added a noticeable reluctance to treat Medicaid patients on the part of many physicians. And this from a profession that alleged it willingly treated poor patients gratis only five or six years earlier—that is, before 1965.

Conclusions

The original 1970 conclusions of this study included the confident prediction that "Medicaid as it is known today is destined to be phased out during the next decade." We were wrong. Medicaid is still with us—together with many of the problems identified by 1970: still grappling with federal standards and state diversity; with budget crises and disputes over reimbursement rates; and with broader questions of how to provide health care to the "medically indigent," now more politely called the "uninsured" and "underinsured." In 1970, however, there did seem some immediate possibility for change. Bold proposals from the Nixon White House were calling for a Family Health Insurance Program as part of the administration's Family Assistance Plan, in order to cover what Medicaid then covered for young, low-income families. The combination of this with an expanded and more effective program for the elderly and disabled under Medicare might have reduced the need for other forms of medical assistance among the most needy population groups. It also seemed possible at the time that Medicaid would be replaced by something more exclusively "medical," through the development of comprehensive health services provided through some form of national health insurance. The Health Security proposals then being sponsored by Senator Edward Kennedy were an example of such an approach.

In 1970, Medicaid was an instructive museum of ideological conflict and organizational deficiencies. Title XIX of the Social Security Act as drafted in 1965 confused welfare and health care goals. The combination of an expansionary program of health services and a program of cash assistance provoked Medicaid's initial dilemmas of costs and rapid political recoil. Whether Medicaid was a health care program or part of a broader program of income maintenance was contentious; the "intention" of Congress, as lawyers and policy analysts have long known, is at best a slippery process. Some legislators intended to provide a new concept in medical care. Others, even among those who were in favor of title XIX, saw no need for any radical change from earlier policies under which health care was purchased from private vendors on the same basis as other goods (bedding, pots and pans, and so forth) purchased for cash assistance recipients. Some supporters saw a radically new health program, which might cover a large proportion of the uninsured (as initially proposed in New York), and the purchase of extensive health services in the private sector (as in California)—an important step toward universal comprehensive health coverage. For others, Medicaid was a logical, incremental, defensive move *against* threats of national health insurance.

The lack of clearly stated national goals for Medicaid in 1965 seemed a major and reverberating deficiency to many by 1970. Congressional errors were transmitted down the line as the programs were developed in the states—leading to conflict in interpretations of Medicaid between powerful committees in Washington and the legislatures of major states, state budgetary crises, and the sometimes selfish behavior of medical providers. In that sense, any villains portrayed in these pages were themselves the victims of confusion in the Congress.

Why was there this initial confusion about the purposes and goals of Medicaid? There can have been few legislators who were unaware in 1965 that Kerr-Mills was somewhat less than a success. That program had already demonstrated characteristics that were later to plague Medicaid: the transfer of funds by states from one public pocket to another under the stimulus of greater federal matching funds; the unevenness of programs from state to state; the implications of attaching a system of medical vendor payments to an administrative structure of grants-in-aid that relied on minimal federal direction; the interpretation of "medical indigency" as a rather rigid test of means, albeit at a somewhat higher average level than for cash assistance; the greater interest by the state legislatures in balancing their budgets than in reorganizing medical care; and, in the state bureaucracies, the inadequate administrative expertise for running a major medical program. Yet title XIX was developed under similar principles.

Those loath to ascribe confusion as a natural attribute to Congress might assume that the adoption of the Kerr-Mills strategy for the much larger Medicaid was predicated on deliberate doctrine, founded perhaps on recondite principles of marginal gain or of greater chaos, out of which ultimately clarity might emerge. Medicaid brought medical care to many thousands of persons, with less individual financial anxiety than if the program had not been developed; in this sense the gains were real by 1970, though marginal and expensive, and the balance sheet should be so interpreted. In this scenario the major defects of Medicaid lay in the lack of adequate cost projections and cost-benefit analyses. Those favoring a doctrine of greater chaos—a try-anything-and-see-what-happens approach—might point to Medicaid's intrinsic social importance in accelerating congressional and general concern over the costs and provision of health services in the 1970s and beyond—a necessary element, perhaps, in some future rationalization of health services in the United States. Built on the rhetoric of the past rather than the realities of the late 1960s, Medicaid proved that politics is the art of the possible, legislatively speaking. From a policy perspective, title XIX can be seen as a necessary and useful, if expensive and somewhat painful transition from the 1940s to the 1970s.

In shape as well as intention, Medicaid began with inbuilt deficiencies. The assumption that effective and economical medical services could be provided through existing structures of health services and public assistance was challenged almost as soon as the program was implemented. The parallel implementation of Medicare in 1966 made Medicaid's struggles starkly visible in several ways: in the early efforts to tie Medicaid with Medicare's then generous reimbursement rates; in the cumulative impact of the two programs as they hit providers simultaneously; in the equation of both programs with a doctrine of bringing the otherwise uninsured into the "mainstream"; and, by seeming to abolish provider "charity," in redefining hospitals, nursing homes and health professionals as players in a medical marketplace. The stage was set for rampant entrepreneurialism in health care from the late 1970s on into the twenty-first century.

Unlike other forms of assistance, Medicaid was asked to do more than fill a gap or provide a backup service for reasonably effective programs (such as jobs or housing) in the private sector. Other programs were insufficient. If Medicare, designed to provide health care as an entitlement to the whole population over age sixty-five, had been sufficiently comprehensive, Medicaid's substantial and growing commitment of services to the elderly would have been unnecessary. If private health insurance had effectively covered the working population (including continuing coverage for survivors and dependents, and in times of sickness and temporary unemployment) the concept of medical indigency need not have been invented—and decades later we would not still be struggling with the problem of the "uninsured." Medicaid, with its uncontrollable budgets and rising costs, was a reflection of broader deficiencies in health insurance coverage and health care organization.

Over and above basic inconsistencies in the philosophy of vendor medical payments, Medicaid tested, and found wanting, the traditional federal grant-in-aid when it applied to a service rather than a cash payment program.. In its first few years Medicaid showed that if a primary purpose of Congress was to bring medical care to every person in the country—raising vital issues of equal protection—control of these services could not be left to fifty states. In 1970 the proposed Nixon Family Assistant Plan seemed to be moving towards nationwide standards and administration. We predicted that there would be tighter federal regulation over providers of care and increasing federal standards for services in the future as an essential part of public purchase of services in the private sector. In any event, the Nixon proposals went nowhere, and Medicaid continued as a collection of state programs with federal funding but without national standardization or strong federal direction. A political football, Medicaid became part of a national cost problem as far as Congress was concerned, and part of continuing budgetary and service crises in the states.

Two basic assumptions marked the adoption of vendor medical payments in Medicaid in the late 1960s. The first was that services were more likely to be available and of better quality through purchase in the private sector rather than through the development or expansion of publicly financed and controlled hospitals and clinics. Prevailing problems in public hospital systems (of which New York City was a notable example) seemed to bear out this assumption in 1970. Moreover, many states and local governments, having relied for years on vendor medical payments, did not have a ready-made public system for development. And when they did, some were happy to offload a local tax burden—as when Philadelphia closed its city hospital in 1977. A second assumption, at least in Medicaid's first two years, was a social ethos of equal opportunity in medical care; that is, a commitment by many reformers to provide medical services to the poor of roughly the same quality as those provided to other members of the population. This was interpreted as meaning provision of services through one set of providers rather than espousing a separate-but-equal philosophy for medical care. Medi-Cal was the most publicized example of this "mainstream" approach, in that state administrators embarked on a deliberate program to break down California's separate public hospital system as the locus of medical care for the indigent. Taking Medicaid as a whole, however, it proved impossible to overthrow centuries of poor-law mentality, let alone shoulder the increased costs. How quickly realities intervened!

Medicaid thus began with major problems. But it would be wrong to conclude without considering some of the benefits of Medicaid that were evident by 1970. In most states, for those on Medicaid the provision of care was better than it was before 1965. At least in established health facilities there was probably less of a gap between the services provided for the poor and the non-poor than there was before. Even in the most conventional hospital, the notion of the "welfare patient" (as of a lesser class) was less rampant (though it still continues to some extent). There was increasing realization of the fact that health services should be divorced from the cash payments in the welfare system—now generally recognized through Medicaid state contracts with managed care organizations. Medicaid continues to be a rich resource for social negotiation about the nature and scope of health care, which services should be covered and for whom, how they should be provided, and how costs can be controlled. Medicaid, more than Medicare, also offers a platform for service innovation at a time of continuing budget cutbacks, particularly in serving patients who need multiple services for chronic conditions in a largely uncoordinated health care system.

Legislative and institutional lessons can also be learned from Medicaid's implementation. To have an effective government medical care program, it must have the support of the administration (both in Washington and the states), in the legislature and in the executive. There must also be a commitment on the part of the providers and recipients to make certain the program is efficient, and fairly utilized. Providers have to be convinced that the program is not a license to print money—though many providers now complain that Medicaid is bleeding them dry instead. The pendulum may have swung too far in the other direction, creating unwilling rather than willing vendors. Professions have to recognize that they are professions because they owe a peculiar fiduciary responsibility to the public (an ongoing task). Recipients have to be assured of sufficient dignity so that they treat the program with respect. Federal supervision, and perhaps control, may have to be far more effective than it was between 1965 and 1970, if the program is not going to be bankrupted; and the medical providers have to learn to live with such control.. Medicaid is still fascinating, still important—and still a work in progress.

I have ruthlessly adapted this chapter from its original, much longer and more detailed version: Rosemary Stevens and Robert Stevens, "Medicaid: Anatomy of a Dilemma," *Law and Contemporary Problems*, Health Care, Part I, 1970, XXXV (2): 348-425.

Serious students of Medicaid history are advised to go to the original, which includes additional source materials, discussion, and references (no less than 358 legal-type footnotes), particularly for discussion of federal and state administration. See also Robert Stevens and Rosemary Stevens, *Welfare Medicine in America: A Case Study of Medicaid*. New York: Free Press, 1974, republished with updated introduction, New Brunswick, NJ: Transaction Publishers, 2003.

Notes

1. For figures, see U.S. Department of Health, Education and Welfare, *Social Security Programs in the United States* 14 (1968).
2. U.S. Department of Health, Education and Welfare, *Medical Services Available to Meet the Needs of Public Assistance Recipients.* H.R. Rep. No. 1799, 87th Cong., 1st Sess. 31 and passim (1961). Hereafter cited as *Medical Resources.*
3. Subcommittee on Health of the Elderly of the Special Senate Committee on Aging, 88th Congress, 1st Sess., *Medical Assistance for the Aged, the Kerr-Mills Program 1960-1963*, p. 75 (Comm. Print 1963). Hereafter cited as *Medical Assistance for the Aged.*
4. *Hearings on H.R. 3920 before the House Comm. on Ways and Means,* 88th Cong., 1st and 2nd Sess. 31 (1963-64). Hereafter cited as *1963 Hearings.*
5. New York State Department of Social Welfare, Office of Medical Economics, *Medical Care Expenditures for the Aged in the United States Under the Federally Aided Public Assistance Programs, January-March 1963* (1963).
6. Testimony of Wilbur Cohen, *Hearings on H.R. 6675 before the Senate Comm. on Finance*, 89th Cong., 1st Sess. 166 (1965). Hereafter cited as *1965 Hearings.*
7. Testimony of Edmund Brown, *1963 Hearings*, p. 920.
8. See, for example, Burns, "Some Major Policy Decisions Facing the United States in the Financing and Organization of Health Care," 42 *Bull. New York Acad. Med.* (2nd ser.) 1972, 1080 (1966); Werne, "Medicaid: Has National Health Insurance Entered by the Back Door?" 18 *Syracuse L. Rev.* 49 (1966).
9. *New York Times*, May 1, 1966, p. 1 col. 2.
10. The *New York Times* reported these various opinions and events. For detailed footnotes see Stevens and Stevens, "Medicaid: Anatomy of a Dilemma," *Law and Contemporary Problems*, Spring 1970, pp. 366-370.
11. 112 Cong. Rec. 20,267 (1966). (Remarks of Senator Saltonstall.)
12. House Ways and Means Committee, *Limitations on Federal Participation under title XIX of the Social Security Act*, H.R. Rep. No. 2224, 89th Cong., 2nd Sess. 8 (1966).
13. Ibid. The total cost (federal, state, and local) if all states adopted a New York-type plan was estimated at $6.4 billion annually. *New York Times*, October 24, 1966, p. 23, col. 1.
14. *AMA News*, January 2, 1967 (Dr. Joseph D. Giovino).
15. Ibid., January 16, 1967.
16. *Medical Tribune*, August 28, 1967.
17. *New York Times*, January 20, 1967, p. 88, col. 1.
18. See M. Greenfield, *Medi-Cal: The California Medicaid Program (Title XIX)* (1969); A. C. Barnes, *A Description of the Organization and Administration of the Cali-*

fornia Medical Assistance Program: Title XIX (1968); and for detailed footnotes on California's implementation of Medicaid, Stevens and Stevens, pp. 370-373.

19. Tax Foundation, Inc., *Medicaid: State Programs after Two Years* 70 (1968). Hereafter cited as *Medicaid*.
20. Greenfield, *Medi-Cal*, p. 53 and passim.
21. House Comm. on Ways and Means, Social Security Amendments of 1967, H.R. Rep. No. 544, 90th Cong., 1st Sess. 118 (1967). Hereafter cited as Amendments of 1967.
22. *Hearings on H.R. 12080 before the Senate Comm. on Finance,* 90th Cong., 1st Sess. 217 (1967), pp. 1591-92. Hereafter *1967 Hearings.*
23. Ibid., p. 497.
24. Advisory Commission on Intergovernmental Relations, *Intergovernmental Problems in Medicaid* 33-34 (1968), pp. 34-35.
25. R. Myers, *Medicare*, pp. 282-285 (1970).
26. *1967 Hearings*, pp. 275-276.
27. *Hearings before the Senate Comm. on Finance*, 91st cong., 1st sess. 6-7 (1969). Hereafter *1969 Hearings.*
28. U.S. Dept. of Health, Education and Welfare, Social Security Administration, *Research and Statistics Note* (November 7, 1969).
29. Ibid., June 18, 1970.
30. P.L. 89-97, sec. 1902(a)(19), 1965.
31. U.S. Dept. of Health, Education and Welfare, Social Security Administration, *Research and Statistics Note* (July 16, 1969).
32. U.S. Dept. of Health, Education and Welfare, *Handbook of Public Assistance Administration*, Supplement D, para. D-5340 (1966).
33. Ibid., para. D-5330.
34. *AMA News*, January 13, 1969.
35. Tax Foundation, *Medicaid*, p. 42.
36. *1969 Hearings*, pp. 8-9.
37. *New York Times*, August 13, 1969, p. 33, col. 5.
38. *AMA News*, various issues.
39. Ibid., July 1, 1969.
40. Testimony of Dr. John Knowles, 25 Congressional Quarterly Service, *Congressional Quarterly Almanac* 850 (1970).
41. *Washington Report on Medicine and Health*, April 14, 1969.
42. P.L. 91-172, designed for other purposes, also amended sections 1902 and 1903 of the Social Security Act.
43. 25 Congressional Quarterly Service, *Congressional Quarterly Almanac* 203 (1970).
44. Task Force on Medicaid, *Interim Report*, 1969; *Report of the Task Force on Medicaid and Related Programs* (1970).
45. Staff of the Senate Comm. on Finance, 91st cong., 1st Sess., *Medicare and Medicaid: Problems, Issues and Alternatives (Comm. Print 1970)*, p. 245 and passim.
46. 35 Fed. Reg. 8780 (1970).
47. Task Force Report, p. 104.
48. *1965 Hearings*, p. 681.
49. *New York Times*, January 25, 1968, p. 26, col. 1. For other references in this paragraph and elsewhere, see Stevens and Stevens, "Medicaid: Anatomy of a Dilemma."
50. Quoted in *This Week for Hospitals*, February 17, 1969.
51. *AMA News*, July 21, 1969.
52. Ibid., March 10, 1969.

53. *1969 Hearings*, pp. 161-162.
54. *New York Times*, September 22, 1970.
55. Ibid., January 28, 1967, p. 26, col. 2.
56. *AMA News*, December 14, 1969; Lavin, "What to Expect from Washington Now," *Med. Econ.*, January 20, 1969, p. 21.

6

Governments and Medical Care: Comparing the U.S. and Great Britain in 1977

The provision of medical care has become inextricably intertwined with government, whether one has a health service under public management, as in the United Kingdom, or subject to public subsidy and regulation, as in the United States. Yet there are serious concerns on both sides of the Atlantic about the proper role of government. We have come to appreciate that resources for medical care are finite; that the costs and benefits of medical care should be spread reasonably over the whole population, and that this can only be done through taxation or government regulation; that increasing expenditure on medical care does not necessarily mean concomitant increases in value received; and that in some respects, we may run the risk of becoming an "over-medicalized" society, to our own detriment. Decisions on many aspects of medical resources are political and economic: the result of social decisions rather than of individual judgment, or even the judgment of physicians to which individual decisions have traditionally been delegated.

This is a good time to ask, in Britain as well as the United States, whether, given the common pressures of modern medicine—which impose on governments both financial and ethical choices of how resources ought to be distributed—different countries are moving to common solutions. Is the government role in medical care one that we can generalize about, at least in the next decades? Are we all moving in similar directions, so that eventually our health services may look quite similar? I will argue that the government role in Britain and the United States is in some ways moving in similar directions, but only up to a point. There are definitional problems here: Americans and Britons use the same vocabulary but often mean quite different things. Both "government" and "medical care" have culturally specific meanings. The customs and traditions of government relations between government agencies, as well as between government and private groups, provide a predetermined context for the developing role of government in medical care. But medical care, too, may have quite different meanings in different places. Thus, while there may be great value in future comparisons of medical services, differences will undoubtedly remain in the scope and nature of government intervention in medical care on each side of the Atlantic—not because the technological processes are necessarily different, but because distinctive patterns of behavior have been slowly built up over the last two hundred years.

The Government Role in Britain

The United Kingdom and the United States have been divided by ideological expectations as well as language over the past thirty years, expressed in the lingering rhetoric of Britain as a welfare state and America as the bastion of private enterprise. However, beneath the ideology the role of government has been changing in each country. Old labels no longer suffice; indeed, each country is looking warily at the earlier concepts of the other. In Great Britain the National Health Service (NHS) is moving away from its earlier centralization of management toward decentralized health services, and to a greater use of what in the United States are called consumer organizations. Meanwhile, in the United States, a system originally distinguished by decentralized private controls is moving to one with a much firmer government relationship.

Some scholars are now using the phrase "contract state" to describe changing relationships between government and private groups in both Britain and the United States.[1, 2] Contract usefully (if perhaps confusingly) suggests both a commercial and fiduciary relationship between government and the private sector. Taking into account the noticeable increase in public use of private and quasi-public agencies, government may be seen as purchaser and private groups as sellers in a marketplace. However, contract also suggests a pact, as in the term social contract, with expected roles and responsibilities assumed by private organizations that act as government's agents. To understand how far the two countries are (or are not) becoming similar, it is worth looking at their concurrent developments since World War II. Interestingly, health services in both countries have gone through three distinct phases of development since the ideological debates of the 1940s.

In Britain, the NHS began with a period of nationalization, moved to a period of administrative consolidation during the 1950s and into the 1960s, and with reorganization in 1974 began a third period of change. The first stage was one of political idealism and practical success: Comprehensive health care was to be assured and provided by a democratic government and largely paid for out of general taxation. Looking back to the 1940s, the achievement was astonishing. Hospitals were nationalized and grouped into regional and local consortia; consultants and specialists put on salary and given specific assignments in geographical regions; virtually the whole population signed up with general practitioners; and local governments provided ambulances and other supportive services. The structure was in many ways unwieldy, but it worked.

The middle-class population came rapidly to accept medical care as a right, as natural a privilege as free education. The medical associations lost the embattled shrillness of the earlier parliamentary debates; the NHS became an essential plank in the Welfare State. By the early 1950s, there were few calls from anyone for a return to a private system.[3]

The second stage of development was under way by the time I entered the NHS as a hospital administrative trainee in 1957. The services were being consolidated with remarkable success. I remember sitting in the offices of the Sheffield Regional Hospital Board reading, as one of my first assignments, the reports of the hospital surveys, which had preceded the NHS little more than a decade before. It was extraordinary how quickly the old non-system of independent hospitals and itinerant specialists had been harnessed into an organized hospital service. The system looked as though it had been there for generations.

This second period of consolidation was beginning, however, to be seriously challenged by 1960 as success began to give way to smugness and to criticism. Smugness was apparent not only in self-congratulation within the NHS—self-congratulatory comparisons with the United States were only too evident—but also apparent in the less than dynamic management by professionals, and by voluntary members of the hospital management committees. While some managers and board members were undoubtedly effective, others appeared to be little more than rubber stamps, or administrative conveniences for participating physicians. But there were, of course, many other problems in the NHS as it was developing. For political and pragmatic reasons the NHS had been designed as three separate operating parts: hospital and specialist services, general practitioner services, and local government services. The awkwardness of the tripartite structure of the health service inevitably led, through years of debate, to pressures for major reorganization of all health services into integrated local units. Broader reforms in local government, as well as organizational changes in community nursing services, and reform in the social services, provided the final impetus for major change. Thus the third stage of the NHS began in 1974 with a reorganization of health services that appears in 1977 as historic and imaginative a development as the original National Health Service Act of 1946.

Despite the gloom cast upon reorganization by lack of funds and inevitable problems of morale among professional staff whose careers were suddenly shifted, reorganization has had effects that are important in an international perspective. First, the deliberate attempt to create a unified comprehensive, area-wide health service in which hospital, family practice, and community health services were to be combined, subtly redefined the concept of a health service. In theory, at least, the new health boards were freed from blinkered constraints, and able to look at health services as a whole, on a population basis. The personalities, power structures, budget allocations, and politics inherited by the new agencies obviously made the process incremental rather than revolutionary. Nevertheless, the underlying message and challenge of reorganization was to redefine health services, and decide which services were appropriate, within a given budget, for a given population. The potential power was there to achieve change because of single payer funding.

In contrast to the initial expectations of local health planning in Great Britain in the 1970s, in the United States concurrent talk about area-wide planning, community health services, health maintenance, and the like seemed rhetoric rather than reality virtually from the beginning. This was not for lack of effort. Notably, the privately funded National Commission on Community Health Services worked hard during the early 1960s to develop a plan for local health services in the United States. Its final report[4] offered a series of recommendations for the development of comprehensive health services at the local level. However, there was no commitment to such a change in real-world politics, nor were there coordinated money streams through which such change might be accomplished. Americans might well be struck by the language of the British reports, for example the so-called Green and White Papers for reorganizations in Scotland, for those simply assumed that health services ought to have a demographic and epidemiological base; that is, that the nature, amount, and distribution of health services depended on how many old people there were in a specified geographical area, how many children needing specialized services, and so on, and that any plan for services should be built on this basis.[5, 6, 7, 8] In the United States, debates tend to assume that a health service is defined, rather, by its resources; that it is, in effect, a collection of buildings, equipment, physicians, nurses, and other personnel; that medical care is an industry; and that this industry is dominated by entrenched organizations, competing power centers, inventive entrepreneurs, and Machiavellian interest groups.[9, 10] In its simplest form, one concept is population-oriented; the other, producer-directed. In one the goals could be characterized as mutual; in the other, competitive.

A second important element of reorganization of the NHS evident to the outsider—and one made more striking by Britain's general economic situation in the early 1970s—was the reaffirmation of government's responsibilities to assure and to provide health services to the whole population: services that are both universal in terms of population coverage and (within budgetary limits) comprehensive. The uncompromising language of the 1946 National Health Service Act created public expectations of what government ought to provide. Health services were part of a package of supporting services for individuals: a floor from which individual initiative would supposedly flourish. In a welfare state, private enterprise might (or might not, of course) lose its most ruthless edge. The NHS made a strong egalitarian political statement in providing opportunities for rich and poor alike, as of right, without a means test. In theory, at least, all social classes would pay for, and benefit from, tax-supported health services. The underlying purpose of the welfare state in Great Britain was not, however, primarily what Americans might suppose it to be, assuming they bought into the NHS at all; that is, to provide equal economic opportunity as a ground rule of democratic capitalism, so that anyone could go out in the manner of Horatio Alger or Samuel Smiles to make a fortune in the world. Rather, the welfare state symbolized a struggle to provide for everyone a certain quality of life that, in theory at least, made Britons proud to be British. The NHS had collective rather than individualistic goals.[11]

The British stance was undoubtedly in part a reflection, in the postwar years, of a desire to sweep away the old prewar class inequities and to restructure the various elements of society. But the result was that the ideology of the early welfare state was not primarily economic, but was rather visionary, humanistic, and egalitarian. In the United States, in contrast, the ideology of government provision of health services was, and has continued to be, economic and/or strategic. Change, where it does take place, is through crisis, compromise, tradeoffs, and pressures.

In the 1970s, health services are regarded as a necessary part of the British fabric of life, and the government role is to provide them. While the economic rhetoric in London is toward a deliberate attempt towards private enterprise generally, and a downplaying of the welfare sector, the most important effects on the NHS promise to be restricted budgets rather than any massive changes. The most important changes may have already taken place. Reorganization emphasizes, in its structure, area-wide responsibility for planning and managing health services. Continued belt-tightening may push the various health authorities to define new priorities more starkly than before, and to assume much more real authority than the early governing boards were able to exercise, but these changes may prove all to the good. The basic point is that the initial goals and aspirations of the NHS remain.

In terms both of defining medical care substantively (as deriving from specific population characteristics) and ideologically (as government guaranteed), the NHS has pointed to directions that, in the context of area-wide and regional planning ideas that are widespread in the United States, may also be relevant there. British health services had developed another characteristic by the late 1970s that had more than a parochial interest in the United States: the decentralization of responsibility for health services from London (for England and Wales) or Edinburgh (for Scotland) to area and district agencies. In thirty years the NHS had moved from a largely centralized service based on preexisting power formations and institutions, to one that is, at least in theory, community-based, integrated at the area-wide level, and imbued with substantial local and private initiative.

National government's role in medical care in Britain began as a dominating force, but has lessened by the late 1970s. Prevailing signs promise increasing authority to the private groups of individuals who make up the health authorities and councils, and to professional administrators, including physicians, who run the service on a day-to-day basis. What foreign observers have seen in Britain in the first thirty years of the NHS are both a shifting of responsibility from central government to local agencies and a shift from parliamentary decisions to decisions made on the local level. The various processes of consultation between health boards, local groups, health councils, professional advisory committees, local governments, and social service agencies make decision-making much more open or pluralistic than was true of the initial NHS, when it was, in effect, largely run as a professional service by health professionals.

The new health boards in Great Britain and the newly developing health systems agencies in the United States have some surface similarities. Each is responsible for planning health facilities in geographical regions. Both will be forced to grapple with the distribution of scarce resources, the guarantee of minimum benefits versus the demands of powerful hospitals for new departments or equipment, and the balancing of priorities among competing and righteous interest groups. Substantively, ideologically, and structurally, then, policy developments in Great Britain and the United States make the government role in medical care much more relevant for comparison than at any time in the past history of the two nations.

Central government's role in Britain in the late 1970s may be broadly classified under four heads. The government is first, and most critically, the financial manager of health services, raising taxes and disbursing them. Second, it is responsible for the regional distribution of resources; third, for general standards of administration and infrastructure (construction and so on); and fourth, for overall regulation. Stretching the point a bit for the sake of argument, these elements of the governmental role are not too dissimilar from the situation in the United States in the 1970s.

The Government Role in the United States

This is so because opposite processes have been taking place in the two countries. While the NHS has been trying to decentralize its organization, U.S. health services have increasingly been subject to central (federal) standard setting.

In Britain, at least since 1948, government has a decisive and unquestioned role in the provision of all aspects of medical care. In the United States, until the 1960s and 1970s, enormous efforts were made either to ignore the government role altogether or, where it clearly did exist, to justify government intervention in terms that were only peripherally concerned with providing medical care. Government provision of health services has had, as a result, an uneasy history in the United States. The two large government programs, Medicare and Medicaid, were both established by legislation in 1965, with economic rather than humanitarian aims; Medicare being designed to protect the income of the elderly from devastating hospital bills, Medicaid to stop the continuing cycle of poverty and ill health for those who those already indigent. Medicare provides insurance benefits and hospital care, doctors' bills, and certain other health services for twenty million Americans, chiefly for Social Security pensioners. The federal government collects the taxes and manages the insurance funds, and pays bills by arrangements with recognized private insurance agencies. Both Medicare and Medicaid subsidize medical bills; neither guarantees comprehensive service.

The government role in the United States is subordinate to other goals. Health services are provided to the military and to veterans in vast government service systems. The Federal Health Employees Benefits System provides fringe benefits to public servants. Numerous other government programs developed from the mid-1960s, to deal with the construction of facilities, or the provision of services for special population groups. As with Medicare and Medicaid, these were typically generated by goals that were not primarily to provide health services. For example, health services were provided to migrant workers as part of an overall package of benefits to improve the economic conditions of this group. There is no overall health service ethos as such.

Yet, cumulatively, the U.S. government role has rapidly become extensive. By the mid-1970s, federal, state, and local government funds combined accounted for about 40 percent of all monies spent for personal health care in America. And Congress was concerned about how public money was being spent. Thus, in the three periods of development in the government role in medicine in the United States after the end of World War II, there was, first, a period that joined experimentation in methods of health insurance with federal subsidy of research and health care institutions. The insurance sequence went as follows: congressional flirtation with the idea of national health insurance in the late 1940s, its rejection as national policy in 1950, and a huge concurrent buildup of private health insurance to the working population through the cooperation of employers, whose participation was encouraged by government though the provision of tax incentives. Most new government programs funded directly by taxation between 1946 and 1963 were directed toward institutional subsidy and investment in biomedical research; that is, building the health care infrastructure. This was the time of the expansion of the National Institutes of Health (NIH), and of subsidized construction of private hospitals in rural areas, and later in urban areas, under the Hill-Burton program, which provided earmarked federal grants to states.[12]

Both sets of policies, for insurance and subsidy, used federal action to stimulate action in the private sector. Tax incentives to employers increased employer demand for private health insurance on behalf of their workers—and private insurers (not-for-profit and commercial) were only too happy to oblige. NIH funds flowed to private as well as public universities (while building a vast government campus for NIH in-house research close to Washington, in Bethesda, Maryland). Hill-Burton funds went to states for hospital planning, but their main targets were local groups seeking to establish a rural hospital and willing to take the initiative and responsibility to do so. (In this they were somewhat similar in effect to the much earlier state system described above in chapter 1).

Between 1963 and 1966—signified by President Lyndon B. Johnson's Great Society programs—there was a second stage of development. Based on public goals to eliminate poverty and improve general social conditions, numerous social programs were developed in a very short time, including Medicare and Medicaid. For comparative purposes, two points are particularly relevant here. First, these public programs had many characteristics of the private sector, and second, they were not "health services" in British terms; that is, they did not usually provide direct patient care. Medicare, for example, was more similar to commercial fire or car insurance than the British NHS. Its primary purpose was to protect individual income against financial catastrophe. Medicare's structure and form mimicked those of Blue Cross and Blue Shield (then organized as an array of not-for profit corporations) and commercial medical insurance policies.

In the 1970s Medicare primarily covered the enormous costs of hospital care in the United States. It did not cover services that might be regarded as important for the quality of life in Britain, including preventive and routine primary care, dental care, services to improve hearing, eye care, meals-on-wheels, and many other home care services. Nursing home care was (and is) only available under Medicare for those who have been discharged from a hospital. Benefits outside hospitals require the beneficiary to meet a deductible (i.e., the first set of charges on each year's bill) and coinsurance (i.e., consumer responsibility for part of the bills incurred for covered services) and there are specific limitations on services. From its beginning, Medicare was a complicated program based on monetary risks. It also carried political risks. As the cost went up, benefits might be cut, or charges and contributions increased.

If the role of government in medical care in the United States in the 1940s and 1950s had been to stimulate investments in health service resources (new buildings, more research, additional professionals), in this second period the government role was that of an entrepreneur, enabler, and fixer. Those members of the population who were clearly dependent and could not provide for health services out of their own pocket were helped through publicly organized or subsidized schemes, chiefly under Medicare and Medicaid, provided they fell into classified groups: the old, poor, migrants, and other special groups. Government also had an enabling role in encouraging private initiative in health services, in what was becoming known as the health care industry. Medicare was implemented through for-profit and non-profit-making health insurance corporations. Profit-making nursing homes, home health services, and private laboratories sprang up in response to the promise of government spending. Many professionals incorporated as private businesses: groups of physical therapists or respiratory therapists, for example. But all independent health practitioners benefited in some way from federal largesse.

One result of the Great Society programs in medical care was enthusiastic endorsement by leaders of private organizations who saw the potential for profit-making at government expense—in some cases, at government's decree. The number of private nursing homes rose rapidly, while hospitals added staff and equipment, and physicians' fees increased. A related result was a patchwork of overlapping medical care programs, with presumed problems of waste and inefficiency. Spiraling rises in government spending were accompanied by relatively little cost regulation.

In this situation of government involvement without accountability, medical care became a vast, disorganized industry, employing four million people by the mid-1970s, spending each year an average of over $500 for every woman, man, and child in the country, with costs moving inexorably upward. As the combined impact of the Great Society programs took full effect, congressional committees got tougher. A short period of expansion in the late 1960s was rapidly followed by one of recrimination, breast-beating, and retrenchment. Instead of enabling the private health sector to expand further, the congressional mood shifted to repression and regulation of health providers in an effort to rein in rising costs.

There is now abundant evidence of maldistribution of resources geographically, as well as inequality in the receipt of medical care by area, racial group, ethnic group, and economic group—trends apparently exacerbated rather than reduced by government activities. Though equality of health care was never a goal, the vague, more slippery word, "equity" appeared as an additional trigger for congressional debates, and buzzword for the growing ranks of health care experts. In the late-1970s the United States is being forced to face questions that are quite similar, substantively and ideologically, to those of any welfare state. Cost control implies the development of standards and priority setting, while equity presupposes some recognized principles of fairness, if not egalitarianism, and the means to implement them.

This third stage of government involvement in American medical care post-World War II is thus geared towards regulation of the still largely private medical care sector: nonprofit hospitals, profit-making nursing homes, private medical and other practitioners. Since the late 1960s, congressional committees have become increasingly concerned about fraud and abuses in Medicare and Medicaid, not only by patients but chiefly by providers. The new development of an extensive system of Professional Standards Review Organizations (PSROs) is designed to monitor the extent of care and the cost of care given to patients in hospitals under public programs. Government has become much more concerned over the distribution and organization of medical services, and the new health systems agencies are designed to review and monitor health services on an area-wide, local basis. In ideological terms, what is now happening in the United States may prove to be similar to what happened in Britain during the discussions preceding the NHS. The situation in wartime Britain in generating the NHS may be paralleled by the current chaos in American public programs, by discoveries of widespread abuse, rising costs of medical care, and the lack of public accountability. In this sense, there is a strange quality of déjà vu.

While Britain is struggling generally to revitalize its profit-making sector and downplaying the role of the welfare state in the 1970s, the United States is searching for its own version of a welfare state. The government role in medical care in the United States seems already so potent that some broader guidelines will soon be essential. As in Britain, the government role in the United States may be classified under the headings of financial management (tax policy and disbursement for Medicare, Medicaid, and other programs), distribution of resources (more equitable and efficient provision), development of standards, and regulation. In these respects, the government role in the United States seems much more similar to that in Britain than was true thirty years ago. Naturally, the question arises whether and how far the two systems are converging—or at least, how far they may ultimately be more similar.

Are Governments Moving in Similar Directions? In Some Ways, Yes

The developing government role in Britain and the United States does suggest some convergence. It seems clear that future governments will be responsible for assuring a minimal level of health benefits to the whole population; for keeping a lid on total national spending for medical care; for defining priorities in the medical care system; for ensuring an organizational framework through which medical resources could be distributed across the population with reasonable equity; and for training an appropriate number and mixture of professionals. Given the pressures of modern specialized medicine, government clearly has a role as paymaster, policymaker, and regulator, whether there is a national health service or not.

It can also be argued, up to a point, that medical care poses certain common dilemmas for government, which may ultimately lead to similar solutions in very different national contexts. Specific problems raised by the existence of modern medical technology may require some common answers. Increasingly specialized services, to work well, require organization. Modern medicine has flourished because of specialization: specialization in research, among members of the medical profession, and in the development of new health professions, hospital departments, and clinics. But no specialized service can work well unless it is well organized and efficient: and it is here that government is drawn in. There must be coordination among the specialists, plus access by patients to the system so that they can reach the appropriate specialist; otherwise the value of specialization is lost. On both sides of the Atlantic, such considerations lead to discussions of primary care, family practice, health centers, and multispecialist coordination.

Concentration of specialized services and equipment in major hospitals leads to considerations of regional specialty centers, emergency services, and regional or area-wide hospital networks. In both countries, too, movements to decentralize the management of medical care to local agencies, and to recognize the role of private decision-makers, including decisions made by patients about their care, have brought the "consumer" into the picture. The NHS has always included boards made up of private citizens. But the development of local health councils purportedly representing the consumer has added another feature; they take the nationalized service another step away from being a streamlined, standardized public agency. Meanwhile, the United States is relying increasingly on groups of private citizens to take on government responsibilities (boards of health systems agencies are a case in point). There seems to be an emerging, generic governmental role whose primary impetus is to dissociate government funding of medical care from strictly governmental management. Control by politicians and civil servants of day-to-day decision-making in medicine is not on the horizon in either nation. Yet the ultimate checks and balances in the public and private sectors are not fully developed yet; meanwhile, movements in each country raise fascinating questions of the accountability of government for public expenditure. Already, though, it seems clear that while governments may delegate responsibility for managing medical services, delegation has to be accompanied by increasing government regulation. Management has superseded ideology as the prime purpose of reform. The British pin their hopes on private management of a public system, while the Americans grope toward better public regulation of a private system.

But how far, in fact, is convergence a reasonable conclusion? Even if health care were purely a technocratic system for which standard organizational, regulatory, and economic rules applied, "government" and "medical care" would continue to have variable meanings across the two cultures. Broad-brush similarities there may be in the organizational roles of government; but this is a quite different observation than leaping to the conclusion that eventually the British and American medical care systems will look the same. It may seem over-obvious to remark that medicine is only part technology, and that a good part depends on cultural norms and social traditions. But while the point may be obvious, it may also need stressing. The term "medical care" means something quite different in Britain and the United States; and, I think, this difference will continue.

The American governmental role is distinguished by rhetoric that the federal role is, and should be, weak. Yet there is a strong federal role in setting standards for private industry compared with Britain. American society has long accepted a strong governmental regulatory role; indeed, American industry is remarkably responsive to pressures for standardizing industrial techniques and labeling products, whether dangerous drugs or breakfast cereals. Reporting of information to federal agencies by government units and by private industry is much more stringent than in Great Britain. In Britain, there is, on the face of it, strong centralized direction in the nationalized sectors, including the NHS.

Yet, there is also pride in "muddling through": decisions tended to be taken informally and independently, both in government and in industry.[13]

These practices spill over into the government role in medical care. The American governmental tradition still discourages any appearance of a national health service but allows for tough federal controls on hospitals and physicians. In Britain, on the other hand, a national health service is readily accepted, but there has been long resistance to detailed standards, reporting, and monitoring of services.

Such differences are not academic; they are readily visible in the 1970s. To British eyes, American hospitals, physicians, and health care organizations are remarkably closely regulated. Private groups of physicians work on behalf of the federal government in new professional standards review organizations (PSROs). These organizations were designed to develop computerized sets of information about the diagnostic and treatment methods of individual physicians with respect to hospital care of patients in publicly subsidized programs: approximately one-third of all general hospital patients. These profiles, together with special studies, will go directly to Washington. Physician fees and increases are already monitored, and patients staying in hospital beyond a specified number of days for each condition are automatically tagged for review as to whether a prolonged stay is necessary. Even in areas outside public programs, strong regulatory patterns are evident. American general hospitals, while largely under private ownership, are under almost constant inspection from public licensing boards or quasi-public accrediting agencies. Complicated formulae are being developed for approving the building of new hospitals or nursing homes in each state, or major expansion of existing facilities. Decisions that in Britain might be taken on a common sense or rough-and-ready basis are translated to industrial type complexity.

In contrast, to American eyes medical care in Great Britain in the 1970s seems oddly under-regulated; its standards unspecified; its techniques for planning underdeveloped; its lines of responsibility muddled with committees. Running expensive health services by boards of health service employees working in committee is as alien a concept to American eyes as detailed "peer review" may be to eyes looking in the other direction.

But if governmental roles and styles are different, so too are perceptions of "medical care." In Great Britain in the 1970s health services have a holistic meaning. Health, like housing, is still a social service accepted as such by both government and the population. It seems logical that social workers should work closely with health workers at the local level. Patients do not hesitate to ask their family doctors about housing conditions, meals-on-wheels, or residential care, and family doctors expect to have at least some knowledge in these areas. Such an interlocking of personal care services is virtually unknown in the United States, where efforts to deal with mundane aspects of everyday life are confined largely to a few experimental health centers for the poverty-stricken—survivors from the War on Poverty of the mid 1960s. Middle-class America does not expect its doctors to find wheelchairs, nursing homes, or placement for an invalid patient. There are numerous other agencies to do these things for the poor; the middle class, for better or worse, are expected to rely on their own initiative.

Medical care in America is not holistic, but limited and technical, a basket of consumption goods. For most of the population medical care in the United States is not an expected service but a purchasable commodity. While financial risks are usually shared through health insurance, there is no such thing as "comprehensive medical care" as understood in Britain. There are neat, often cryptic lists of benefits made available under specific health insurance policies (for example, so many days of hospital care for specified conditions, with the insurance covering 80 percent of expenses up to a specified amount). Physicians hold out their services for a fee, reinforcing the purchasing image. Angry patients sue when they feel cheated in these transactions—whether righteous, disappointed, or merely unrealistic—as they would in purchasing expensive merchandise. The system of medical malpractice, under chronic stress by the 1970s, vibrates with the buzz of litigious patients, in large part because of the continuing commercial imagery of American medicine. Medicine is part of the market system. Richard Titmuss, in his book *The Gift Relationship* (1971), has neatly described blood transfusion services as a symbol of cultural differences in society in each nation, with the American system built on more commercial principles than the British.[14]

The distinctions between the United States and Great Britain are not merely a result of a postwar welfare state in one society, the lack of one in the other, but can be traced well before then. Even in the nineteenth century British medicine had a flavor quite distinct from its American counterpart, and these distinctions have survived the ideological debates. Two examples illustrate the distinctions. The first relates to concern about "exploitation" in medicine in the late nineteenth century. In Britain the concern centered on the exploitation of physicians in contract practice with public and private agencies; in America, there was more concern about exploitation of the public by physicians. Such concern has surfaced again in the 1970s with the unmasking of doctors cheating public programs by making fraudulent claims on Medicare or Medicaid. In the United States, advertising, kickbacks in the form of fee-splitting, holding out as a specialist in dubious fields, and other forms of greed were engaging professional leaders in debates about the apparent commercialization of the medical profession in the late nineteenth century, but appear to have been far less important in Great Britain.

A second example relates to the comparative development of hospitals. From the 1870s and 1880s until World War I, hospitals sprang up in America to provide surgical care for middle-class Americans. British hospitals were, on the whole, of an older, charitable tradition, owing their primary allegiance to the more numerous working class. Basically, the British hospital, for all its faults, came out of a tradition of care for the dependent; while the American hospital, warts and all, grew up to sell a professional product: surgery in the new gleaming operating rooms. There are, of course, many other distinctions in the professional development of medical care in the two countries: the role of the primary physician, different developments of the two nursing professions, of dentistry, and of other institutions. There is a risk of oversimplification. Nevertheless, the general point sticks. Even before national health insurance came to Britain in 1911, the character of medical care in the two countries was different.

Medical care has continued to have a different connotation in Britain and the United States. British visitors are constantly surprised at the relative disorganization of medical care in America, the onus put on the consumer to select a doctor—to "shop around" for care—the assumption that the best medical care in the world is available, providing you can pay for it. American visitors to Great Britain are surprised at the degree to which health services are accepted as an integral element of cultural life, and sometimes alarmed at relatively inferior physical facilities—no deep-pile carpets in doctors' offices, the folksy simplicity of some GP surgeries, the willingness of the middle class to sit for hours, if necessary, in cavernous and dismal outpatient departments, and the assumption that the British consultant (medical specialist), like the British judge, is the only person in the drama whose time is valuable.

British visitors to America might be surprised to find that even in the new, consumer-oriented middle-class health clinics of the 1970s, the so-called health maintenance organizations (HMOs), the emphasis is on luxury, marketing, and salesmanship. In Britain there has been little questioning of the assumption that excellent care can be given in terrible surroundings; indeed, there may be some perverse pride in making do in draughty basements. Not so in the United States. No self-respecting health maintenance organization would open its doors without hotel-type furnishing and the latest in equipment, even if the results in costs of services will inevitably be high. The commodity orientation of medicine has struck even (or especially) here. Some of these may be surface differences, of course. The actual care given to an individual patient with a given diagnosis may be quite similar. Nevertheless, the distinctions are by no means frivolous. It is a matter of considerable importance in untangling the various relationships between governments and medical care to recognize that medical care has no constant definition. The phrase encompasses no single package of attitudes or benefits.

Now, as in previous centuries, there is no general rule for government involvement in anything save, perhaps, following John Stuart Mill, a rule of general expediency and the hope that whatever government does, it will not do mischief.[15] But if there is no common principle about what the government role will be, or ought to be, in medical care, let us at least celebrate our achievements and learn from our distinctions. The United States might benefit from the British experience in running a medical care system, if only by contrasting the limitations and potentials of area-wide planning. Comparisons are also useful in medical care regulation, including quality assessment, computerized reporting systems, medical audit techniques, and in other areas. While there has been fruitful interchange of ideas, knowledge, and skills in medical education and biomedical research in the past, in the future we may learn to appreciate the most interesting organizational and managerial elements of each health care system. It is salutary to recognize, too, that our vocabulary is not always readily interchangeable.

"Governments and Medical Care" was originally published in *Medical Care: A Scottish-American Symposium*, edited by Gordan McLachlan (London: Oxford University Press for the Nuffield Provincial Hospitals Trust, 1977), pp. 157-175.

Notes

1. Bruce L. R. Smith and D. C. Hague, (eds.), *The Dilemma of Accountability in Modern Government: Independence versus Control* (London: Macmillan, 1971).
2. D. C. Hague, W.J.M. Mackenzie, and A. Barker, *Public Policy and Private Interests* (London: Macmillan, 1975).
3. Rosemary Stevens, *Medical Practice in Modern England: The Impact of Specialization and State Medicine* (New Haven: Yale University Press, 1966).
4. National Commission on Community Health Services, *Health is a Community Affair* (Cambridge, Mass., 1966).
5. Department of Health and Social Security, *Administrative Reorganisation of the Scottish Health Services* (London: HMS0, 1968).
6. Scottish Home and Health Department, *Reorganisation of the Scottish Health Services*, Cmnd. 4734 (Edinburgh: HMSO, 1971).
7. Scottish Home and Health Department, *The National Health Service and the Community in Scotland* (Edinburgh: HMSO, 1974).
8. Scottish Home and Health Department, *The Health Service in Scotland, The Way Ahead* (Edinburgh: HMSO, 1976).
9. Robert Alford, *Health Care Politics* (Chicago: University of Chicago Press, 1975).
10. Douglass Carter and Philip R. Lee, *Politics of Health* (New York: Medcom Press, 1972).
11. Richard Titmuss, *Essays on the Welfare State* (Boston: Beacon Press, 1969).
12. Rosemary Stevens, *American Medicine and the Public Interest* (New Haven: Yale University Press, 1971).
13. Andrew Shonfield, *Modern Capitalism, the Changing Balance of Public and Private Power* (London: Oxford University Press, 1965), chap. 13 and passim.
14. Richard Titmuss, *The Gift Relationship: From Human Blood to Social Policy* (New York: Pantheon Books, 1971).
15. John Stuart Mill, *Principles of Political Economy* (Toronto: University of Toronto Press, 1965, reprinted).

III. Buzzwords, Rationality, and Dreams: 1968-1986

Introduction to Section III

A shifting role for government according to the perceived exigencies of the moment demands, in parallel, constant shifts in political rhetoric to justify, rationalize, and mobilize change. Otherwise health policy might lean too far in one perceived direction or the other and become, for example, too "socialized" in the views of some, or too indigestibly "market-oriented" for others. Alternatively, policy may get stuck in stalemate. The five pieces included in this section illustrate aspects of this movement through some of the efforts to define, critique, or influence policy in which I was engaged between 1968 and 1986.

The big expansion of federal health programs in the 1960s and 1970s created expectations about the possibility of effective federal leadership in health care. "Having the power, we have the duty..."—a quote from President Johnson's introduction of the Economic Opportunity Act of 1964—was the title of a DHEW report in 1966. The new programs also added an army of health care experts to policy debates: in the emerging fields of health services research, health care management, health planning, health law, and bioethics. These were heady times for members of these groups. The prevailing mood was idealistic, opportunistic, and optimistic. As potential pundits, experts provided a fertile field for rhetorical innovation, and might actually influence events. Perhaps constructive change could be achieved. In this hope, analysts and would-be reformers spent countless hours in meetings, doing studies, writing reports, and making presentations. Acronyms proliferated, designating new special fields for policy expertise. Among them: RMPs (Regional Medical Programs) and CHPs (Comprehensive Health Planning agencies) in the 1960s; HMOs (Health Maintenance Organizations), CMHCs (Community Mental Health Centers), HSAs (Health Systems Agencies, which superceded RMPs and CHPs under 1974 legislation), AHECs (Areawide Health Education Centers), PSROs (Professional Standards Review Organizations) in the 1970s; DRGs (Diagnosis-Related Groups, codes used for hospital reimbursement under Medicare), and PPOs (Preferred Provider Organizations, distinguishing a private health insurance network of selected providers) in the early 1980s.

Like many others, I was a product of federal funding, having trained in health services administration and public health under a U.S. Public Health Service traineeship in the early 1960s, and then, through 1976, doing university-based research (on medical specialization in England and the United States and related topics) that was heavily subsidized through peer-reviewed grants from the National Institutes of Health, as well as through private foundations. Federal initiative seemed potentially benign—indeed, necessary in the absence of massive private initiative, if health care were to become better organized and more efficient. It was starkly evident by the late 1960s that the United States, for all the money it was spending, had no national health policy, and that throwing tax money into a multitude of unconnected efforts was profligate and inefficient. "From the viewpoint of the city or neighborhood," I wrote in *American Medicine and the Public Interest* (1971), "the federal health establishment offers a maze of almost incredible entanglement" (p. 506). Primary goals were to get a grip on organizational chaos, and thus improve efficiency and effectiveness and reduce costs, while improving access to care across the population.

There was no single or simple approach to change. As Herman and Anne Ramsey Somers had pointed out in *Doctors, Patients and Health Insurance* (1961), health care had become a huge industry, representing an entrenched, internally-differentiated mass of power centers, organizational cultures, and agendas. Though remaining on the table as a potential force for rationalizing (or reorganizing) the health care system, universal, government-sponsored health insurance had been rejected time and again. A mass of perceived problems in diverse constituencies called for a variety of efforts to create and influence policy. These five pieces illustrate some of them. They address calls for a better national data and research infrastructure; a national role in organizational innovation to be implemented in the private sector; regional policy and planning for the distribution of the health care workforce across areas and regions; enhancing access to health care for individuals through civil rights and other legal protections; and last but by no means least, inventing and diffusing motivating rhetoric, as a basis for doing any of these things.

In 1968, on the basis of my first book, *Medical Practice in Modern England: The Impact of Specialization and State Medicine* (1966), I became a founding member of the scientific and professional advisory board of the new National Center for Health Services Research and Development (NCHSRD), which was directed by Paul J. Sanazaro and located in the Department of Health, Education and Welfare. The board's chair was Kerr L. White, a world leader in the development of health services research, including health care organization and services evaluation. (The board was initially called the scientific and technical advisory board, but this was changed when a member pointed out that the acronym was STAB, not exactly an auspicious designation.) The National Center was set up ostensibly to recognize the importance of health services research, and to provide a central focus for this within the federal government. However, as is often the case, legislative goals provided unclear markers for implementation.

For the advisors the inclusion of "development" as well as "research" in the title of the center suggested a promising new role for federal stimulation of organizational innovation in the private sector. Paul Ellwood, a member of the committee, was to make this promise explicit two years later through inventing the concept of the "health maintenance organization" as a private, federally-assisted health care corporation that would compete with other HMOs to provide health-oriented (rather than just disease-oriented) services to a local population. (The HMO Act of 1973 was to provide a partial trial of the model.)

The purpose of my paper (chapter 7), written as a discussion document for the NCHSRD advisory board in 1968, was to raise possible, alternative strategies the new center might pursue in the absence of clear goals. My paper is that of an agent provocateur. I must admit to being slightly shocked at the light, flip, even arrogant tone of the presentation of this relatively junior committee member, compared with the somber analyses that pass for policy papers in our present. I also refer to Machiavelli in a positive way, reflecting my Britishness rather than the more negative American gloss on the name—and I would not do now, as a fully acculturated American. I include chapters 7 and 8 to recreate the sense of opportunity that existed in policy discussions in the late 1960s.

No doubt it was politically unrealistic, even at that time, to expect this (or perhaps any) federal organization to mobilize as a change agent. NCHSRD's subsequent history was disappointing and dismal, as least for it advisors. Support for the center dropped away in the 1970s. The term "development" was excised. Through a series of name changes and functional shifts, the center eventually became the Agency for Health Care Policy and Research, renamed again the Agency for Health Care Research and Quality (AHRQ). AHRQ plays an important research role in quality and outcome studies in our present. My purpose here is to provide some of the flavor of the late 1960s: the enthusiasm for "what might be" that distinguishes ideas for change every time a plausible new one glitters on the policy scene.

Chapter 8 is drawn from a discussion document about the potential federal role in the development of HMOs, when that concept took flight in 1970. Beverlee Myers, then a senior administrator in the Office of the Director of the Health Services and Mental Health Administration (part of DHEW), asked my Yale colleague, David Pearson, and me to work with her to tease out general principles and strategies for federal engagement. We wrote two connected papers; this is part of one of them. I appreciate David's encouragement in my selecting from and editing the paper as it appears here. After leaving DHEW, Beverlee Myers served as director of the California Department of Health Services, and then as professor and chair in the School of Public Health at UCLA; she died in 1986. I think she would have been amused at having our labors resurrected.

From the perspective of our more jaded present, some of the points made in chapter 8 are obvious, overly optimistic, and naive. Within government, at least, policy thinking about federal roles in stimulating change was then relatively new. I include this chapter for its historical relevance as part of the discussions about the HMO as federal policy, but also to illustrate the kinds of questions and potential challenges that were being addressed in

1970—and, of course, the willingness of bureaucrats to seek advice on very general questions.

At the time the terms "laissez faire" and "regulation" were being tossed about as alternative national strategies (or buzzwords around which reformers might rally and debate could take place). HMO policy, as originally conceived, would supposedly cover the nation with private, multi-specialty health systems, each competing with the next (via laissez-faire competition), thus providing Americans with a locally organized, private solution to the alternative of government-sponsored national health insurance (via top-down regulation). As we point out (and it needed to be pointed out), regulation is a necessary condition of market enterprise, in health care as in any other sector. If a competitive market were going to work well, federal regulation would be necessary to build active consumer participation and reliable information. These were not remotely new ideas, but newly expressed in relation to HMO political rhetoric. Decades later, well into the twenty-first century, we are still debating similar questions about the "market," "regulation," and "consumer directed care."

The theme of chapter 9 is that top-down regulation does not work without the regulatory power to go with it. In the case of workforce distribution, as in many other policy areas, it was difficult to see where this would come from. My paper on the "regionalization of health manpower," in the terms then used, was given at a federally supported national conference on regionalization and health policy in 1976 organized and chaired by economist Eli Ginzberg, who edited the subsequent report, a DHEW publication (1977). The policy question was how to improve the distribution (or alleviate the "maldistribution") of health care resources, which were (and still are) very uneven from state to state and place to place. I was invited to give the manpower paper.

Explicit and implicit assumptions about standardization and rationalization infused the regionalization debates. Researchers could (and did) provide estimates for the "ideal" number of hospital beds for a population of 100,000, and for the ratio of physicians in different fields. As I show here, there was, however, no consensus in Congress or elsewhere for planning or regulatory mechanisms that had teeth. The numbers were thus largely empty gestures, though they were useful for drumming up federal assistance for "shortage" fields and geographical areas. Theoretically, efficient regional networks or organizations could have developed through federal funding or through the private sector. But the latter was not a viable possibility in 1977. As an aside, in retrospect the rush of hospital and health system corporate mergers in the 1990s might be viewed as a market-based continuation of the regionalization debates.

Chapter 10 shifts gears to the question of civil rights legislation and enforcement as a health policy lever. Much has been written about the welfare rights, civil rights, and disability rights movements of the 1960s and beyond. By 1981, when the Institute of Medicine published its report, *Health Care in a Context of Civil Rights*, which I chaired, the Office of Civil Rights of the new

Department of Health and Human Services (which replaced DHEW) was more concerned about subtle patterns of discrimination represented by disparities in access, different sources, and differing results of care, than by overt, readily identifiable racial discrimination. There were marked differences, for example, in the use of nursing homes (which were heavily dependent on Medicaid) by race and ethnicity, and concern that the growing health policy preoccupation with health care cost control might reduce the availability of care for groups for whom federal civil rights protections were most critical: racial and ethnic minorities, and persons with disabilities. The full report is well worth reading today; Bradford H. Gray was study director. Here I include my own prefatory remarks to highlight the difficulty (now as then) of grappling with questions of parity and disparity of care in terms of scientific evidence of discrimination that stands up as evidence in a court of law.

In the world of policy formation, beliefs and rallying cries have proved at least as important as evidence in stimulating change—an underlying theme of chapter 11. If there has been a search for a holy grail in health care policy, it has been the hope of finding a concept—a word—that would rally diverse points of view to a single cause: the word that would reform health care around a well understood principle and meet the political agenda of all parties concerned; or shift prevailing attitudes about promising directions for change; or position specific changes as inevitable and/or necessary; or at least provide temporary consensus. "Equity" was such a word, suggesting broad but reasonably applied, real-world notions of fairness.

I gave a number of talks on the "right to health" and "equity" in the early and mid 1980s. Chapter 11 was written for an international conference on "health care provision under financial constraint," held at the Royal Society of Medicine in London in 1986. (I was honored to receive the Royal Society's medal on this occasion.) The paper was published in 1988. As invited, my topic was "The U.S. View." I chose this paper for the chapter here because it tries to elucidate the implicit goals of the U.S. health care system, as I saw them then. Economist Uwe Reinhardt, who also participated, thought I was too critical in assuming lack of social opprobrium in the face of inequities; and, indeed, I may have made that point too strongly for effect. On the other hand, arguably the proof is in the pudding: Look not at what they say (or think), but what they do. Whatever the well-known inability to mobilize America's unwieldy political system, the average international observer might well assume, as I do here, that lack of attention to the uninsured implies a state of callousness or lack of caring.

By 1980 the experiment with federal leadership in health policy was dead—if, indeed, it had ever been strong enough to deserve the moniker, experiment. Its legacy was disorganization and runaway costs, rather than organizational and distributional effectiveness. Now the "market" sprang to the forefront as an alternative experimental force for rationalization, regionalization, efficiency, and equity.

7

The Federal Role in Health Care Research: Thoughts for Discussion and Development (1968)

Conceptually, it is useful to think of two justifications for government-sponsored health services research: 1) investment in research as a process of intellectual investment from which new knowledge and ideas will flow; and 2) research as the purchase of specific items or factors of knowledge that are directly related to improving a particular organizational process or system. The biomedical research sponsored by NIH has tended to follow the first assumption, focusing largely on undirected, peer-reviewed research grants and projects, and on the development of individual research interests. The systems-directed research of NASA has, in contrast, followed the second assumption. It has set out specific targets for development, and research has been directed toward these ends with the expectation of an identifiable payoff.

The assumptions underlying health services research are in some respects analogous to both the investment and the purchase models. Most recently, however, emphasis has been on the latter. The argument goes as follows. There exists a health service system or industry of vast proportions, employing four percent of the civilian labor force, and devouring six percent of the gross national product. This system is apparently inefficient and ineffective in terms of costs, manpower utilization, and the distribution of services, and these problems can be seen as amenable to systematic analysis and perhaps solution. In these respects the task of health services research can be viewed as somewhat similar to the NASA model. The mandates given to the National Center for Health Services Research and Development for controlling costs (or, more realistically, for increasing the value of health services), and for improving health services for high-risk groups, fall directly within the definition of research as the purchase of knowledge and techniques that have a definite organizational payoff. The implicit purposes of these mandates are that well-directed research will make the health industry both more efficient and more equitable.

It was in this context of focusing and catalyzing research for utilitarian or industrial purposes that the National Center was established. To quote Assistant Secretary of Health, Education, and Welfare Philip R. Lee:

> The ultimate goal of the Center is to aid practitioners and institutions involved in health services to improve the distribution and quality of services and to make the best possible use of manpower, funds and facilities. It seems to me that the mission of this Center is really the essence of what we are talking about when we refer to the formulation of public policy in the area of medical care.[1]

The primarily utilitarian assumptions of reducing costs and distributing service were, however, to be directly imposed upon an ongoing pattern of research support to individual investigators that followed the undirected NIH research model. It may not be realistic to expect the old research grants system to meet the imposed utilitarian expectations. Indeed, in some respects, as has become evident, the assumptions conflict. Grants to academically-based researchers do not necessarily result in developmental-type research of immediate practical use. Where—and how—the two types of research can be mated within one organization is a matter of immediate urgency for the Center.

Two possibilities for clarification suggest themselves: 1) The research grant process might be modified—through direction, encouragement, or stimulation—to encourage research to be done on specific problems. This would assume that the Center developed its own overall plan, which would relate knowledge deficiencies to the priorities of service needs. 2) Alternatively, the research grants system might be left as it is, and a second structure of contracts developed in parallel, to plug the gaps in industrial research needs. The Center would need an in-house analytical process to discover and decide what these needs might be.

Can the research grants process, with its inbuilt mechanisms to stimulate quality through peer review, and its assumption that research is a process of investment—in people, in institutions, and above all in ideas—be adapted to the problem-solving inherent in the industrial complex? The broad answer would appear to be No. Some of the knowledge gained in academia is of course directly relevant to industrial application; for example, studies of utilization review, costs, or task analysis. Some, in its long-term application, can be thought of as "basic research," in the sense of developing new theories, systems, and tools; for example, identification of the variables associated with regional manpower distributions or hospital use, or the creation of econometric or sociometric models. Other research may be viewed as part of the constant intellectual process of organizing, integrating, and communicating existing knowledge, and thus of helping to diagnose, to interpret, and perhaps to guide the human condition.[2] But the combined result of the grants process, as in biomedical research, is an accretive mosaic of knowledge, rather than the purposeful thrust that is the basis for technological advance. It is unrealistic to expect that this system of itself will automatically meet the research expectations of the health service industry.

The biomedical research experience provides a vivid illustration of the boundaries of undirected research. After many years of vast financing, the biomedical establishment is still groping toward methods of applying what is already known, toward identifying research gaps, and toward defining biomedical research in relation to social goals or public accountability.[3] Nor is there any reason to suppose that the output of biosocial research (which is, I take it, the broad definition of the Center's relationship with the universities) would be different.

Aware of the dichotomy of interest, the Center has attempted to approach the two underlying assumptions—the utilitarian and the academic—through the concept of a grid. Seven program areas have been built around disciplinary divisions (economics, social analysis, bioengineering), areas of broad health services interest (manpower, institutions, organization), and basic research information (data systems). These divisions provide a useful approach to handling the research being undertaken through the research grants system; to pointing up the gaps in research in each area and thus ideally stimulating curiosity among researchers to undertake needed studies; and to building a cadre of researchers in various disciplinary and interdisciplinary fields. At the same time, to meet its mandates to improve health services, the Center has set up task forces: for example, on improving health care for the disadvantaged, problems of hospitals, data systems, economics, and outcome criteria. The process of interaction between the task forces and the program areas, while not yet formalized, is conceptualized as a grid.

How effective is this format? Is it an uneasy compromise between two conflicting assumptions, or does it offer a constructive approach in which opportunities in academic research and in industrial R&D will be fruitfully joined and therefore optimized? The answer is conditional on the various possibilities inherent in the present structure, and in evaluating the relative weights to be given to directed versus undirected projects.

It is in this context that the meaning of "Research and Development" in health services has to be defined as a central element in the Center's mission. Does R&D mean Research *for* Development? If it does, the R in R&D is not really synonymous with the R of academic-based research. Alternatively, does Development mean activism? That is, the development of service rather than the development of research? These are open questions.

Unfortunately there seems to be little of direct value for health service R&D in the experience of other federal departments. The Department of Defense, in attempting to identify specific research factors that have contributed to the development of new weapons systems, found that only a small proportion of the technological foundations for development rested on knowledge contributed by pure or undirected research, as against the directed or applied research of the last twenty years.[4] But the health service system is not directly analogous to weaponry. The DOD model may hold true for health services in definable technological areas—for example in cost accounting techniques, computerization, coronary care units, or biomedical engineering. Indeed, there is much to be said for developing a strategy of concentrated research geared toward technological goals in relation to a deliberate, directive master plan. However, the major deficiencies in the health service system are not primarily technological; they are largely conceptual, strategic, and managerial.

In conceptual terms, the Center's grid approach makes sense. It offers on the one hand a potential channel for maximizing the products of the undirected grants process; and on the other, the purchasing of research, through contracts of many different kinds, for making good the gaps and deficiencies in the health care system. Its potential is sufficiently wide, in other words, to encompass both Research *for* Development, and also academic research at the theoretical, integrative, and applied levels. If, however, the grid approach is to make sense as a realistic, as well as a conceptual, mechanism, some practical decisions must be made in relation to the respective roles of the program heads and the central staff, on the uses of grants and contracts, on the development of information, on the encouragement of university and non-university constituents, on the relationship between the Center and other national agencies, and on a system of evaluation of the Center's work in both undirected R and directed R&D.

This comes back to the core issue for clarification, which is the specification of the Center's research assumptions. Currently, the exigencies of grant-supported research are taking the major part of the time of the program staffs and of the small core group. The development of priorities in the industrial sense—that is, identifying what needs to be known and done to make the health service system better—is falling largely to ad hoc groups. Staff does not yet exist to do this on an ongoing, interpretative, intramural basis, but in the long-term it would be logical to think in terms of regular evaluation of research through a communications and analysis division within the Center.

By being based on a system of research, rather than on a system of industrial development, the impact of the Center on health services will not be immediately apparent. NIH is going through some turmoil as to outlays of money for biomedical research in terms of economic, social, and human values. Health services research, by being more clearly applied (less "basic") than biomedical research, will in future face similar problems. The Center could decide to be the hub of ideas and assumptions for future health development. It could finance developmental projects without necessarily building in research components; that is, act as a specific catalyst for change. It could provide managerial and other forms of technical assistance. Indeed, a number of possibilities for industrial development have been raised in the Center's various committees.

To accept some or all of these assumptions as primary goals would, however, require a future modification in the staffing roles of the Center, a different use of contracts, a much greater need for extra-academic support, and a different mechanism for internal evaluation. More immediately, the identification of research priorities and strategies depends on how the Center views itself in the long-term as well as in the short-term, and what it hopes to accomplish in the next five, ten, or fifteen years. These assumptions are not clear-cut. Moreover, they offer real problems of definition, synthesis, and implication.

The following five models are offered for discussion. Each makes certain assumptions, and outlines certain strategies in relation to these assumptions. None is discrete, nor is the list exhaustive. The models represent choices open to the Center in planning for the next few years.

Model A: The Machiavellian

Assumptions: The Center is the focus and catalyst of health services research. It is, however, only one source of funds (and thus influence) in such research. Its primary task is to develop a pervasive influence, through a unique informational system, authoritative pronouncements about research needs, and gentle but persistent efforts to catalyze relevant research that will be financed by others.

Strategy: The core of the Center would be an informational and analytical service. This would include an intramural (or extramural) think tank, capable of generating appropriate ideas, and an intramural staff capable of putting such ideas into action. The research grants process would remain as it is now, but as a virtually independent arm of the Center. Such grants would be seen as an investment in ideas and processes, with some payoff; but the grants would not be manipulated to ensure that payoffs occurred.

Each program head would be involved in a constant analysis of research in a defined field of interest, in conjunction with the central analytical staff. Such responsibilities would involve the program heads (as well as the central staff) in a constant system of communications with the health service industry. In the process, each program head would become an informational expert, able to offer service on ongoing developments, as well as to catalyze new projects. In this sense, the Center would act as the conscience (ombudsman) of health services research.

The system of grants and contracts under the Center's own auspices would be relatively unimportant. Contracts would be used as seed money to stimulate other institutions to undertake specific projects, and to further the Center's total informational and analytical effort on various issues from different angles, and even with different conclusions. Contracts would fund part of many research and developmental activities (some successful, some unsuccessful), rather than focus on three or four major channels for research and development. The thrust of the strategy would be toward information exchange, the creation of a dynamic climate of ideas, and organizational innovations.

Model B: The Octopus

Assumptions: The Center will only act as a focus and a catalyst if it has direct lines from Washington to the outside world. It has the unique opportunity to develop population studies, and to study the health service system in microcosm. Therefore the most practical approach is to add to the process of undirected research a deliberate (and separate) strategy of R&D in selected areas.

Strategy: Existing health service research centers would be utilized as extensions of the operation of the Center. They would be seen as experiments in the provision of on-the-ground utilitarian/developmental research. In addition, selected projects would be funded through contracts from the Center (or in conjunction with other agencies) to stimulate developmental experiments in auspicious locations (e.g., funding to develop a health care system in a new town or urban sector) or relevant research areas (e.g., funding of two or three major projects in cost-benefit analysis).

In this model, grants would continue as before, and the program directors would be primarily concerned with the smooth operation of the research grants process and its analysis. Task forces would generate the system of contracts, the major thrust of the Center. Contracts would be carefully selected to pinpoint effort in a few important areas.

Model C: The Academician

Assumptions: The Center would accept that, like the NIH, strength of performance in medical care research lies in the advancement of high quality research in health services, no matter to what specific areas it is directed. Research grants offer a well-tried approach. There will be gaps, and the gaps may be plugged or partially plugged by contracts. But, in its desire to stimulate quality, the Center would go out of its way to be the focus and catalyst of research excellence.

Strategy: The activities of the Center would be directed toward the research grants process as its major long-term research investment. The program directors would be concerned with the type and quality of personnel undertaking research under all federal projects, and with making sense of the end products of research from a global point of view. Questions to be decided would include the appropriate balance of federal funds between grants given to institutions for local allocation (blanket subsidy) and grants awarded to particular investigators (selective subsidy); the coordination and simplification of the research grants process from the institution's point of view; the impact of the pattern of grants and contracts on recipient institutions as a whole, and the desirability of developing "centers of excellence" (pace the NSF); types of research systems to be funded, including the potential of independent research agencies, health service research centers, and social science or policy institutes; types and amount of training to be developed, at what levels, and at which institutions;

and the potential for analyzing and stimulating research through the publication of position papers, both inside and outside universities.

Contracts would be used for purposes of "selling" the Center (i.e., for securing initial visibility while consolidating long-term aims), for furthering the specific suggestions of task forces, and for giving increased flexibility and responsibility to the program staffs.

Model D: Troubleshooter

Assumptions: The Center cannot hope to solve all the problems and issues of health services research, and must be realistic in defining its given goals and mandates. Recognizing its responsibilities as a focus and a catalyst, and expectations that it will attack problems of health service costs and health service distributions, the Center's primary aims should be to launch a major effort to engage in problem-solving, through systems analysis and through other techniques that are designed to improve the operation of industrial systems.

Strategy: The Center would be the RAND of health services, offering specific services at different operational levels, from advice on regional or urban planning of health services to analyses of specific groups of personnel, departments, or pieces of equipment. The strategy would be designed to attack systematically the deficiencies in the health service system, including existing and potential health service policies.

At the core of the Center would be a specially-selected RAND-type staff, with its own carefully-developed system for stimulating projects, supplemented by the use of consultants, experts on sabbatical, and Ph.D. students. It would extend its intramural functions through a major use of contracts. A project could either be assigned to an individual, or could be assigned competitively to multiple programs.

Model E: The Jeremy Bentham

Assumptions: It is unrealistic to look at health services in a void; they are creatures of society and responsive to the prevailing social mood. Health itself is relative; it means different things to different societies or sectors of society, and to the same society at different times. The Center, as a focus and catalyst of health services research and development, is in a unique position to act both as a unifying and as a critical force, poised between the fragmented, often arbitrary development of the health service industry, and the evolving problems of health and disease in society. The Center would thus act as the conscience or ombudsman of the public, rather than of health services research.

Strategy: The research grants process would continue as before. In-house, training, and contract efforts would be geared toward analyses: 1) to define health in terms of other social programs; 2) to measure health and the impact of health services through end-result studies; 3) to encourage interdisciplinary and cross-disciplinary research through grants and contracts for research and for training programs; 4) to build bridges with other federal and local agencies to do joint studies of health-welfare, health-education, health services in the urban setting, etc.; 5) to analyze the impact of different governmental and private policies in the health sphere; 6) to conduct cross-national comparisons; 7) to build a core philosophy in health that, in its interpretation of the social and human condition, will lay foundations for further public and private development. This model would provide a depth of thought that would act as a catalyst for change, rather than provide the mechanisms of change itself.

* * *

In an ideal situation it might be possible to take the assumptions of Jeremy Bentham, the tactics of Machiavelli and the Troubleshooter, the goals of the Octopus, and the methods of the Academician, and accomplish all at once, in an organization of dynamic (and perhaps confusing) complexity. But situations are rarely ideal. The question of how far the Center should establish its own research priorities depends on whether it wishes to put its major stress on undirected academic research (thus investing in creativity and excellence) or on directed research with an organizational payoff. The question of how far the Center can promote "health" depends, similarly, on the primary model for development, as do questions as to who should look at relationships between health and welfare, or health and poverty. Under Bentham, both would be priorities. Under Academician, the latter might be defined through the encouragement of interdisciplinary research systems.

The purpose of the models is to emphasize that questions on the future directions of health research and on the type of contracts to be awarded are contingent on the crystallization of the Center's primary assumptions. This essayist has a leaning toward Model A (Machiavelli)—that is, the use of contracts to provide seed money for the stimulation of improvement in the organization of medical practice, urban health services, and other utilitarian-type studies, and the use of grants to stimulate excellence, inquiry, and reflection. The seed-money approach would demand access to new, non-academic constituencies. The analytic process, acting as a pivot, would attempt to take the findings from research; the core staff would decide what to do with such findings and thus put more seed-money into potentially fruitful service development. Such a system would be expensive in terms of staff, and is perhaps impossible in the short run. But the short-run and long-run priorities may be different in terms of social needs, political demands, and economic restraints.

As a new organization, the Center has yet to crystallize its assumptions in terms of objectives. Until these are defined, and the boundaries of effective action are therefore recognized, the Center's potential will remain largely unfulfilled.

From "Approaches to the Grand Assumptions in Health Care Research: Thoughts for Discussion and Development." Unpublished report prepared for the National Center for. Health Services Research and Development, U.S. Department of Health, Education and Welfare, November 25, 1968.

Notes

1. Philip R. Lee, quoted in *Group Health and Welfare News*, July 1968, p. 6.
2. For development of these themes, see Harold Orlans (ed.), *Science Policy and the University* (Washington D.C.: Brookings Institution, 1968); Richard Titmuss, *Commitment to Welfare* (New York: Pantheon Books, 1968).
3. See, for instance, "Research in the Service of Man: Biomedical Knowledge, Development and Use," a conference sponsored by the Subcommittee on Government Research and the Frontiers of Science Foundation of Okalahoma for the Committee on Government Operation, U.S. Senate, November 1967.
4. See Chalmers W. Sherwin and Raymond S. Isenson, "Project Hindsight," *Science*, June 23, 1967.

8

The Federal Role in Relation to HMOs: Laissez Faire versus Regulation (1970)

Rosemary Stevens, David A. Pearson, and Beverlee A. Myers

Just as laissez faire has generated its own series of accepted clichés, many of the values relating to democracy in general and the "right" to health in particular are rarely examined in detail. Bernard Shaw once spoke of England and the Untied States as two nations divided by a common language. Semantics are equally problematical in probing beyond the well-worn phrases that have become associated with acceptable values for medical care. The phrases themselves obstruct efforts to define what they actually mean.

What, for example, does "planning" mean in health? What is "regulation"? What are the supposed advantages and limits of competition? Even the concept of the "public" appears simple until the question is asked, Who is the public? American government works chiefly through a series of interest groups and lobbies; public opinion is chiefly those issues defined as important in the press; and congressional attitudes appear to be related in some cryptic way to reams of documentation amassed in the congressional record. The "public" is not pressing for welfare reform, nor for that matter for health maintenance organizations. We [the authors, Stevens, Pearson, and Myers] have defined public acceptability [for the purposes of the larger paper of which this is a part] in the rather watery way it is often defined in politics: as acceptance rather than rejection. Indeed, we would remark that democracy in practice is a largely negative operation, working through checks and balances rather than initiative. The public voice is more articulate in voting somebody out than voting someone in, and in stopping existing policies (e.g., the SST—funding for the development of supersonic transport) rather than generating grassroots innovations. Most innovations come from special interests.

Consumer participation in health services or (especially) health insurance is almost nonexistent. If HMOs are to be successful as competitive organizations, public apathy must be translated into public expertise through making adequate information available about health services, and through broad participation in decision-making. In health, a "public" needs to be created.

HMO policy objectives should recognize the strengths of public-private association with recognition of a proper balance of federal involvement through development, implementation, and evaluation of minimal standards and regulations. The ideal design of HMO program activities might not be feasible or desirable for implementation at the onset. Therefore, implementation of benefits might be phased to allow evaluation of technique, format, and fiscal viability. To this extent, there must be requirements for data and information to allow for evaluation of program effectiveness.

Economic objectives include two major categories:

1. *Fiscal Viability*: At present both consumers and providers are deeply concerned with rising costs. Policy objectives should allow for appropriate cost controls: Distinct incentives should exist to control costs. Fiscal viability and cost controls are also associated with efficient program operation and administration, and the HMO should be structured for efficiency.
2. *Financing*: The use of public monies should be so structured that the method of financing is equitable; that is, no segment of the population should contribute more than its ability. Further, the price to the consumer for HMO services should also be equitable. Funds should be obtained from Congress to provide long-term support at appropriate levels that will allow effective program operation.

Consumer choice and information are priorities. Effective choice of purchase (whether of a record player or health maintenance organization) assumes that the consumer has relevant information, including guidelines for evaluation. This would seem a necessary prerequisite of any form of competitive health insurance, including the form that now exists.

One striking fact of American medical care as presently organized is that adequate information is *not* available. This is true of insurance provisions (the most notorious deficiency), the relative quality of institutions and practitioners, and even information about the availability of health services in an area. The consumer has few "rights" to health care that can be brought to adjudication inside or outside the legal system. Consumer protection is minimal. In this area as well as in the area of consumer participation, American health services as now designed fall far behind the "socialized" European systems. When, therefore, nods are given to the values of American capitalist democracy as an argument in favor of HMOs, it should be realized that many of the values discussed [notably, the existence of informed consumer choice] are in fact alien to the present system of medical care in the United States.

A market system of competing HMOs would presuppose a new informational network about health services and entitlements. Such a network is not currently available in the average American community. This could be provided in part through the marketing departments of individual HMOs. Assuming, however, that in health, demand will always exceed supply, the marketing itself may not be very aggressive. Nor, of course, may it be pitched toward socially optimal information (e.g., HMO A might seek to attract enrollees by the décor in its waiting room and its gleaming equipment, while HMO B might actually provide extra service). Additional foci for information will thus be necessary, whether through Better Business Bureaus, consumer watchdog agencies for health, or local or federal regulation. Whatever the vehicle, encouragement of consumer choice explicitly demands the regulation of information.

In this as in other ways, the basic issue is not about laissez-faire *or* regulation, or even of federal *versus* private regulation, but of the government (or private) regulatory role being effective in achieving market goals.

This point needs elaboration, given our present confusion about the proper role of government in the United States. In theory the government *is* the people; thus, the more that government power is exercised, the more the aims of democracy can be fulfilled. Set against this is a fear of a powerful government oppressing the people, limiting individual freedom, and destroying the values of the free market system. Unless one assumes that the "people" are hapless pawns in the political process (and this may be true), these two sets of values are basically inconsistent. They have been resolved at the federal level—and this is particularly true of health care—into a simple formula, which might be stated thus: Federal intervention is often necessary in the workings of the private enterprise system, but as far as possible such intervention should be inefficient. The curious result of this policy is that the federal role in health has been one of minimal public accountability and minimal consumer protection—even in relation to programs that are federally financed.

The administration of Medicare is a case in point. The federal role would have been much more effective on behalf of consumers if it had been exerted from the beginning to protect the interests of Medicare patients, by ensuring that their dollars were used wisely. This could have been done through consumer information services, local ombudsmen, independent audit, local Medicare committees, or through other means. The governmental role in consumer protection under Medicare has been virtually nonexistent. Medicare was in theory a program of minimal governmental control; it has developed in fact as a program of government irresponsibility.

Irresponsibility is not the same as laissez faire. The words have, however, too often been interpreted as if the two ideas had similar meaning. The government role does not necessarily have to be "monolithic" or totalitarian. A strong governmental role does not necessarily mean centralization. It does however assume basic elements of public accountability. Nor does a weak government role necessarily encourage the virtues of a private enterprise system. When large sums of public money are involved the result may be quite the reverse. Again Medicare is a case in point. While the insurance intermediaries have been following the goals of private enterprise in maximizing profits, the process does not appear to have led to efficiencies in the health payment system.

For HMOs to succeed as a general, market-oriented policy, a *strong* governmental regulatory role is necessary to promote

a)   decentralized control of health services;
b)   competition among health systems;
c)   adequate public information; and
d)   other measures desired for consumer protection.

It may be stated as an axiom that the weaker the government role in health in the 1970s, the more power will accrue to other groups (such as insurers) or be dissipated.

Source: Edited extracts from a longer, unpublished paper by Rosemary Stevens, David A. Pearson, and Beverlee A. Myers, "The Federal Role in Relation to HMOs: Laissez Faire versus Regulation." A Report of an Inquiry into the Issues. Prepared for the Office of the Director, Health Services and Mental Health Administration, U.S. Department of Health, Education, and Welfare, December 15, 1970.

9

Regionalization and Health Manpower
(1977)

The federal government has become a major contributor to health manpower: directly in grants to health manpower education and indirectly through subsidizing professional incomes in massive federal reimbursement schemes for medical care, notably Medicare and Medicaid. Since some geographical areas and populations have far more health care available to them than do others, one might expect a strong governmental interest in the regional and interregional distributions of health manpower that may have resulted from its investments—even the ultimate regulation of the numbers of personnel in all major health occupations and geographical areas. In fact, government has shown a reluctant interest in this phenomenon. Yet politicians can no longer accept that as inevitable. There is a tussle between the rhetoric of equity, implying as it does a reasonably even spread of health professionals across the population, and the diffused power structure of the health care system.

Health services are, of course, complex organizations. The U.S. health care system is a congerie of thousands of independent interest groups and competing bureaucracies, each pressing its own policies. Decisions on the supply, entry standards, curricula, and competence of professional workers are usually delegated by government to—or just assumed by—the professions. The leading professional associations thus have a major impact on policies in the manpower field. A second important set of interests has arisen in the steady expansion of hospital facilities, with their large employee groups and training programs, and in the interchange of interests between hospitals and health care planning groups. Government is a third force to be reckoned with as public investment in health care has risen to the present 40 percent of all expenditures. The question this paper deals with is, How far do, and should, hospitals, health planning agencies, and government intrude on the traditional arrangements where manpower distribution lies solely in the discretion of the professions?

Regionalization of health manpower, in the sense both of distributing appropriate manpower with reasonable equity and efficiency across the face of the United States and of ensuring adequate care at the local level, has become a topic enmeshed in the broader power plays of health care development. Congressional committees see professional monopolies as villains constricting the free operation of the market system. Hospitals and other organizations compete with each other for prominence in the local health care scene and for control of regional health care planning agencies. Professional associations and professional schools often see hospitals as presumptuous and government as a monster encroaching on hard-won prerogatives. It is against this richly woven background that the "regional" questions must be dissected, for one sector's "regionalism" may be anathema to the next; and the motivations behind each may be quite different.

Regionalization of health manpower is of central importance to any discussion of regionalization of health services. Yet there is no structure or authority for the development of coordinated health services at the regional level. Thus government manpower policies to date have been largely indirect. Meanwhile, the partial efforts that have been made and those now being considered have imposed peculiar stresses on the health professions, notably on the organization and independence of the schools of health sciences and of the various associations of the medical profession.

Ducking the Regionalization Issue: Buildings Do Not a System Make

Health care facilities have cast a spell over the way we tend to think about modern health services. The very phrase, "the health care industry" inspires images of vast hospitals and disciplined teamwork between work crews and equipment. Death is translated as a pinpoint of light faltering across an EKG machine. Cure becomes the happy coincidence of drugs, therapy, research, and effective machinery. For those for whom less dramatic metaphors are applicable, there are other institutions: nursing homes for the elderly and chronically sick, community mental health centers, state psychiatric hospitals, neighborhood health centers, health maintenance organizations. Health services have become a world of buildings. It is only a step from here to the notion, implicit in all health planning legislation to this date, that the regulation of buildings will lead to regulation of the entire health service industry.

That notion would have considerable appeal if the buildings—the institutional framework of medical care—were also the employment centers for the 4.4 million persons who actually work in the health care system. In that case, one could encourage a health care system through clusters of institutions in each region or area. Physicians, nurses, therapists, technicians, attendants, secretaries, and other members of the army of 200 or more health service occupations would either be employed by an organization or would have full-time contracts for specified services. Employers would thus decide how many personnel were required in each category to serve a particular population, and would hire, fire, and remunerate accordingly.

In an employment-based system, the allocation of funding through a regional health consortium, channeled through its institutions, could have a direct impact on the distribution of health manpower in that area. For example, a regional health agency might decide to employ more nurse practitioners as a partial substitute for physicians in primary care. Since, under this scheme, the organization would have an effective monopoly of the job market in medical care, this decision would expand the demand for nurse practitioners in the area and reduce the demand for primary physicians. In areas in which the demand for primary physicians was met, there would be no job openings; physicians would have to practice somewhere else. In aggregate, there would thus be a shifting of personnel within and across regions according to the supply of available jobs.

How neat and tidy all this is. However, it bears little relation to the way in which health manpower is actually influenced and distributed. Hospitals do, it is true, employ about 2.9 million of the 4.4 million persons engaged in the health care industry, and the numbers have been rising year by year. Indeed, the 7,000 hospitals in the United States reported a net gain of almost 1 million employees between 1965 and 1974, a major reason for the escalating costs of hospital care. But to depend on health care facilities to provide a rational distribution of personnel for health services is a distorted view of the power structure of the industry.

While hospitals are the major employers of health employees, they are by no means the only employer. Health workers are employed in the country's 20,000 nursing homes, in health maintenance organizations, in home health agencies, in the Veterans Administration, in Indian Health Services, and in many other services, programs, and institutions. Many health workers are self-employed: pharmacists, dentists, optometrists, physicians. The combined result is not an industrial employment situation that could be rationalized into national, regional, and local units through the structure of employment. It is rather a hodgepodge of professionals, technicians, clerical workers, and others, clustered in different settings. The physician in his or her private office, the pharmacist in the drugstore, the nurse in a visiting nurse association, the laboratory technologist working for a private laboratory service, the dentist and dental hygienist, the podiatrist, the optometrist, and others in their offices are all essential elements in the provision of comprehensive health services, and all are elements that cannot be effectively regulated through health care buildings and facilities.

The dichotomy between the rhetoric of "planning" and the realities of private enterprise is an essential element underlying any discussion of regionalization. Robert Alford, in his book *Health Care Politics*, describes regionalization as part of the language of "corporate rationalization"—part of the platform of those who would extend (and manage) health services through hospitals and other health care facilities. The phrases that health care planners, often hospital-based, use to describe changes in the health care system, tend to assume an expansion of their own institutional territory rather than to reflect changes in a system composed of complex and conflicting interests.

Physicians in particular are largely immune to the changing politics of hospital planners. While the number of physicians employed by hospitals has been going up, such physicians are still in the minority. Of 360,000 physicians in non-federal practice in the United States in 1975, only 21 percent were in hospital-based practice, the great majority of them working in residency training positions. Most full-fledged physicians are private practitioners; indeed, most of the elite members of the health professions are organized outside the hospital. Appropriate patterns and distribution for private practitioners in any field cannot be achieved through the same channels that may regulate the bricks-and-mortar of health care facilities. Control of the distribution of health manpower through the job market, that is, through employment by health care institutions, remains a possibility, but one that would require substantial changes in the health care system. Such a shift would assure the virtual disappearance of the private practitioner.

Axiom: Political Boundaries and Regions Are Frequently Antithetical

A second factor that is sometimes forgotten by the more enthusiastic proponents of regionalization is that health professions and occupations are not regionally organized. There is no general recognition of medical service areas on a prescribed geographical basis. Perhaps the state comes closest to providing a geographically defined territory for health manpower, overseeing and coordinating programs in higher education within the state and licensing thirty or so health care occupations. Yet states are far from ideal planning units. In some respects, especially in terms of bringing medical care to the people, they may be too large, while in other respects, as in the training of professionals, they may be too small. Most states are too large geographically to define the supply and distribution of health manpower with precision. New York State, for example, has a relatively large supply of physicians, but they are concentrated in New York City, and there are recognized shortages in counties upstate. Yet there are both professional and political limitations on any state attempting to redress these balances.

There has been little analysis of interstate health manpower differences and what, if anything, these mean. Though differences in the interstate distribution of physicians are generally appreciated, little work has been done over the whole array of health professions. According to the U.S. census, New York, at the top of the range, had 210 physicians for a population of 100,000 in 1970, whereas Idaho, at the bottom, had only seventy-six, almost a threefold difference. It is possible, of course, that the physician count may not be as important as the total array of health personnel available. Yet no benchmark measurements are available to evaluate the total supply of health personnel from state to state, or from place to place. And even if one were able to redress balances intrastate, how would one redress balances within a state?

Current political boundaries may bear little relationship to the actual service area for health professions; however, since we do not have readily defined "service areas" we must rely on the geographically defined information that does exist. Such information reveals considerable differences in manpower supply from place to place. For example, according to the 1970 census, Wichita, Kansas had 112 physicians for a population of 100,000, a figure well below the national average of 138. Perhaps to compensate for that, the city had a relatively generous supply of nurses (637 practical and registered nurses per 100,000 people compared with a national average of 525) and was relatively rich in pharmacists and optometrists. Its proportion of dentists, however, was almost half that of the national average, and it had only one-third of its national "share" of podiatrists.

Miami, Florida had dentists, optometrists, nurses, pharmacists, and podiatrists at rates similar to those for the whole nation. It had, however, an apparent overabundance of physicians (231 for a population of 100,000, compared to the national average of 138). It can be argued that Miami has attracted both retired physicians and immigrants. (Florida has, in particular, a relatively large supply of physicians who are Cuban refugees.) But if so, why does the argument not apply equally to dentists?

Detroit shows an average pattern in the major professions, with the exception of its supply of nurses, which is somewhat low: 458 per 100,000 as against the national average of 525. Chicago also has a below-average nurse ratio but is relatively rich in optometrists and pharmacists. Baltimore, in contrast, has only half as many optometrists as the national average. Nashville has an average supply of optometrists and pharmacists, an above-average physician supply, and a very generous supply of nurses, but has well below the expected supply of dentists. New York City has an average supply of nurses and optometrists, above-average quotients of pharmacists, and a well-above-average supply of physicians, dentists, and podiatrists. Relatively speaking, there are more than twice as many physicians and dentists in New York City as are available in cities like Wichita, Mobile, or Jersey City.

Geopolitically, of course, city boundaries make no more sense and frequently make less sense than state boundaries as areas for health manpower planning. Economic catchment areas and the domain of city hall rarely coincide. Yet there is probably no "perfect" planning area. One may conclude from these illustrations that there are wide differences in health manpower from region to region, according to available measurements, and that the differences are not necessarily internally consistent across all professions. Within broad categories—the richer states and areas having a more generous health manpower supply, the poorer the least generous—each place reveals its own idiosyncrasies.

Such patterns are hardly surprising, reflecting as they do an assorted combination of influences. Environmental factors combine to play some part in the patterns of manpower distribution. These include climate, the general income of an area, expected professional income, professional connections, previous experience in the area (for example, as a student in a local professional school, or in postgraduate training), the availability of facilities, medical expectations of a population, coverage of particular services under a state Medicaid program, job openings in fields such as nursing, and other factors. There is no single overarching element. Since there has up to now been no regional agency responsible for medical care in a defined service area, assessments have not been made of what overall distribution of manpower is appropriate to a specific population or place. The age distribution, socioeconomic distribution, and health status of the population are obviously important bases for any future health manpower projections. But traditional patterns of health service and professional behavior may also play some part with respect to the types of patients and conditions seen by different types of health workers, the volume of work, and professional incomes.

Tallying up numbers, evaluating workloads, providing forecasts and plans, predicting shortages in one field and excesses in the next, are tasks the new health system agencies (HSAs) set up under the 1974 health planning legislation (Public Law 93-641) may perform admirably. These are, however, empty exercises unless coupled with a will to improve the actual array of health manpower or with authority to implement agreed-on changes. Since there is no single employer of health care workers at the local level but, rather, a myriad of occupational situations, authority cannot be exerted through the direct actions of a powerful employer. The scope of action is therefore limited. Efforts can be made via the HSAs to supply health workers to places where there are clearly deficiencies. This relatively non-controversial approach exists in the federal National Health Service Corps, which supplies personnel (usually physicians) to "medically underserved" areas. Efforts to upgrade shortage areas are also built into planning and Health Maintenance Organization (HMO) legislation as a priority, and into educational programs through manpower legislation. But dealing with identified shortages is one thing; tackling the much broader question of regional distribution of health care personnel is another, requiring as it does fundamental approaches to the power structure of the industry. It is here that battle is joined between the health care institutions, the health professionals and—increasingly—federal agencies that are heavily subsidizing manpower production.

The present [1977] situation is one of unclear goals and diffused responsibilities. The fact that members of the affluent middle class have available to them relatively much more service than do the poor, and that suburbanites have more than inner-city residents or the rural population, is generally regarded as "maldistribution." Federal programs in the last decade, if anything, appear to have exacerbated the situation. Yet, the goals of the social programs and the general (expansionary) use of tax funds suggest that the direction rather should be toward equalizing health care opportunities.

As far as practical priorities go, the major task at the federal level is to devise mechanisms where at least the new graduates of federally sponsored educational programs will be encouraged to work in needy areas and discouraged from entering the richer sectors.

The Parameters of the Problem and Possible Solutions

How are new graduates to be persuaded to work in inner cities and rural areas, and—perhaps of more impact—persuaded not to work in the richer parts of attractive cities? Even such limited goals pose problems of federal initiative.

Outright direction of health manpower, no matter how life has changed, is alien to the traditions of American medical care. Other possibilities may well become part of the U.S. health care system. At one end of a range of future options, proxy "employers" could be developed to cover virtually all the health occupations: The number of practitioners could be limited in each state, city, or health services area by, for example, controlling licenses, hospital staff privileges, or permits to receive funds from Medicare or even from private health insurance.

Regional control of access to health care occupations is technically possible under existing arrangements: through the states' power to license hospitals and professions and regulate the insurance industry, and through the power of the federal government to require conditions from hospitals, HMOs, and other agencies participating in federal programs including Medicare and Medicaid. For example, a hospital could be required to offer admitting and other staff privileges to physicians, and only to those physicians, whose presence could be justified on the basis of specified community "need," defined, for example, by each local Health Systems Agency (HSA).

Since most physicians rely on hospital affiliation, such restrictions could be potent. If a physician seeking to practice orthopedics in a particular area were denied a hospital staff position, he or she would be bereft of the means to pursue a career. The alternatives would be to change specialty or go elsewhere. Doctors would be discouraged from entering practice in specialties and/or locations well supplied with physicians. Regionalized medical services would be achieved, relatively painlessly, and responsibility for planning would be clearly assigned to HSAs.

Alternatively, the power to license physicians, dentists, pharmacists, optometrists, and others might be made contingent on practice in specified agencies or locations. National licensure arrangements might also be developed with specified manpower goals in view. In well-served areas the available licensing "slots" would be used up and practitioners would be deflected to work elsewhere. Such arrangements would have the advantage of recognizing the existing system of private practice or self-employment of many health professionals and not move to the more extreme possibility of a national health service in which all health service workers are employees.

Yet, if efficiency is the talisman, why not go all the way? Once the federal government has distorted the market system by intervening in the field in as massive a way as it has done, the logical answer to rational distribution might well be complete federal control of professional locations. Whatever the form of regulation, the most effective way of insuring that health manpower is relatively evenly and efficiently spread across the population would be for government or its agents to monopolize health care jobs. In a national health service, jobs would be made available only where justified by regional economic priorities and/or planning criteria.

Such control could, of course, come in various forms. In a universal, comprehensive national health insurance program, control might come through government monopoly of health care incomes, with a predetermined amount of insurance funding funneled through regional agencies, and amounts earmarked for specific purposes. In a location with twice as many physicians as another, relative to the population, physician incomes from national health insurance theoretically would be half as much. This factor might discourage independent practitioners from settling in generously served areas and might make the relatively needy areas more attractive.

To have any noticeable effects on distribution such a system must depend on three important factors: first, on relatively large numbers of new professionals entering the system and making such choices (otherwise, little change would be evident); second, on unified insurance funding to a region, to be reallocated among the manpower groups; and third, on insurance funds representing the major part of professional incomes. An effective monopoly of health care incomes could do away with pressures for government monopoly of health care jobs.

None of these solutions is currently palatable to the professional associations or to Congress. Instead, at the other end of the range of options, there is continued federal tinkering with various elements of manpower distribution, notably those most susceptible to government influence and those least threatening to the professions. Regional concerns about the numbers, costs, and quality of health manpower are implicit in identification of "shortage areas" as a priority for various forms of federal assistance. These concerns are expressed also in proposals to restructure health care through the marketplace by the development of health maintenance organizations (HMOs), thus developing closed-staff service systems where jobs would be regulated by independent agencies. Encouragement of community hospitals to become area health education centers as a focus for coordinated education and training programs at the regional level is another way that regional concerns are expressed, as are Professional Standards Review Organizations (PSROs) to monitor standards for institutional care in local areas, and a series of proposals to influence the selection and education of applicants to professional schools and the location of physicians in graduate education.

Congressional Concern with Health Manpower Distribution

The federal government has become heavily involved since the early 1960s in subsidizing health-profession education. While frequently ducking the issue of demand, the Congress has become involved piecemeal with supplying health manpower on a massive scale.

The Health Professions Education Assistance Act of 1963 (Public Law 88-129) provided construction grants for expansion of schools of medicine, osteopathy, and dentistry and authorized loans for students in these professions. Federal loan provisions were extended to students of optometry in 1964, the same year provisions for nurse training were extended in a new Nurse Training Act (Public Law 88-581). These and other programs have been extended since the mid 1960s into major federal involvement in the production of health professionals. Federal support of such training through the Department of Health, Education, and Welfare rose from $24 million in 1960 to $533 million in 1974. Since much of that aid has been tied to a requirement that the schools expand their enrollments, the federal government has contributed to an expanded manpower supply, and thus to increasing health care costs. Current [1976] health manpower legislation (Public Law 94-484) continues the process by maintaining or expanding manpower supply.

If one major result of federal programs to subsidize medical care and professional education has been to expand the supply of health manpower, a second has been to emphasize preexisting patterns of distribution. The richer states, not the poorer, gained most from federal matching grants to states for Medicaid programs for the poor. Medicare coverage has been of most use to the elderly in areas well staffed with health professionals. Figures for 1969 (the most recent available) show that the number of persons receiving physician services under Medicare ranged from 386 per 1,000 enrollees in the North Central States to 510 per 1,000 in the West. Studies developed by Columbia University suggest a similar pattern for Medicaid.

Since both Medicare and Medicaid reimburse for health services on the basis of services provided without specifying in advance how many services should be provided or where these services should be given, the programs have had a cushioning effect on health manpower distribution. While some practitioners have been enabled to establish "Medicaid practices" in low-income city areas such as in Harlem or the Bronx, most independent health practitioners and employees in health care institutions have been funded to do whatever services they have felt to be necessary. Medicare's payment of usual, customary fees has encouraged uneven provision of manpower from state to state, city to city, and urban to rural area, and between inner city and suburban areas. In turn, Medicare and Medicaid have had a ricochet effect on congressional interest in manpower supply and distribution.

Numerous examples of maldistribution of health manpower were presented in hearings on health manpower legislation in 1974 and in congressional reports in 1974 and 1975. The president of the American Medical Association, Dr. Malcolm Todd, posed the problem with respect to physicians: "To say we're eliminating the shortage of physicians is playing with words. It won't make any difference if we do have 440,000 physicians in 1980 because they won't be where we need them. Unless we can come up with acceptable incentives for rural practice and inner city practice, we're going to have the same [distribution] problem in 1980 that we do now."

Where Have the Professionals Gone?

Physician population ratios have generally improved in the last decade, but, as might be expected, they have improved most in already well-served areas. The number of physicians for a population of 100,000 rose from 132 in 1959 to 156 in 1970, an 18 percent increase, but the West North Central States (Iowa, Kansas, Minnesota, Missouri, Nebraska, and the Dakotas) showed an increase of only 8 percent; and the East South Central States (Alabama, Kentucky, Mississippi, Tennessee), only 13 percent. In 1970 the West North Central States had an overall physician population ratio of 135 per 100,000; the East South Central States, of only 105. In contrast, New England and the Middle Atlantic States, which had improved their ratios by 20 percent and 23 percent respectively between 1959 and 1970, showed 190 physicians for a population of 100,000, almost twice as many as in the "poorest" states. While states in the South Atlantic region (Delaware down through Florida) and the Mountain States (Arizona, Colorado, Nevada, New Mexico, Utah) increased their low physician supply at relatively faster rates than average, the overall fact remained that there were wide discrepancies in apparent supply by major regions—at the very time federal aid to education and service was being extended. The difference in the average physician-population ratio between the richest and poorest regions in 1959 was seventy-seven physicians for a population of 100,000; in 1970 the difference had extended to eighty-five physicians for a population of 100,000. For every 100,000 residents of the Middle Atlantic States there were on average eighty-five more physicians than were available in the West Central States.

What such differences actually mean in service and health care needs in different areas would require detailed analysis of manpower and working patterns in relatively homogeneous, defined health service areas or with respect to specific populations. Yet the gross regional discrepancies are extremely important in assessing the political aspects of manpower development. Health manpower planning is a highly political field; the scope and volume of federal funding inevitably make it so. These differences are of increasing significance with respect to federal policies toward health manpower regulation, and to functional realignments among governmental agencies, health care planners, professional schools, and the professional associations.

Interregional and interstate differences are, however, only one gross reflection of differential distributions in manpower supply. Urban-rural distributions are uneven, and apparently worsening. The number of counties without a practicing physician grew from ninety-eight counties in 1963 to 132 in 1970; reportedly, the major characteristics that hampered counties in getting physicians was a small total population, a lack of technological facilities, and a lack of medical group practice arrangements (for service coverage, colleagues, and other reasons). A small population implies both a lack of financial support for a physician and practice in a relatively isolated area; there are both fiscal and environmental aspects to be considered in addressing rural services.

"Regionalization" as applied to rural care has two distinct problems: staffing rural and other underserved areas by insuring adequate personnel; and coordinating multi-specialist care within the larger service areas of specialists. Solution to the problem of staffing underserved areas assumes that manpower policies will be developed on a regional basis. Where there are observed deficits, policies can be developed to fill the gaps. Solution to the specialist problem assumes regional communications networks among different practitioners, including patterns of referral of patients—so that a family physician can refer a patient to a specialist—as well as continuing education of all professions.

The need for regional service networks linking personnel in city centers with practitioners in outlying areas has been an idea that has been in circulation for some time, even if it has usually not been translated into fact. The Bingham Associates plan developed in New England in the 1930s provided an early example of such developments. More recently, distribution of health manpower within cities and suburbs has received increased attention. Between 1950 and 1970, the number of physicians in the United States increased by 50 percent, from 219,997 to 334,028. The number of physicians in metropolitan Chicago declined in this period: There were 2,000 fewer physicians at the end of the period than at the beginning. Physicians had moved out of the inner city to the suburbs, typically to clusters of professional office buildings in large commercial centers. The movement was generally toward communities of high socioeconomic status. In the inner city the physician-population ratio fell from 111 physicians per 100,000 in 1950 to seventy-five in 1970.

The movement of health manpower toward high socioeconomic areas appears to have been a general phenomenon. New York State has shown a similar pattern of rich areas getting richer, poor areas poorer during the federal largesse of the 1960s. A recent study by the Board of Regents of the State of New York, the state body responsible for education and licensure, found a tenfold difference in per capita physician supply among New York counties, with particular deficiencies in upper New York State. In New York City, the overall ratio of physicians to population was reportedly the same in 1967 as in 1948, but there were marked differences in supply by the socioeconomic status of different census districts. Other cities, including Baltimore and Boston, have shown similar patterns of shortages in inner city districts, as measured against the overall supply of health professionals, though richer districts are served quite generously. Similar discrepancies are reflected within medical specialties.

In short, available measures suggest that federal subsidies of heath manpower education and services have inflated the volume of care but have had little effect, no effect, or an adverse effect on the preexisting distribution of health care personnel. Congressional committees are quite clear on that point. The report from the House Commerce Committee on the proposed Health Manpower Act of 1975 stated bluntly: "Increases in the supply of health professionals have not led to a more equitable distribution of health manpower, in fact, despite significant increases in total supply, the geographic maldistribution of health manpower has worsened in the past decade."

Puny and Partial "Solutions"

The inherent conflict between congressional rhetoric and political reality makes it unlikely that distributional questions will be confronted head-on. The approaches are experimental, tentative, and indirect. Even where there are real possibilities for improvements in distribution—for example, in establishing a national network of health maintenance organizations—the rhetoric slides off in the direction of less confrontation.

The HMO is a self-contained, locally run health service system. Offering defined health services on a prepaid basis to an enrolled service group, it must balance the costs of its benefits to subscribers against the costs of personnel and other expenditures. There is a built-in planning system in each HMO, which does not exist in other forms of private practice; that is, the incentive to develop staffing patterns to meet limited and specified service for a defined group of patients.

That was part of the appeal of HMOs when the notion surfaced in 1970. If the HMO became the dominant pattern of medical care for all persons in the United States (a hope that was then optimistically expressed), decisions about health care costs and resources would be decentralized to the local level. Staffing decisions would be taken by each organization, and there would be less call for other regional systems of manpower surveillance and/or regulation. If the great majority of the population were served by self-contained health service systems, there would be little or no room for physicians or other independent practitioners above the service requirements of each system. Inevitably, then, HMOs would have some effect on the redistribution of health manpower from area to area and region to region. Blanketed together over the nation, HMOs could form an interlocking network of independent health care systems.

The heady prospects of 1970, however, have had relatively little impact on the real world. Requirements tied to federal construction grants and loans under the HMO Assistance Act of 1973 (Public Law 93-222) have made it difficult, if not impossible, for HMOs to compete with traditional health insurance plans, which are allowed to offer fewer services. By May 1975 there were 173 HMOs in thirty-three states, serving 5.7 million members. A number of these were in financial difficulties. While federal requirements for HMOs may be relaxed in future legislation, a stimulus perhaps to renewed expansion, the HMO has moved conceptually from a potential basis for health care reorganization on a massive scale, to an alternative system of delivery in certain areas. The regional manpower implications of HMOs are, at best, underdeveloped, for even in areas with HMOs there is extensive room for independent practitioners.

Professional Standards Review Organizations (PSROs) take a different stab at regionalism, but one that is also indirect and flabby as far as distribution is concerned. The PSROs are not strictly manpower agencies at all, but utilization review mechanisms, though they too may have some spin-off effects that affect thinking about health manpower at the regional level. Another creature of the 1970s (under Public Law 92-603), PSROs were designed to regionalize the organization of physicians, with appropriate staff, to survey the utilization of health care facilities by inpatients in one of the federal health programs (notably Medicare and Medicaid). As physicians become aware of the patterns of patient care within a particular geographical region and of the existence of marked variations in the use of services by professionals, from person to person and hospital to hospital, eventually a regional consciousness may develop around PSRO functions that could encourage physicians—through PSROs, medical societies, or other channels—to stimulate manpower improvement in the region. At the same time, PSROs may provide a basis for more general consideration of health services by the medical profession within physician service areas. Thus they could help to develop the idea of the service area as an integral base for manpower development. However, with PSROs barely off the ground, such considerations are speculative, to say the least.

Even the new planning legislation (Public Law 93-641), which replaced the previous Comprehensive Health Planning Agencies and Regional Medical Programs with a network of Health Systems Agencies (HSAs), is scarcely more directive. If HSAs concentrate on health facilities planning and coordination, they will have little overall impact on the goals of improving access to medical care and correcting maldistribution—the rationale for the passage of the legislation. At present, it looks as if HSAs will have little influence over manpower distribution. Their primary manpower activities may well be to develop census-type information about manpower in defined health service areas, identify areas that are underserved with respect to aid under federal programs, and provide a forum for discussions of manpower development.

Other federal activities have supported different aspects of regionalization. During their brief life [1965-1976], Regional Medical Programs (RMPs) [established under Public Law 89-293] encouraged the establishment of links between university medical centers and community hospitals with respect to the graduate education of physicians; that is, hospital-based residency training in the specialties. RMPs encouraged, too, the development of emergency medical services on a regional basis, multi-institutional coordination of kidney transplant and dialysis networks, referral and transportation systems for neo-natal intensive care, and coordinated arthritis services. In their last few years, RMPs also sponsored primary care services in underserved areas and funded the training of nurse practitioners, physician associates, and community health workers, presumably to increase the access to and availability of medical care in local areas. In calendar year 1974, almost 20,000 such health workers were being trained under the sponsorship of RMPs.

The 1971 amendments to the Health Manpower Act [Public Law 92-157] encouraged the development of Area Health Education Centers (AHECs), pat-terned after a recommendation in the 1970 report of the Carnegie Commission, *Higher Education and the Nation's Health*. An AHEC is a community hospital located at some distance from a medical school but linked with such a school as an independent health-manpower teaching center. The AHEC, in turn, subcon-tracts with smaller hospitals, educational institutions (for example, community colleges), medical, and other groups within a defined region to provide a base for the coordinated development of training programs for health care personnel. Eleven medical schools are sponsoring such arrangements. Special emphasis is to be placed on the training of primary care physicians, nurse practitioners, physicians' associates, and other allied health personnel. The AHEC has an avowedly regional manpower interest.

Service is much more directly stressed in the National Health Service Corps program, established under the Emergency Health Personnel Act of 1970 (Public Law 91-623), and implemented in 1972. Under this program, and its subsequent amendments, the federal government places health professionals to work in areas identified by state and local planning agencies as having critical manpower shortages. An initial rule of thumb was that such areas must have a ratio of less than one primary physician to 4,000 population (compared with the national average of 1:2,000), and a dentist-to-population ratio of less than 1:5,000. As of February 1975, 981 counties and areas had been so designated. New criteria for shortage areas are now being developed (under Public Law 94-454); the number of such areas will undoubtedly increase.

The National Health Service Corps approach has two important characteris-tics. First, the program deals with filling obvious gaps in personnel rather than with any attempt to distribute personnel across different regions. Second, the Corps attempts to promote private practice in these areas. Communities are not asked to accept charity. Patients are charged fees that are returned to the National Health Service Corps, with the expectation that once the service is established, the community will prove its "financial viability" to support a private medical or dental practice. The National Health Service Corps, buttressed by scholarships to health profession students who agree to serve a year in the Corps for each year of scholarship assistance, may be successful in establishing practitioners where none was available previously. Whether it will promote private practice remains to be seen.

The Corps, like other federal regionalization programs, tackles only a narrowly defined aspect of manpower supply and distribution. In its focus on underserved, often poverty areas, the Corps continues a philosophy of limited aid to upgrade services to deserving groups. Such was the philosophy underlying programs such as the Hill-Burton grants to hospitals [established in 1946], neighborhood health centers, and health services for migrant workers or Appalachians [all products of the 1960s]. Each of these programs has stimulated local health care clinics or services designed to bring these populations more nearly up to the services available to wealthier groups. In all cases the goals were modest, in that no attempt was made to redistribute services within regions composed of all socioeconomic groups.

The federal approach to the regionalization of health manpower through regional health services has thus been both spotty and coy. Regional planning agencies (HSAs) promise to be exhortative rather than directive. Regional health care systems (HMOs) may be of limited application. Regional qualitative review agencies (PSROs) may or may not serve as a focus of interest for physicians. Regional educational centers (AHECs) may produce additional numbers of personnel required in their service areas but will not redistribute health manpower overall. Nor will the promise of manpower to underserved areas through the National Health Service Corps have an effect on the health manpower available to the general population. These approaches are partial attacks on different elements of regionalization. [And there is no single definition of a "region."]

Against this backdrop, congressional concern over the distribution of health manpower is growing. Federal aid to increase the supply of health professionals and to develop experimental, "innovative" programs, such as the sponsorship of physician assistants, has led to increased services for some population groups. But it has also led to increased costs without concomitant general improvements in the equity or efficiency of medical care. Lacking the will, the temerity, or indeed the capacity to organize middle class medical care on a regional basis, congressional committees have focused their attention on the producers of health professionals; that is, on the educational institutions that have swallowed up millions of federal dollars with unquestioning alacrity in the last few years, and on the professional associations whose policies have affected, in particular, the number and distribution of independent practitioners.

Since physicians are the prime example of such practitioners and since their decisions have a ripple effect on the use of all health care services (physicians making the key decisions about treatment and hospitalization and directing most other health care workers), it is the medical schools and other professional structures of medicine that are now receiving the most searching attention. Introducing the 1974 report on health manpower from the Senate Committee on Labor and Public Welfare is a quotation from then Assistant Secretary of Health Dr. Merlin Duval: "Medical schools have received $1,083,740,000 since direct federal aid to medical education began in 1964. There is now reason to believe that the quid pro quo is at hand..." Collisions between Congress and the medical profession raise the question of medical school responsibility, on behalf of the public, for regional service and education.

Professionalism under Stress

Until recently, the interactions between the American Medical Association (AMA), the medical schools, state licensing boards, and other professional organizations provided a complex private governing structure for determining how many physicians would be trained and who would enter the profession. The American medical profession has long prided itself on its independence from corporate or government influence. Private practice, selection of specialty and practice location, and the virtual right to a hospital staff appointment have been part and parcel of that history. Any question of government control of physician distribution thus faces the resistance of the medical professional organizations. The professional monopolies are challenged on the one hand by institutional bureaucracies (the hospitals and planning agencies), and on the other by government agencies seeking value for subsidies to professional education. The current situation is one of uneasy maneuverings. Everyone wants high quality medical care available at reasonable cost to the whole population, but there is no agreement on how goal can be met.

Traditional antagonism by medical societies to a medical care system run by hospitals or other medical care corporations probably rules out the expansion of hospitals or hospital-sponsored organizations as the organizing focus for regional medical services. AMA policy is quite clear that hospitals should have a single standard of eligibility for hospital medical staffs, based on quality rather than on any numerical criteria, and that hospital medical staffs should function as independent entities with "professional prerogatives...to establish their bylaws, rules, and regulations." Such policies imply that all trained physicians in an area should have hospital staff appointments, even where there is an excess of physicians in certain specialties. For the near future, unless there is overriding federal legislation, hospital medical staffs promise to remain open to all qualified local physicians, whether there are too many such physicians or too few. Hospital medical staffs will not develop, of themselves, as closed-staff corporations, which would provide a functional approximation to actual employment.

While opposing limitations on the job market by hospitals, physicians have also continued to oppose national health insurance proposals that would have obvious organizational effects on the health care system. The most notable examples, the Wagner-Murray-Dingell bills of the 1940s, if passed, could have had enormous effects on both the regional and the specialty distribution of physicians. Such proposals are still possible. A system would be devised whereby each member of the population would have a personal physician who would act as point of access to and, coordinator of, health services for the patient. Such physicians could be paid on a contract or capitation basis. Overnight, there could be incentives for physicians to be recognized as primary care physicians and insurance funds to reimburse them, spread relatively evenly across the population. Specialist services would not be reimbursed unless ordered by a primary physician, a provision impacting in turn on the distribution of specialists, depending on regional variations in the referral patterns of primary practitioners. Without any direct employment of physicians or other limitation on where individuals might practice, national health insurance could encourage both a network of services based on primary care and a diffusion of physicians more nearly appropriate to population distribution.

Even without national criteria for specialists, a health system built on primary care might have important geographical implications. Surgery is the area of medicine in which physicians are probably most dependent on patients being referred from other physicians. A recent study by the American College of Surgeons and the American Surgical Association found that surgeons were much more evenly distributed than, for example, internists. (The least evenly distributed specialty is psychiatry.) A universal health insurance system that required every person to have a primary physician by whom virtually all health care would be orchestrated is one way to avoid an increased direction of physicians into certain specialties and geographical areas.

Yet that is precisely the type of national health insurance most firmly opposed by the professional associations. While the establishment of primary care is a major professional goal—indeed, the AMA has recommended that half of all physicians be in primary care—the current manifestation of the Wagner-Murray Dingell bills, the so-called Health Security proposals, are the least likely of all the major heath insurance proposals to gain the support of the majority of physicians. The right of physicians to control their place of work, including the freedom to establish a private practice wherever they wish, is perhaps the most jealously guarded of professional privileges. Instead of sponsoring proposals that would center medical care on the primary physician and encourage the distribution of specialists in referral networks from primary physician to specialist and back, the official professional position is to promote extensions of existing forms of private health insurance that would encourage a continuing maldistribution of physicians.

The medical profession is thus in some respects in a box. If the professional associations were more machiavellian or able to set their sights on the longer rather than the shorter view, they might well decide to support national health insurance to avoid more irksome forms of regulation in the future. If the structure of health care is not to be touched directly, inevitably regulation of the medical profession will fall more heavily from other directions. The result of an unwillingness by Congress (or anyone else) to regulate the socioeconomic environment of practice, and resistance by the profession to any such control, may be increasing government influence over the medical schools, including selection of students and curricula, the number and distribution of physicians in specialty training, professional licensing, and standards of clinical work through PSROs.

These questions are central to regionalization, for if there is little likelihood of direct regional organization of medical manpower, there will be increased efforts to manipulate regional distributions in indirect ways. Health manpower legislation was enacted by Congress as this piece was being completed (Public Law 94-484). The proposals leading up to the legislation differed, but the basic thought was the same. The number of physicians is to be limited by controlling the immigration of foreign-trained physicians. The supply of physicians will then rest largely on the output of U.S. schools, which is now largely controlled by federal grant programs to the schools; almost half (45 percent) of the total budget of U.S. medical schools came from federal support in 1974, with another fifth (21 percent) from state and local funds. Geographical distribution and specialty distribution of physicians are also to be tackled through leaning on the medical schools. As a condition of receiving capitation grants, medical schools will have to designate 50 percent of first year residency positions in primary care by 1980. The schools are also required to accept an unspecified number of U.S. citizens who are now training in schools abroad. These proposals do not go as far as others, including those that would require schools to select a specified proportion of students who guarantee to enter primary care or apply for work in an underserved area. Nonetheless, they represent substantial inroads into medical school responsibility for selecting students and providing a curriculum. Medical schools have not been so vulnerable to pressure since the shackling of standards and curricula by the profession and by state licensing boards from the time of the Flexner Report (1910) into the 1920s. In some respects it seems that Congress has taken out its frustration with the medical profession by attempting to restructure the medical schools.

Medical Education and Regionalization

The pressure is also on at the level of graduate medical education. There are considerable imbalances in the relative geographical and specialty distributions of residency trainees from place to place. Relative to population, New York trains almost four physician residents to every one trained in Mississippi or New Jersey. (The 1972-73 figures were, respectively, forty-four residents per 100,000 in New York, and twelve in New Jersey; the number for Mississippi was eight.) Almost a third of all interns and residents in training in the United States are graduates of foreign schools but they, too, are spread unevenly across the U.S. population. Foreign medical graduates (FMGs) represent at least half of all physicians in residencies in Rhode Island, New Jersey, New York, Illinois, South Dakota, Delaware, West Virginia, and Puerto Rico; but less than 10 percent in Maine, Vermont, Mississippi, Arkansas, Colorado, New Mexico, Utah, California, Oregon, and Washington. If the supply of FMGs is reduced in the future, some states will evidently suffer more than others. There will also be considerable geographical implications for the distribution of residencies, unless U.S. graduates are guided into training in states in which they have had little interest in the past. Changes in the total number of physicians and in the balance between U.S. and foreign graduates—both the result of federal initiatives—have long-lasting regional implications.

Because of the availability of residency positions, U.S. graduates have been remarkably free to choose a residency and a specialty in their preferred geographical location [with foreign physicians acting as a backstop]. The result of these preferences is evident in the figures. Between 1967 and 1973, Alaska and Arizona increased their supply of U.S.-trained physicians by more than 60 percent; Florida, Hawaii, Nevada, and New Mexico by more than 30 percent; California, Oregon, Washington, Colorado, Idaho, Utah, Maine, New Hampshire, Vermont, North Carolina, and South Carolina by at least 20 percent. In contrast, several states suffered a net loss of U.S. graduates between 1967 and 1973, including West Virginia, South Dakota, Ohio, and New York. Others showed virtually no change: Iowa, North Dakota, Pennsylvania, Illinois, and Michigan.

These changes do not follow changes in the distribution of the U.S. population. Nor were the states with the largest increases necessarily those with the greatest number of medical schools. For example, there were no medical schools graduating students in Alaska, Hawaii, Maine, or Nevada between 1967 and 1973, yet those states were relatively high gainers. Other states relatively well served with schools, including New York with twelve, showed losses or less-than-proportionate increases. If past patterns are a guide, the majority of U.S. graduates will choose to practice in states that are different from the state of their medical school. Assuming the continuation of a relatively large supply of residencies compared with the number of U.S. graduates, the shifts will continue to be toward the relatively "attractive" states, and any major reduction in the supply of foreign graduates will make these regional shifts much more evident.

Among the ten states with the largest population, Illinois, Michigan, New Jersey, and Ohio have proved relatively unattractive to U.S. graduates. Compared with the national average of 138 U.S. medical graduates for a population of 100,000, Illinois has a ratio of 104 per 100,000; Michigan, ninety-eight; New Jersey, 106; and Ohio, 103. All of those states have supplemented their supply of physicians with a steady stream of foreign graduates. If the supply of foreign graduates is withdrawn, or reduced substantially, and if the residency training slots and insurance reimbursement mechanisms remain the same, encouraging U.S. graduates to set up practice where they wish, these states will lose ground rapidly. States such as California, with 200 U.S. graduates for a population of 100,000 in 1973, will continue to gain doctors, and the existing interstate maldistributions will widen. Federal policies to increase the number of U.S. medical students will further skew the distributions.

The logic of all of this, in terms of protecting federal investment in medical schools of almost a billion dollars by 1972-73, is to control the distribution of residencies so that physicians will choose regions and specialties in patterns more appropriate to service needs. Such proposals are appearing in congressional debates on manpower legislation. The Kennedy proposals of 1974 (S. 3585), for example, would have established both a national council and a regional council on postgraduate physician training for each region of the Department of Health, Education, and Welfare, in order to develop a program to certify first year residency positions by specialty, the total number not to exceed 110 percent of the number of U.S. medical graduates in a given year. While direct government control over residency training may never come to pass (the emphasis in the legislation was on studies), the combined effect of the debates is one of increasing pressure to assess the number of positions to be offered, by specialty and location. Government pressures on the medical schools would thus be extended to the graduate level.

The most likely course of events is for some reduction in the number of foreign medical graduates entering the United States, but not immediately large enough to encourage the medical societies of Illinois, Michigan, New Jersey, or Ohio to insist on a major limitation of residency slots throughout the nation, so that U.S. graduates would be "directed" to those states. There will probably also be some limitation on the number of residencies by the professional accrediting groups but, again, not enough to have a marked effect on geographical distributions. Medical schools will encourage primary care more than in the past, and there may well be an increasing proportion of physicians entering the primary care specialties; there will also be some decline in the proportion of graduates entering surgical specialties. In each case the changes will be relatively small and incremental; they will not lead, of themselves, to major regional redistributions.

Meanwhile, the medical profession's monopoly over entry to the profession and education will have been weakened. In some respects the profession has become the villain of deficiencies in a health care system that Congress is unwilling to reform directly.

Conclusion

One basic conclusion of this analysis is that there can be no comprehensive attempt to plan health manpower on a regional basis (that is, with a reasonably equitable distribution of personnel among regions and a reasonably effective distribution within each region) unless such manpower is part of a regionally organized service system. The classic national-regional-district model of planning is possible when: (1) governmental structures are authoritarian, for example, in health services of the U.S. armed services or Veterans Administration; (2) health services are developed in virgin conditions, in areas or to populations that have not had adequate health care before (and where professional organizations are weak), for example, the provision of services to medically underserved areas through the National Health Service Corps; (3) physicians and other personnel work as employees or quasi-employees (for example, under exclusive contract), as in health maintenance organizations. These are not the predominant patterns of organization of physicians and other key managers of medical care in the United States.

The distribution of health manpower in various parts of the country, between urban and rural areas and within the sectors of major cities, has been debated ad nauseam in health manpower hearings. Lacking the means to influence the major health professions to accept regional manpower planning voluntarily, and lacking the desire to confront and override the major health professions, Congress has chosen to exert its influence indirectly. The result has been a series of "chippings" at the edges of the system.

The impact of indirect regulation over professional activities promises to have little effect on the distribution of health professions across or within specific regions. But while the location and function of independent practitioners remains a jealously guarded professional prerogative, other traditional privileges of professional monopolies are being eroded. As a result of indirect efforts to redistribute physicians, medical schools are now firmly tied to government direction on the grounds that they are "national resources." In the current climate of anti-professionalism, the work of individual practitioners promises to be much more heavily scrutinized than in a direct health service system. Licensing will probably be made more stringent, surgeons watched for "unnecessary surgery," physicians for hospital admissions, all for potential malpractice liability.

While the effect of indirect regulation taken as a whole may be to control aspects of practice other than the location and population served, the primary problems seen by Congress will continue to be the maldistribution of personnel and the need to ameliorate that maldistribution in the interest of equity. There is a basic conflict between action and rhetoric.

In present circumstances, no single regionalization policy for health manpower is likely to be effective as a means of providing interregional balances or regional service networks, though the development of educational centers in underserved areas may have some impact on regional service systems, and some on manpower distribution. Detailed federal regulation of medical schools, however, carries the danger of rigid entry patterns and curricula without concurrent service advantages: Entrenched systems are rarely changed by tinkering with entrance and education. Programs involving loans to students that can be paid back by service in needy areas have yet to prove their worth. Taken together, the programs may lead to marginal improvements in distribution but no more than that.

Major redistribution of manpower on a regional basis will have to await fundamental changes in the health care system or in insurance reimbursement mechanisms. There may never be equity and/or efficiency in the health care system. However, three potential forms of regional control are long-term possibilities: These may be termed employment, quasi-employment, and restrictive regulation. A marked shift of independent practitioners to employed positions would create a job market in which the controlling force would be health care employers, including hospitals and HMOs. Distribution would be managed through job opportunities and job restrictions. Passage of a national health insurance scheme with specified funds channeled through regional reimbursement agencies could create a different form of market. Distribution might then be controlled through the flow of funding to private practitioners. Instead of a monopoly of jobs, there would be a monopoly of professional incomes.

Restrictive regulation is a third possibility. State licensing boards or regional planning agencies could simply prescribe how many practitioners, of what kind, would be permitted to practice in given areas. Such mechanisms would be similar to certificate-of-need requirements for the development of facilities. Health insurance that required each individual to register with a primary physician is another potentially interesting restriction that could have major effects on the distribution of care. Each of these three approaches is administratively straightforward. HSAs provide a potential structure for implementation. While the HSA may not be the appropriate "region" for all manpower considerations, and while data sources clearly need developing, the delay in reaching regional manpower goals is not one of governance or ignorance, but of political ambivalence.

Medical students are more aware of questions of distribution than were their predecessors a decade ago; indeed, the Student American Medical Association has been calling for a draft of all medical graduates into underserved areas. The American Medical Association is working with HEW to provide physicians on a voluntary basis to relieve National Health Service Corps personnel for meetings and vacations, and is developing national guidelines as a basis for regional standards of hospital care for PSROs. The PSROs themselves provide new regional groupings. Specialty groups are concerned about the number and distribution of residency positions in their specialties; a concern stimulated in part by congressional investigation. States are moving to reform their licensing boards before the federal government does it for them. Regional concerns are implicit in all such activities.

Yet, while there is a general commitment to the ideals of regionalism by all concerned—government, institutions, health professions—there is reluctance to approach the ideals or the ideas directly. Meanwhile, apparently unintended effects of indirect regulation may affect the long-term situation. For example, regulation of independent medical practice may become so oppressive that physicians and others will prefer employment in groups, if only to facilitate records review or to provide group malpractice insurance coverage. Any such move would have obvious regional connotations.

Such thoughts are, at present, only speculative. The professional monopolies are under stress, but that does not mean the development of regional health care systems. Independent practitioners may well have most to gain by supporting a comprehensive and uniform health program in which they would emerge with increased power through professional organizations, but emotional and political signposts point in other directions. Debates over regionalization promise to continue. At this point we, like Jimmy the Greek, can only offer odds on or against certain modes of regionalism, or perhaps, in a more scholarly tradition provide—as I have tried to do here—outlines of the implications of current developments.

This chapter (edited here for clarification where necessary) was originally published as one of eighteen invited chapters on regionalization policy in a publication from the U.S. Public Health Service, Health Resources Administration: Rosemary Stevens, "Health Manpower," in *Regionalization and Health Policy*, edited by Eli Ginzberg, DHEW Publication No. (HRA) 77-623 (Washington, D.C.: U.S. Government Printing Office, 1977), pp. 107-119.

How could the American health care system (or non-system) be reformed to give better care to the population? Regionalization was one answer, at least in theory, through the 1970s. Passage of the National Health Planning and Resources Development Act at the end of 1974 gave the topic practical and political relevance—though, as it turned out, for a very short period. As I try to show here, governmental action as a positive lever for organizational change was an unrealistic prospect even in 1976, when the final manuscripts for the volume were submitted.

Selected Bibliography

Alford, Robert R. 1975. *Health Care Politics: Ideological and Interest Group Barriers to Reform*. University of Chicago Press.

American College of Surgeons and American Surgical Association. 1975. *Surgery in the United States, A Summary Report of the Study on Surgical Services for the United States*.

American Medical Association. 1973. *Measuring Physician Manpower: Contributions to a Comprehensive Manpower Strategy*. Center for Health Services Research and Development, American Medical Association.

American Medical Association. 1975. *Physician-Hospital Relations, 1974*. Committee on Private Practice and Council on Medical Service, American Medical Association.

Comptroller General of the United States. 1974. *Congressional Objectives of Federal Loans and Scholarships to Health Professions Students Not Being Met*. Report to the Congress, General Accounting Office. Report No. B-164 031 (2).

Crowley, Anne E., ed. 1975. *Medical Education in the United States 1973-74*. 74th Annual Report, American Medical Association.

Dewey, Donald. 1973. *Where the Doctors Have Gone: The Changing Distribution of Private Practice Physicians in the Chicago Metropolitan Area, 1950-1970*. Illinois Regional Medical Program.

Halstead, John Philip. 1975. *Examining the Examiners: An Investigation of the Licensure Examination Practices and Policies for Florida's Boards of Dentistry, Medical Examiners, Podiatry Examiners, and Veterinary Medicine with Recommendations for State and Federal Action.* State of Florida, House of Representatives, Committee on Regulated Industries and Licensing.

Institute of Medicine. 1975. *Controls on Health Care.* Papers of the Conference on Regulation in the Health Industry, January 1974. National Academy of Sciences.

Johnson, Walter L., Rosenfeld, Leonard S., and Fernow, L. Carol. 1974. *Physicians' Staff Appointments in Southern New York.* Health and Hospital Planning Council of Southern New York.

Martin, Beverly C. 1975. *Medical School Alumni: Professional Characteristics of U.S. Physicians by Medical School and Year of Graduation.* Aspen Systems Corporation for American Medical Association.

Mullner, Ross, and O'Rourke, Thomas W. 1974. "A Geographic Analysis of Counties without an Active Non-Federal Physician, United States, 1963-71." U.S. Department of Health, Education, and Welfare, *Health Services Reports*, 89: 256-62.

Pearson, David A. 1975. "The Concept of Regionalized Personal Health Services in the United States, 1920-1955." In Ernest W. Saward, ed. *The Regionalization of Personal Health Services.*

Public Accountability Reporting Group. 1975. *Regional Medical Programs: Developing Local Health Resources and Services for People: Accomplishments of the Nation's RMPs 1974-75.* Boise, Idaho.

Regents of the University of the State of New York, Task Force on Medical School Enrollment and Physician Manpower. 1974. *Interim Report and Synopsis of Findings to Date.* New York.

Stevens, Rosemary. 1971. *American Medicine and the Public Interest.* Yale University Press.

U.S. Congress, House. 1974. Conference Report on S. 2994, *National Health Planning and Resources Development Act of 1974.* 93rd Congress, 2nd Session, Report No. 93-1640.

U.S. Congress, House. 1975. Committee on Interstate and Foreign Commerce, Report on HR 5546, *Health Manpower Act of 1975.* 94th Congress, 1st Session, Report No. 94-266.

U.S. Congress, Senate. 1974. Committee on Labor and Public Welfare, *Health Professions Educational Assistance Act of 1974.* Report on S.3585, 93rd Congress, 2nd Session, Report No. 93-1122.

U.S. Congress, Senate. 1974. Committee on Labor and Public Welfare, Subcommittee on Health, *Health Manpower, 1974.* Hearings on S.3585, 93rd Congress, 2nd Session.

U.S. Department of Health, Education, and Welfare, National Center for Health Statistics. 1975. *Decennial Census Data for Selected Health Occupations: United States, 1970.* DHEW Publication No. (HRA) 76-1231.

U.S. Department of Health, Education, and Welfare, Social Security Administration, Division of Health Insurance Studies. 1975. "Medicare: Use of Physicians' Services by Geographic Region, 1969." *Health Insurance Statistics*, DHEW Publication No. (SSA) 75-11702.

10

Health Care in a Context of Civil Rights (1981)

This [Institute of Medicine] report is peculiarly American. The committee [which I chaired] was brought together at the request at the Office for Civil Rights, Department of Health and Human Services, to review information about observable disparities or inequalities in health care affecting two large, dissimilar, and distinctive groups—members of social/ethnic minorities and handicapped persons—whose only link is through civil rights legislation. Minority groups are a primary target of legislation under Title VI of the Civil Rights Act; handicapped individuals under Section 504 of the Rehabilitation Act. We were asked not to draw conclusions as to whether and in what respects members of these groups were subject to racial discrimination or discrimination by virtue of handicapping condition. Nevertheless, the choice of these two groups—whose conjunction would make little sense in considering policies in any other country's health care system—was clearly generated by interests as to whether and in what respects civil rights procedures ought to be extended in the health care system.

As a committee we have tried to be objective in the collection, analysis, and presentation of our data. Yet the subject matter of this report is value-laden. The ambiguities, complexities, and tensions in American health care make discussions of equality particularly difficult. Who is to say what is fair or unfair in the receipt of health services in the United States, and on what basis? There is no consensus, at least as yet. What disparities in the receipt of care are to be regarded as just or unjust? What differences are to be legally prohibited under civil rights legislation? Nearly all Americans would claim that at least some health services should be available to all members of the population or even perhaps that, as far as possible, health services should be distributed "equitably." But how does one approach questions of equity? Does equity mean equal numbers of visits for all groups? Equal length of life? Because the structure of the American health care system is not designed to deliver services equally to all members of the population, it makes little sense to assume that, with a little tinkering, it would.

Moreover health is not the same as the receipt of medical care. Factors extraneous to the health care system, such as income, diet, smoking, genetic heritage, and stress, may powerfully affect an individual's condition. Even in countries where equality of services is a goal, as in Britain, there remain striking differences in the health of different groups.[1] Britain's analysis of health by social (occupational) class raises a yet further set of uncertainties. Discussion of social class differences is faintly un-American; race and handicapping conditions provide more urgent classifications, as reflected in civil rights concerns. Even the choice of groups for study (and available data) reflects cultural beliefs.

Yet it is precisely *because* the questions are difficult and value-laden and because of the empirical complexities of investigation that this report has been undertaken. If serious discussion about equalities and inequalities in American health care is to take place, review of available evidence about disparities in American medical care is obviously essential. Members of this committee agreed to give their time to this study because of concern about the adequacy of care to various members of the population, signified here as care to minorities and handicapped individuals. Equity is an important value in the society in which we live. Access to health care ought to be assured to all members of the population. This study reveals serious imbalances in care received by different groups. As financial resources for medical care become more limited, particularly in programs, such as Medicaid, that disproportionately affect needy individuals, it becomes correspondingly more important to articulate the social goals of health care programs and to measure their effects on different populations. By arraying available evidence about disparities in health and health care—scanty though this evidence often is—this report is a beginning of a process of discussion and debate (and better data collection) out of which health and civil rights policies can be more openly addressed.

Civil rights approaches also need considerable discussion and clarification as they apply to health care issues. We do not mean to imply in this report that disparities in care in and of themselves are civil rights issues in the legal sense. If the law's objective is to eliminate purposeful discrimination on the basis of race or physical handicap in the delivery of health care, then it will not suffice simply to discover or show that there are significant disparities in the use of, or access to, health care. As one of our legal critics pointed out, many observers believe that the major civil rights problem today is not conscious and overt discrimination, but rather the more subtle problem associated with a pattern of racially neutral decisions that have racially disparate consequences. The problem here may be a structural one of institutional indifference or insensitivity to the concerns of racial or ethnic minorities or other constituencies not represented in the decision-making process. From this standpoint, perhaps the most effective regulatory action would be to require the decision-makers, in various health planning contexts at least, to assess the likely consequences of proposed actions on access to and utilization of health care services by racial and ethnic minorities or other disparate groups.

This and similar points of debate can only be reached persuasively, however, after careful review of available evidence. We show here the evidence on disparities that now exists and note the serious shortcomings (sometimes conflicts) in this evidence. Adequate data are prerequisites to civil rights enforcement activities under present legal obligations and to the continuing process of definition of disparities that are to be regarded as unreasonable or illegitimate in terms of civil rights legislation. We need better data in order to think more clearly about civil rights and health policy development.

Yet it would be a paltry excuse to use the absence of good data to avoid raising policy issues at all. What we have done here is to identify (1) areas in which disparities appear to exist in the health care of members of ethnic/minority groups and handicapped populations compared with the general population, and (2) areas in which better information is particularly needed. For analytical purposes we have assumed that any evidence of disparity deserves investigation as a potential health policy or civil rights issue.

Given the committee's mandate and time constraints, the report is inevitably "unfinished." Reviewers consulted by the Institute of Medicine and by the committee have chided us, *inter alia*, for failing to specify empirical questions or conceptual frameworks; for being insufficiently critical of the complexities in health care (and in American society in general) that may well lead to disparities in care; for failing to disentangle the effects of socioeconomic status; for not providing adequate definitions of "ethnicity"; for lack of discussion on the ethical implications of disparities in care; for suggesting that disparities may imply discrimination.

Some of these criticisms arise from serious inadequacies in the basic data. For example, ethnicity (or handicap), health care, location, and social class are mutually dependent variables *all* of which need to be understood in assessing how real and how general differences in health care actually are. Middle-class blacks may have better health care than lower-class non-blacks; poor people may feel discriminated against whether or not they are from a minority group; persons with hearing problems may report different health care experiences in different cities. Unfortunately, as this report shows, most existing studies do not array data (or do not collect data) by all these variables. We need studies of what different subgroups think about health and illness, whom they go to for care, and with what satisfaction and apparent results. Useful classifications of handicapping conditions are only beginning. In many ways the inadequacies in the data reflect a general unwillingness to think about the policy issues. This report is designed to stimulate action on both the policy and the informational fronts.

Some of the criticisms stem from the committee's mandate. We have not developed empirical questions or conceptual frameworks. We have presented an overview of current research findings and survey data, on which others may base further investigations. We have assumed that disparities are "problems" in American health care, whether or not these disparities might prove to be quite reasonable in the light of further empirical investigation or interpretations. Some of the criticisms stem from the committee's biases and perceptions in areas where there are differences of opinion. Some errors of presentation or judgment undoubtedly remain. In our thanking a particularly helpful (if feisty) panel of reviewers, it should be observed that it is precisely this continuing process of clarification, dissent, and discussion that this report is designed to provoke.

This chapter originally appeared as the Preface to *Health Care in a Context of Civil Rights, Report of a Study*, Institute of Medicine, publication IOM 81-04 (Washington, D.C.: National Academy Press, 1981), pp. vii-x.

Note

1. *Inequalities in Health*, Report of a Research Working Group (chairman, Sir Douglas Black) (London: Department of Health and Social Security, August 1980).

11

Health Care "Equity": Slippery Concept, Elusive Goals (1986)

As ideology, the concept of equity is useful for pinpointing inequalities and deficiencies in the health care system and for rallying reformist interests. For policy, though, the idea of equity can only exist in a specific framework of politics, organization, power, and money. Just as British notions of equity are bounded by the structures and assumptions of the National Health Service, so American approaches are tempered by the inertia and momentum of health care organizations, the practical tradeoffs of everyday life, conflicting interpretations as to who should be served and how, and the immediate agendas of powerful interests.

Americans are struggling to define and "operationalize" equity in the 1980s—specifically, to come up with programs or incentives that meet three potentially conflicting goals: first, to provide at least a basic, adequate floor of health services to the whole population—this goal in principle is non-controversial; second, to allow individual consumers of health services (and health insurance), as far as possible, as much freedom to purchase medical care as they have to purchase other goods and services; and third, to leave the working of the health service, as far as possible, in private hands. Questions of equity intertwine with each of these missions.

I will look first at some obvious anomalies and inequities in the present U.S. health care system, then raise questions about values and goals, as evidenced in the U.S. system as presently structured, and finish with some nuts and bolts questions of strategy.

Anomalies/Inequities: Dimensions of Debate

Depending on how comparisons are measured, the U.S. system spends between two and four times as much per head on health services as the British system.[1] One obvious anomaly lies in the observation that the richer the resources, the greater the number of Americans apparently denied access to them. An estimated 45 million people are either uninsured or underinsured.[2] Private health insurance is almost universally tied to organized workplace arrangements—a historical legacy that, curiously, is rarely questioned, which was born of the selling of voluntary hospital insurance in the Depression and of government fringe benefit incentives to business and industry in the 1940s.

Anyone can, of course, buy insurance as an individual, but individual policies are relatively expensive (and it is easy to put off the decision or spend the money on something else). Large numbers of Americans thus gamble with the system: those with part-time or temporary jobs, or new employees who are not entitled to health insurance as a fringe benefit, or those between jobs or otherwise unemployed. More than one-fifth of the population under age sixty-five has either no automatic protection for medical bills or grossly inadequate protection should they fall sick—either from private or government programs.[3] Not surprisingly, equitable access to health insurance has become a major political issue in the United States—exciting federal policymakers, state legislators, and major businesses, which are, in turn, being pressed to extend their coverage to laid-off workers.

An outside observer looking at U.S. health insurance arrangements who is unaware of the quirks of history might assume that present American insurance patterns were a natural outgrowth of the equity assumptions of industrial capitalism, with benefits designed primarily to protect worker productivity—and little concern about anyone else. However, here we come to another anomaly. The U.S. government is, in fact, heavily involved in guaranteeing medical service provision to selected groups of persons who are "unproductive" and socially dependent, primarily the elderly and the poor.

Through Medicare, the federal government oversees an enormous system of transfer payments from the working population to the elderly (those sixty-five years of age and over), to provide national hospital and related services insurance. The program also covers the disabled and—by virtue of effective interest group lobbying in 1972—patients with end state renal disease. One might say, as a result, that kidney disease is a "Cinderella" service, using British terminology. It was (and still is), the one and only chronic condition singled out for U.S. government national health insurance coverage.[4]

In the twenty-one years since the Medicare legislation, the federal government has backed into a huge national health insurance program of health care, which is limited in very large part to services for the elderly. Americans tend to take this for granted. Medicare has become an accepted part of Social Security. But this choice of a priority population is in fact extraordinary. The U.S. is the only country in the world that has begun a national health insurance program by concentrating on the oldest generations. Ninety percent of Americans over the age of sixty-five are covered by Medicare hospital insurance, part A. Virtually all of these also subscribe to part B, a federally subsidized insurance program that concentrates on doctors' bills and other professional medical services.

As is the case with private health insurance, care is not provided directly, but purchased for patients on a contractual basis from hospitals, doctors, and health care systems that are largely under private ownership.

In terms of access to acute care, Medicare makes an important social equity statement. The elderly are now better covered, for hospital care at least, than younger members of the population. In financial terms, the Medicare program is also quite generous. In 1984 Medicare spent on average about $3,000 (£2,000) per beneficiary. Indeed, it can be argued that in purely financial terms the United States is doing more by way of health protection for its elderly than the United Kingdom.

Within the United States, meanwhile, there are claims that elderly members of the population are receiving more of their "fair share" of health care resources, in terms of the distribution of public funds to different population groups, particularly in comparing the elderly with children. It is, indeed, easy to argue that the United States has made a set of private and public choices in the last two decades that have "dramatically altered the age profile of well-being," with gains for the elderly being made at the partial expense of services for children, which have been in turn a casualty of reduced tax expenditures.[5]

The internal distribution of Medicare funding is also open to serious criticism, both in terms of allocation to different services and in geographical distribution. Despite its cost, Medicare pays less than half of the total health expenses of the elderly, is heavily weighted toward acute medical services, and is a long way from comprehensive. For example, it excludes essential services such as dentistry, hearing aids, meals on wheels, and basic residential care. Although major efforts are being made to incorporate Medicare patients into organized, private health care networks (the move toward health maintenance organizations), where a mix of preventive, maintenance, and curative services might be provided, and although there are a few experimental programs linking health and social services for the elderly, Medicare is far from being a *health care* system. Its strength has always been to protect the income and capital of the elderly in the face of huge, unexpected hospital bills. And this it does quite well.

After achieving reasonable success in income protection for the older generations in the face of acute, catastrophic illness, with the major exception of patients requiring long-term care, Medicare is finally having to face the slow and difficult transition from a program of health insurance to a more rounded program of health care provision. Costs alone will make this transition essential.

Federal/state programs for the poor (Medicaid) pose other organizational, distributional, and equity issues in the 1980s. Medicaid's byzantine eligibility barriers daunt all but the truly desperate, however needy. These barriers include requirements that beneficiaries be children (and their parents) or elderly, blind, or disabled, as well as poor; and that they meet stringent, detailed means tests requirements. The able-bodied unemployed, per se, are not included. Medicaid represents, in direct descent, nineteenth- and early-twentieth-century welfare values, with programs targeted to recipients whose poverty was unimpeachable: children, the blind, disabled, or the elderly. It says something for the administrative ingenuity of American systems that the confusing matrix of Medicaid eligibility requirements and services, which vary state to state and are nowhere comprehensive, is taken so readily as a bureaucratic given, spawning great "bibles" of administrative regulations.

Medicare's primary contribution is to hospital care of the elderly. Medicaid programs, too, are skewed. They play a particularly important role in medical care of destitute children and in supporting institutional care of the impoverished elderly over and above Medicare benefits. Since many of the impoverished elderly are members of middle-class families who have become impoverished by spending their savings on nursing home care, there is an important middle-class constituency in favor of Medicaid programs for the elderly. Over three-quarters of all payments made under Medicaid in the mid-1980s are for hospital or nursing home care.[6]

Medicare and Medicaid, together, have brought the federal government firmly into national health care policymaking: in seeking cost containment policies, in detailed scrutiny of doctors' behavior through clinical records analysis and policing hospital lengths of stay (to an extent that might well not be tolerated in Great Britain), and in standardized prospective payment systems. Payment for hospital care under Medicare according to Diagnosis-Related Groups (DRGs) began in 1983. Taken together, Medicare and Medicaid, plus a third major federal program for armed service veterans, strongly emphasize institutional over non-institutional medical care. Hence, almost all the regulatory interest in resource distribution in the 1970s and 1980s has been centered on hospital provision, with little effective government influence over other types of care.

The scope of government involvement in the United States should be stressed. Government funding as a whole represents over 40 percent of all health care expenditures. In the three major federal programs of Medicare, Medicaid, and the Veterans Administration, U.S. government agencies spend more per head than is spent in Britain per head on the entire NHS. Yet, in the United States services continue to be partial, spotty, and far from comprehensive.

Goals and Values of American Health Care

What, then, are the goals, assumptions, and values underlying the provision of health care in the United States in the 1980s? And how do these relate to the equity question? The first and most obvious observation of the American scene is that there is no mainstream movement toward more egalitarianism in health care. Indeed, present discussions about equity in terms of fear of "rationing" health care almost invariably decry the limitations on an individual's freedom to purchase expensive medical care that might be incurred in a more equal system. Discussions about distributing scarce resources across the United States deal not so much with the value of righting inequities, but alarm at the possibility of creating new ones. The poor are deprived of services only because they cannot pay. Under a rationed system the rich might face arbitrary service restrictions.

Hence, the sense of alarm expressed in such phrases as "tragic choices" or "painful prescriptions"—and the tendency to project resource decisions directly at the potential impact on fee-paying individuals. Implicitly the fee-paying patient has a right to consume. For those who cannot pay there is no government or constitutional obligation to provide or pay for medical care. As a result, the health care system is inherently and deliberately unequal, favoring those who can afford to pay most or have the best insurance coverage. The lawyers put the issue quaintly but succinctly: "Wealth is not a suspect classification."[7]

Meanwhile the realities of exclusion and deficiencies in the American health care system provoke relatively little passion or interest, whether one is talking about the distribution of health insurance, health status, or utilization. There are obvious correlations between self-assessment of health and family income in the United States, and white Americans are much more likely to rate their health as excellent than black Americans.[8] Although the average number of doctor visits per person per year is more or less equal by social group, there are distinctions in place and type of care.[9] Poorer members of the population and minority groups are more likely to see doctors in hospital outpatient and emergency rooms; others in the offices of private doctors.

Such observations are likely to be seen as intrinsic features of the U.S. system rather than as major criticisms. Arguably, Britons might be more outraged than Americans that fifteen states refuse to cover poor working-class children in their Medicaid program;[10] that over one-third of all American children one to four years are not currently immunized for measles, rubella, DTP, polio, and mumps;[11] or that the transfer of patients from one hospital to another for economic, rather than medical, reasons has become an accepted commonplace.

The underlying point, of course, is that the goals of the U.S. and British health systems are quite different. And this is not merely because one has a national health service and the other does not. While there are no explicit or unified goals for health care as a social good in the United States, implicit goals and value assumptions infuse the American health care system. For the sake of illustration, let me suggest the following seven:

1. To protect individual income from the economic hardship of massive medical bills.
2. To support private enterprise, including the health care industry, through facilitating employment, capital development, industry expansion.
3. To encourage productivity in the health care system.
4. To support scientific and technological innovation.
5. To develop healthy workers.
6. To aspire to social justice via a minimal floor of medical benefits for all.

7.   To avoid major political and organizational confrontations.

Other American critics of the health care system might come up with a different array. However, these points are useful in making three major observations that may be helpful to British and other foreign observers who seek to make sense of the American system.

First, government agencies have become involved in American health care largely to protect individual income and to support the private health care enterprise. Medicare and Medicaid speak for themselves. Beyond this, government agencies have not generally become involved in funding medical care primarily for the purpose of health enhancement. This is obviously an essential point in understanding discussions of equity in the 1980s. The wording of the President's Commission for the Study of Ethical Problems is frequently cited; namely, that society has an "ethical obligation to ensure equitable access to health care for all."[12] However, this statement is significant in two respects. It defines adequate, equitable access in terms of a minimal rather than an optimal level of care, thus laying the basis for a two-class or multi-tiered health care system. At the same time it limits equity to the question of access to services; there is no effort to insure equity in health status or health care outcomes. The philosophy suggested is a policy of equality of access to minimal services but not for equality of results.

A second observation is that the goals and values I have listed are not ascribed specifically to government agencies or the private sector. The history of medical care in the United States has been for a closely intertwined process of policymaking. The flavor of legislation tends to be pragmatic rather than based on egalitarian or other ideological commitments. Employers have had a major stake in government policy because of the central importance of workplace arrangements in the collection of private and public premiums for health insurance. It seems possible that some form of universal national health insurance may be established in the United States in the short-term future, and if so, it will most likely come through joint corporate and government efforts.

Third, the American health care industry is more than an industry in name. It *is* an industry—one of the largest in the United States. In the mid-1980s it provides income for approximately 8 million workers and supports subsidiary enterprises in areas as diverse as medical electronics, computer software, major accounting services, and investment banking. This industry, which also includes the major purchasers of care (employers, health insurers, and government), forms the necessary environment shaping discussions of health care. As a result, equity issues are not limited to questions of the distribution of resources by social class, geography, and race. They also include attempts to include principles of justice that take into account the equity interests of major stakeholders; that is, equity for consumers, equity for decision–makers, and, not least, equity for taxpayers. As a result, there are no simple or obvious directions for resource allocation in health care. Rather, there is array of potential and negotiable strategies, each addressing part of a much wider picture.

Strategies

The growing market ethos of the American health system means regulation of private, often competing entities as potentially the most effective distributional strategy. If equity in Britain is seen in terms of politics and the macro-management of resources, in the United States equity translates, functionally, into micromanagement. Where Britain looks to top-down, regional monetary allocations, special attention to certain neglected, "Cinderella" services, and regional planning, the U.S. approach is necessarily more oblique. This is an important point in considering cross-national U.S./British comparisons.

Four examples of U.S. strategies for "equity" may be helpful in pinpointing the differences as these translate into functional application:

1. Shifting to Enrollment in Private Health Care Organizations such as HMOs
2. Rediscovering (and Emphasizing) Quality of Care
3. Establishing Fiscal (Purchase) Norms
4. Providing Basic Insurance Protection

The first strategy is to develop organizations through which relative priorities in services and across populations groups can be decided. Ideally, decisions would be made on a decentralized basis within a health maintenance organization or service network. In subscribing to a particular organization, the patient accepts, up front, the limitations in the specific coverage offered. These might include rationing services through requiring each patient to have a primary practitioner who acts as a gatekeeper to specialists' services and hospital care; requiring second opinions in cases of major surgery; excluding coverage of services such as liver transplants and limiting services such as long-term psychiatric care; rationing by time (including the length of time it may take to get a medical appointment for all but urgent care); and rationing by encouraging specific forms of patient behavior. This latter point might include, for example, encouragement of self-care and self-diagnosis, consumer education leading to reduced consumption of prescription and nonprescription drugs, acceptance of non-heroic treatments in terminal illness, and, perhaps, even the ability to tolerate minor levels of pain.

There is already an acceptance of variety in third-party insurance coverage in the United States. By putting the onus on the consumer to choose a particular insurance plan or HMO enrollment, the rights of the consumer for optimal care are, in theory, protected in two ways: first, by giving the consumer the option to enroll in one configuration rather than another; and second, by allowing the consumer to purchase services over and above those covered by the insurance organization, assuming such services are available.

Questions of supply have almost always been linked historically with assumptions about the appropriate quality of care. A second fruitful strategy for considering resource distribution in the United States is the use of quality standards as a subtle mechanism for reallocating (and in some cases reducing) services. Outpatient cataract surgery is a case in point. Such surgery has become a major enterprise in the United States, even though there may not be indications for surgery in the vast majority of patients, and even though the case for surgery may vary depending on the visual needs and lifestyle of the individual patient.[13] By suggesting that such surgery may not only be unnecessary but potentially dangerous to patients, the qualitative argument can be used to stem less-than-desirable, market-oriented behavior by both patients and physicians.

Recent publicity about the relative success of coronary bypass surgery, depending on place of operation, extends the qualitative argument one step further. Where a patient goes for such surgery may mean the difference between life and death.[14] It is only a step from here to formal or informal regulation of patient flow to some institutions (centers of excellence with a large volume of such procedures) rather than to others. Suggestions are being made for the development of quality of care ratings for hospitals, for services such as cardiac surgery, somewhat similar to the complex financial ratings that are made by national investment services to determine a hospital's credit rating (and that are, in turn, essential in raising funds on the capital markets).[15] Although the language of such recommendations may be designed to encourage consumers to choose hospitals with the best results, a further result may well be on the distribution of such services across the population. I think we are going to see much emphasis on quality of care as an intrinsic element in the equity debates.

A third point of leverage is the acceptance of fiscal norms; that is, the regulation of health services through standardized rules and restrictions attached to third-party payment systems. The new standardized payment system for Medicare, prospective payment on the basis of diagnosis related groups (DRGs), is a major example of an attempt to standardize Medicare benefits across regions and areas of the United States. Although DRGs were introduced as a market mechanism, one effect was to proclaim that each member of the Medicare population should have a "fair share" of available benefits, according to nationally-defined rules.

The search for norms or rules is also apparent in the increased attention being paid to "small area" variations in health service utilization; variations, that is, that appear to be associated with traditional style of practice rather than with the results of care. For example, coronary bypass surgery shows more than a threefold variation in rates of use between Medicare regions.[16] More generally, there is discussion of the possible development of rates of use for different procedures—rates that might justly be regarded as "right," just as there are already norms for length of stay by diagnostic groups for Medicare patients.[17] The logic of industrial regulation is to make medical services increasingly standardized. In theory, then, the equitable system in the United States would be one that provided reasonable access to a standard rate of use of medical care for all members of the population. Note, however, the detailed regulation and narrow consensus that would have to be established in order to make such a system viable. That is, of course, one of the problems of micromanagement.

The fourth and final strategic example is the evident move toward some basic insurance protection for as large a portion of the population as possible—whether funded by the federal government, the states, by taxes on employers, and/or by taxes on providers. Some of these mechanisms already exist. Major employers might push for increased government protection of the uninsured.

The logic of any strategy for a socially equitable health system in the United States must be based on generally agreed specifications of what should be included in basic medical care, so as to provide an "adequate" level of care as a matter of equity to the whole population. Whether this is possible to do remains a burning question. It appears that those involved in health services research in the United States will be increasingly involved in microanalysis, in an attempt to establish acceptable norms around which a more equitable system can be based. I see no way around the fact, at present, that the United States is heading toward a multi-tiered health care system, with services varying by ability to pay (the "equity," perhaps, of the market premise) though I should like to be proved wrong on this.

To conclude: The goals and values of the American health care system are intrinsically different from those of the UK and thus questions of equity have to be conceived differently. This is more than saying that they have to be approached differently, although this is obviously true. Rather, equity, as principle and strategy, is also different. I believe we are about to enter an extremely interesting decade in the United States, when questions of equity will come to the fore, disguised as organizational, legal, qualitative, or fiscal questions. Two immediate targets will, and should be, the uninsured and children.

Cross-national discussion, such as this, may help to sharpen our relative perceptions. No one familiar with the paradigm national pastimes of British cricket and American football can fail to appreciate the distinctive array of national values: different definitions of solidarity of purpose, technique, the nature of authority, the money nexus, and the role of experts. If Britain is a country that prides itself on fairness, America is a country that prides itself on rules. It is through the micromanagement of rules within a largely private system that basic changes will be made. Equity in the United States means more and more definitional precision—about insurance coverage, payment, services provided, and the quality of care.

In the meantime, the balancing act will continue: a complex, shifting dialogue between conflicting notions of what is fair.

This chapter was initially given at an international conference in London in 1986. It was published in 1988 as "Goals, Values and Equity in Health Care: A U.S. View," in T. B. Binns and M. Firth, eds., *Health Care Provision under*

Financial Constraint. Royal Society of Medicine International Congress and Symposium Series No. 115 (London: Royal Society of Medicine Services, Ltd., 1988). The version presented here is shortened and edited.

Notes

1. A. Harrison and J. Gretton, *Health Care UK*, an Economic, Social and Policy Audit (London: CIPFA, 1984), cited by J. Carrier, "Health," in P. Wilding, ed., *In Defense of the Welfare State* (Manchester: Manchester University Press, 1986): 36.
2. G. J. Bazzoli, "Health Care for the Indigent: Overview of Critical Issues." *Health Services Research* 21 (1986): 362.
3. K. R. Levit, H. Lazenby, D. R. Waldo, and L. M. Davidoff, "National Health Expenditures, 1984." *Health Care Financing Review* 7 (Fall 1985): 23.
4. I would remark, in passing, that studies of the relatively high rates of dialysis in the United States, compared with Britain, rarely point out that these services are financially favored as government policy in the United States, in a unique way. Indeed, kidney dialysis is a curiously inappropriate benchmark of the different "rationing" processes at work in Britain and the United States. It would be more appropriate to look, for example, at the distribution of services for schizophrenia, prenatal and perinatal care, juvenile diabetes, or AIDS. See, for instance, H. J. Aaron and W. B. Schwartz, *The Painful Prescription: Rationing Hospital Care* (Washington, D.C.: Brookings Institution, 1984): 37, 49, 55, 57.
5. S. H. Preston, "Children and the Elderly: Divergent Patterns for America's Dependents." *Demography* 21 (1984): 434.
6. In 1984, Medicaid reported expenditures of $11.8 billion on hospital care and $12.3 billion on nursing homes out of total expenditures of $32.9 billion. These figures exclude the services of physicians attending patients in these institutions, which should be added to these totals. Levit et al., *supra* note 3: 22.
7. R. D. Miller, "Rationing Health Care: The Legal Complexity and Some Guidelines." *Topics in Hospital Law* 1, 4 (1986): 30.
8. Data from the National Health Interview Survey, U.S. Department of Health and Human Services, Public Health Service, *Health, United States 1985* DHHS Pub. No. (PHS) 86-1232, Table 32.
9. Ibid.
10. S. Rosenbaum and K. Johnson, "Providing Health Care for Low-Income Children: Reconciling Child Health Goals with Child Health Financing Realities." *Milbank Quarterly* 64 (1986): 442-78.
11. U.S. Department of Health and Human Services, *Health United States 1985* DHHS Publication No. (PHS) 86-1232 (Washington, D.C.: 1986): 68.
12. Commission for the Study of Ethical Problems in Medicine and Biomedical and Behavioral Research, Securing Access to Health Care, Vol. 1, *Report* (Washington, D.C.: U.S. Government Printing Office, 1983): 4.
13. C. E. Margo, "Selling Surgery." *New England Journal of Medicine* 314 (1986): 1575.
14. "Bypass Surgery May Depend on which Hospital," *Philadelphia Inquirer* (October 12, 1986): 3-E.
15. W. Greenberg, "Information on Quality Will Fuel Competition." *Health Span* 3, 1 (1986): 6.
16. M. R. Cheslin, R. H. Brook, et al. "Variations in the Use of Medical and Surgical Service by the Medicare Population." *New England Journal of Medicine* 314 (1986): 285.
17. J. Wennberg, "Which Rate is Right?" Ibid.: 310.

IV. The Medical Profession: Between Government and Market?

Introduction to Section IV

There is an appealing dualism in setting government and the market in opposition as two, alternative, clashing forces for change. However, as described in the essays here (and in *American Medicine and the Public Interest*, published in 1971), long before the 1970s the medical profession was a further major force in shaping the American health care system, and hospital representatives (see chapter 1) and others were also major policy influences. Each negotiated with government and private "market" players, and sometimes with each other. Indeed, everyone concerned, including those in Congress and government agencies, was to a greater or lesser extent a market player: doing deals with each other, cooperating in writing regulations, inventing strategies advantageous to particular coalitions, and generally engaging in the politics of the moment.

The four chapters in this section illustrate major challenges to the medical profession as a national American enterprise between 1970 and 2001—when the profession was buffeted by change and uncertain of its future role, if any, in national health care policymaking. Though the four pieces were written at different times, for different audiences, certain messages weave through them: growing acceptance in the 1970s that medicine was (is) a business like any other business, accelerated by the passage of Medicare and Medicaid, and thus might naturally look after its own interests before those of society or the public at large; more general shifts toward a business ethos in politics and the culture from the 1970s, stimulating competitive rather than community-oriented policies at the national and local levels; critical (negative) scholarly critiques of the role of professions in general and medicine in particular (see especially chapter 15); the fragmentation of organized medicine into specialty organizations, leaving a power vacuum at the center (an underlying and continuing theme of all four chapters); external threats to medicine's authority, most recently from organizations and agendas in the quality movement (chapter 15); and the search within professional groups for new definitions of professionalism and a new social ethos, given the contextual changes taking place (chapters 14 and 15).

The passage and implementation of Medicare and Medicaid challenged the public role and privileged status of organized medicine, represented politically through the American Medical Association (see chapter 5). Charity to patients by doctors in private practice seemed far less necessary in 1970 than it had before the passage of the Medicare legislation in 1965. At least some doctors and hospitals were demonstrably not behaving "altruistically." Quite suddenly, it seemed, the profession fell from its long-accepted pedestal of unexamined autonomy, trust, and social integrity. Medicare and Medicaid labeled hospitals more overtly as "businesses," with charity redefined in terms of losses to the hospital (for example, through inadequate public reimbursement and private insurance payments and bad debts), rather than as private acts of benevolence. Criticism of doctors engaging in so-called "Medicaid mills," together with the fights for higher fees in government programs, demonstrated to the public only too clearly that doctors, collectively, were human beings.

I wrote chapter 12, "Trends in Medical Specialization in the United States," for the 1970 meeting of the American Sociological Association. Specialization in medicine has long been a major research interest of mine—and still is. The structural fragmentation of the American medical profession into specialties is part of the wider public/private policy story of this book. Organized specialties represent differing organizational interests and diffuse professional power across numerous specialty groups. Unbridled specialization has encouraged, perpetuated, and characterized medicine as an economic, expansionary enterprise in the United States—as George Rosen predicted in his classic text on medical specialization, *The Specialization of Medicine with Particular Reference to Ophthalmology* (1944). Specialization and increasing health care costs have long been interconnected.

Chapter 12 reflected continuing concerns among health policy scholars in the United States, including Rosen (whom I knew), Isidore Falk (my mentor), and Michael M. Davis (cited in chapter 12). That concern, still with us, of course, is how to match fragmentation in professional skills and roles with the delivery of efficient, coordinated, and effective service to consumers. How can a medicine comprised of specialties best be organized, and by whom? The answers have varied from time to time, though none has been fully accepted. Davis and Falk envisaged organized, multi-specialty group practices in the private sector, as did leading exponents of the health maintenance organization at the time chapter 12 was written. The chapter shows that I thought future policy about health care was pretty open in 1970 but that there seemed to be a limited set of long-run choices.

Corporate multi-specialist group practices then seemed an obvious step. Quite apart from the imminent failure of the HMO movement in the form in which it was initially envisaged, I had not counted on the continuation of a reimbursement system (in both public and private health insurance) that actually worked *against* organized group practice. In any event, Medicare, Medicaid, and privately organized managed care insurance were to make it politic for doctors to band together in single-specialty rather than multi-specialty practices in order to protect and further their economic and professional interests. Particularly after the backlash against managed care in the 1990s, consumers were also leery of any restrictions on their freedom to go to a specialist (or specialty group) of their choice.

Predictions made about the future tell us much about the time in which they were written. They include at least a dollop of wish fulfillment, and (sometimes) dire predictions aimed at action in whatever the present then is. The context of chapter 13, written in 1986, was an argument (not mine) that since 1963 federal (and some state) government policies to expand the supply of physicians, through financial incentives designed to increase the number of medical students in public and private medical schools, had actually been too successful. The number of doctors involved in patient care rose from 259,000 in 1965 to 423,000 in 1983. Some signs also pointed to a reduced demand for doctors in the future, especially if the lower physician-population ratios of doctors in organizations like Kaiser-Permanente were extended across the population as comprehensive, corporate health care systems proliferated. This seemed more likely in the mindset of the mid-1980s than it has at any time since.

Had the United States overshot the mark in its concern about a doctor shortage in the early 1960s, and was it soaring toward a doctor glut? Eli Ginzberg organized the Cornell University Medical College conference on health policy at which I gave this paper. He titled the resulting publication *From Physician Shortage to Patient Shortage: The Uncertain Future of Medical Practice*—though avowedly somewhat tongue-in-check.

I started my oration on "The Future of the Medical Profession" with equal alarm, enumerating the joys, or rather the lack of joys, involved in being a physician in 1986, before tempering the gloom with a measure of optimism. Again I was not shy at making predictions, however wrong they might turn out to be. I assumed that physicians would be working in bureaucratic settings in a "job," rather than in private practice as small business owners. Yet the reverse has proved to be the case. The market did not create physician practice organizations that offer one-stop supermarkets of specialist services to medical consumers. Instead it created multiple insurance networks. In the early twenty-first century, most doctors work in small-scale private practices and relate to a barrage of insurers. Most patients are left to coordinate their own care, gather up their medical records from disparate sources when they move or change physicians, and struggle with abstruse and scattered medical bills. Doctors and patients do not seem to be any more satisfied with these arrangements—perhaps less—than they were in 1986.

From the perspective of the organized profession, however, new responsibilities were emerging in 1986 as challenges: assuring physician competence, creating standards of practice, and improving doctor-patient communication. Consumerism was in vogue; I speak of the "end of the era of the passive patient." "Professionalism" was also coming to the fore as an agenda on which the profession might build confidence, manage change, assert leadership, and improve the quality of care—if only they could or would.

One last comment about chapters 12 and 13 before moving on to the theme of professional leadership in chapters 14 and 15. In 1970 the medical profession, the image of the doctor, and the gender of its leadership were overwhelmingly male. Indeed it was commonplace to refer to members of all professions as "he," as I did in the original version of chapter 12. Only 10 percent of the entering class of medical schools were women in the early 1960s; but up to a third were in 1985-86. (The proportion is about 50 percent in the early 2000s.) In the 1980s the increase in women was seen as a godsend for keeping standards competitive in the schools, where the number of male applicants was declining. There was some comment at the Ginzberg conference that women tended to work shorter hours than men did at that time, and this might reduce physician demand. However, there was little or no comment from anyone, including me, that in changing its gender-mix American medicine was embarked on an enormous, fundamental sociological change. It was difficult to see the wood for the trees.

Chapter 14, "Professional Competence and Specialty Board Certification (1999)," addresses the topic of physician organizations, or at least one set of them, as private policymakers. The specialty certifying boards are private, professional organizations that prescribe training and give examinations in medical specialties and subspecialties. The twenty-four independent boards are coordinated through the American Board of Medical Specialties, effectively a board of the boards, located in Evanston, Illinois. I had had a number of contacts with the ABMS over the years as part of my research on specialization. Various members, in turn, had read my work. The ABMS had added three public members to its roster in the 1970s, when there was talk of greater engagement with public policy. I was a public member from 1999 through 2006. Chapter 14 is the keynote speech I gave at a conference on professional competence organized by the ABMS in March 1999. The audience consisted largely of representatives of the specialty boards and other members of the medical profession.

The chapter speaks for itself. My tone of concern about the potential for available medical organizations to get their act together had become more urgent. External pressures on professional prerogatives had become more visible, with particular concern about the quality of care. Though specialty certifying boards and their associated specialty societies were obvious organizations for leadership in establishing practice standards as well as those for education and training, they were moving much too slowly. Would the boards just offer more and more subspecialty examinations on demand and become, in effect, a supermarket for credentials, or could they morph into a qualitative force? In more practical terms, would the boards, marked by a ponderous, turf-ridden decision-making process in the 1990s, lose out because of the more rapid actions of new, non-medical groups with quality agendas?

In 1999 it seemed likely that they would. Competition and strife rather than organizational unity and cooperative agendas marked the discussions of representatives from different boards at ABMS meetings—each concerned about their own specialty jurisdiction and organizational autonomy. As an interested observer of—and by then a vested participant in—the processes of specialty control and the exercise of professional responsibility, this was a fascinating time to be a public member of ABMS.

A major problem for the professional organizations of medicine in 1999-2001 (and beyond) was their virtual isolation from what other policy players were doing in pushing for standards, clinical guidelines, outcomes data, audits, and compliance mechanisms in the broader health care system. The medical profession was marginalized in the fields of health management and health services research, and vice versa. At the national health services research meetings of what is now AcademyHealth in June 1999, I argued in favor of a new public ethos for the medical profession, aided by managers and researchers, as an innovative aspect of "research into action," which was the overarching theme of the meeting. Incredulity was the reaction of some of those present—perhaps associating the "medical profession" solely with the self-interested, union-like behavior of the AMA in the 1990s.

Chapter 15, "Public Roles for the Medical Profession in the United States," published in 2001, was my attempt to articulate the argument more clearly. It is not the most gracefully written piece I have done, nor (alas) the easiest to follow. Its basic points are that there is considerable value to all parties, researchers, managers, and physicians, in working together to support the development of a strong medical profession committed to public goals; and that historical accounts of a profession in decline, overtaken (and even swamped) by managers and market, is only one historical interpretation. Histories are rewritten and recast differently in the context of different times. Thinking about twenty-first-century health care should not be imprisoned by historical myths of any kind.

The decline and fall scenario, suggesting a beleaguered, if not defeated, medical profession, reflected (and ratified) assumptions about health policy that prevailed from the late 1970s through the late 1990s. They were not necessarily appropriate for the new century. Policy agendas of patient safety, quality, electronic medical records, consumer participation in medical decision-making, and clinical measurement techniques required at least the cooperation and, in my view, participatory leadership from the medical profession.

In any event, there was actually remarkable change between 2001 and the time I am writing this, 2006. As noted in chapter 15, in 2000 the boards set up an effective task force on competence, and began to move ahead on a quality agenda and to work with other organizations. All twenty-four medical specialty boards have committed themselves to maintenance of certification through career-long assessments of medical knowledge, professionalism, skills, and practice, and have developed programs to do so. Representatives from the ABMS and individual boards work with, and on, quality assessment groups, and vice versa. These efforts, singly and jointly, have emphasized the lack of applicable research into practice performance standards across specialty and subspecialty fields, and the need for an array of national studies in both surgical and non-surgical fields to act as baseline comparisons against which individual physicians and groups can measure and improve their performance. The roles both of research and enhanced clinical information systems are critical in making this movement work.

There are still a lot of hurdles, and a long way to go. Possibly, though, future historians will write about the end of the twentieth century and the beginning of the twenty-first as a resurgence of medical responsibility in public policymaking, targeted at excellence throughout medicine. Possibly not. I have given up predictions.

12

Trends in Medical Specialization in the United States (1970)

Virtually all the attributes and attending problems of American medicine spring from the gigantic technological achievements in medical science in this century that both precipitated and were facilitated by functional specialization. On one hand there are breakthroughs in chemotherapy or organ transplantation; on the other, acute questions of costs, organization, and, particularly, of management and policy in a system that becomes daily more complex, and whose inequities are ever more evident. Technological excellence presses toward increasing specialization; questions of the availability of services demand increasing generalism at all treatment and planning levels. In a nutshell, the old dilemma of specialism is still with us: how to reconcile a professional structure that is designed to advance knowledge and skills with social expectations for service that are less aristocratic, more egalitarian.

Past Trends in Medical Specialization

Specialization in medicine is by no means new. At least seven reputable medical specialties could be identified even in the 1860s; there was already an "undoubted disadvantage of being what is called a 'general practitioner,'" and concern that in the process it would be forgotten that "[t]he patient is a man; his whole organism is before us."[1] The problems as well as the benefits of specializing have been discussed at length in the medical press since the 1870s. One leading medical educator of 100 years ago, emphasizing the need for practically-oriented family practitioners as well as scientific specialists, compared the attending problems of technological advance that were apparent even then to the equally dubious prospect of more efficient forms of highway traffic: "It has often occurred to me, that if steam power should be substituted on common roads for horse power, collisions would be of hourly occurrence."[2] The analogy was that besides intellectual advance through medical techniques something also had to be done about the disadvantages of specialization.

The collisions attending technological advance in medicine have long been evident. Well before World War I there were complaints that the old family doctor was disappearing and that as a result medical care was being inefficiently fragmented. Health care reformer Michael M. Davis, analyzing what he called even then the "disorganization" rather than the organization of medical services, argued in 1916 for compulsory health insurance that would also redesign health services into effective systems—a proposal that may sound current and familiar.[3] At the same time there were proposals for legitimizing medical specialization by developing standards for specialist recognition and practice. Legislative proposals were made for the licensing of surgeons in at least two states in 1914—a measure that would have excluded general practitioners from the operating room. These same issues—of the role of a personal physician, of multi-specialist networks or groups, of public recognition of who is a specialist—have come up again and again in medicine's history as continuing—and current—responses to increasing professional specialization.

Looking at the developing characteristics of specialization in American medicine, some perhaps obvious but important points should be made. The specialties themselves have evolved in response to the particular scientific and intellectual interests of individuals and small groups at particular points in time, rather than to any set plan. Ophthalmology developed around the invention of the ophthalmoscope in the 1850s, radiology on the invention of the X-ray machine at the turn of the twentieth century, pediatrics around individual interest in the care of the child, which was reinforced by the maternal and child welfare movement of the early 1900s, and so on. And the process continues. In the early 1970s, fields such as nuclear medicine, hand surgery, and pediatric surgery are still seeking professional recognition. There has been no one master strategy for the development of a medical profession stratified into specialties.

It is true that a committee of the American Medical Association set out in 1920 a list of approved special fields.[4] This list, appropriately expanded, formed the basis on which the twenty existing [in 1970] specialty certifying boards in medicine were established, chiefly in the 1930s. But there has been no real attempt within the profession to decide what its internal balance should be—in terms, for example, of the proportion of generalists to specialists, or the relative number of surgical specialists. American physicians have been remarkably free to choose their specialty and practice area, and to sub-specialize. Authority to choose a specialty has been decentralized to individuals, delineation of specialty training to relatively autonomous specialist associations. From the profession's point of view, specialization has been seen in the past as the intellectual prerogative of physicians, not as a framework for developing a specialized service industry.

As part of this process (and, indeed, its rationale for development and the reason for its success), specialization grew around patterns of professional organization that were designed not for a multi-specialty medical care system, but for solo general practitioners. The industrial mass production worker was not expected to know how to put together a whole car. The physician, in contrast, has clung until very recently to the concept that every physician is a "generalist," with specialization as a refinement of a general education, and not a fraction of it. Medical school curricula are only now being modified to reflect specialized tracks and interests. And the medical licensing system still assumes that every physician is a generalist. These attitudes are changing. It should be noted, though, that such change lags far behind the technological actualities.

Finally, in reviewing general characteristics of professionalization, it should be stressed that the structures of medical specialism have been largely determined by professional decisions, not by an organizational rationale or by public definition. A market has certainly operated. It has been a market, however, of excess demand, in which a monopoly profession has controlled physician supply, and restricted other aspects of competition (such as competitive fees and advertising). Practice in large partnerships or health service organizations are still the exception, not the rule. Instead of specialization leading to the logical corollary of coordinated practice systems, the solo general practitioner was largely replaced by the solo or small partnership specialist.

Proliferation of Specialties

The result of this long, largely chaotic process has been the proliferation of specialty identities, functions, and interests. Until recently the American Medical Association recognized thirty-four different specialties in its directory listings; but even this number of divisions proved misleading and insufficient. In 1970, the Association revised its format to include an array of sixty-three specialties. The medical student in considering the future has a plethora of choices. His/her choices lie, moreover, in areas that differ from one another to the extent of being virtually different careers: allergy or therapeutic radiology; plastic surgery or child psychiatry; hematology or aviation medicine; physical medicine or ophthalmology; forensic pathology or family practice. While physicians (and the public at large) continue to regard themselves as members of one profession, conforming to a set of common professional norms, the term "medicine" has become an umbrella for the sheltering of a variety of disciplines.

What is new is not the process and basic problems of specialization but its cumulative effect. As specialty has followed specialty in the advancement of knowledge and pursuit of excellence, as groups of specialists in new fields have formed associations, developed educational programs, and aspired (in the normal process of professionalization) to their own certifying examinations, the stratification of the medical profession has become ever more complex. Who is to say how many specialty divisions should be recognized? What is likely to determine the number of physicians in each specialty?

In the past these questions have been answered within the medical profession as part of a profession's presumed responsibility to determine education and practice standards. Today, in an era of anxiety over the availability and costs of health services, these are also questions of public interest. Costs alone demand it. The American public spent nearly $12 billion on physician services in 1969, the equivalent of $58 a head for every member of the population.[5] Per capita physician expenditures are projected to at least $101 in 1975 and could reach $156 in 1980.[6] This large sum may be seen as a realistic gesture of appreciation of the value of medical care in modern society—a value that is in turn the product of technological specialization. On the other hand, the concept of value itself locks the medical profession into the public domain. If medical care has become sufficiently valuable to be regarded as a necessary service for the whole population—and there is abundant evidence from all sides that health services are now generally so regarded—then the specialty distributions of its major profession are of general concern.

Current Trends in Specialization

In 1968 there were 317,000 physicians in the United States. Of these, 21 percent described themselves as general practitioners; the remaining 79 percent were divided among the various specialties.[7] As far as can be seen, the proportion of general practitioners has been declining rapidly; general practitioners were still in the majority in the early 1950s. But the statement has to be tentative, since one of the characteristics of the American medical system, unlike European medical systems, is that there is still no definitive description of a "general practitioner" or a "specialist." There are, indeed, the specialty certifying boards, each of which issues its own certificates; but there is no compulsion for physicians to take such certification, nor to limit themselves to the boards' descriptions. Physicians may decide to call themselves specialists in any field, irrespective of whether they have appropriate or sufficient graduate training according to the definitions of the certifying agencies. There is thus an initial question of how appropriate is the specialist labeling process.

The self-classification system used by the American Medical Association is, however, the only source of available information on what physicians do. Bearing in mind that from time to time some of the trends may reflect changes in perception rather than job description (for example, a general-practitioner surgeon might call himself a general practitioner on one occasion, a general surgeon on another, and can now call himself an abdominal surgeon), certain observations can be made of apparent trends in specialization. The proportion of physicians in the surgical specialties has been rising. In 1931 only 10 percent of physicians practiced in fields characterized as surgical specialties—general surgery and related specialties, orthopedic surgery, ophthalmology, otolaryngology, obstetrics/gynecology, urology, anesthesiology; the proportion had risen to 26 percent in 1960, to over 30 percent in 1968.[8] In short, nearly one out of every three physicians in the United States is in a field that involves surgery; a number of general practitioners are doing some surgery as well. This increase promises, moreover, to continue. Of all the American graduates in first year resident and fellowship programs in 1968, over 40 percent were in surgical specialties.[9]

In some of the components of the specialties it appears, moreover, that the trends are toward fairly substantial changes. In orthopedic surgery, for example, there are at present 7,000 specialists in practice and another 1,800 in training.[10] There are, in contrast, only about 800 physicians in residency training positions for general practice, and many of these are foreign medical graduates who may not contribute to this country's future manpower pool. Massive infusions of students into family practice will be needed to stem that field's proportional decline. There are a number of other interesting features of recent specialty trends. For example, the number of psychiatrists has doubled since 1960; the number of physicians in the medical [rather than surgical] specialties has been steadily increasing. Nevertheless, the outstanding features of current trends in the United States are the ones remarked: the decline of general practice and the substantial and continuing focus on surgery.

Specialist Manpower Policy Needed

The question must arise: Is this balance appropriate? But the next question must be, appropriate to what? And the next still, who is to make the estimations? And here is the nub of the issue of professional development versus service expectations. From the service point of view, no adequate, detailed manpower projections by specialty yet exist, nationally, regionally, or by area. A number of specialist and service groups have made projections for staffing needs in their own fields,[11] but as yet there is no specialist manpower policy in the form of a master plan. Some such policy is becoming increasingly necessary as a basis for modification of specialist trends—for, in at least the instances of general practice and surgical specialties, there is evidence that the pressures of specialization are running counter to the expressed statements of need for services from both the public and the medical profession.

The importance of primary medical care in a specialist system has been emphasized again and again. Prestigious professional committees, including the Millis Commission[12] and the Willard Committee[13] in 1966, have stressed the desirability of encouraging the development of generalist physicians. And more recently primary care has appeared as a basic feature of several current suggestions for reforming health care programs under public auspices.[14] Yet, such recommendations have had little influence over the choices made by individual physicians; the number of generalists has decreased.

Meanwhile, entry into surgical specialties has continued at a high rate—even though there has been no indication of shortages in surgical fields that would make their current expansion a priority over other specialties. Not only are there twice as many surgeons but twice as much surgery is done in an average

American city than in an English city, with no immediately apparent benefits.[15] Even within the United States, self-contained health service systems—the large prepaid groups—include only half as many surgeons proportionally as are generally available.[16] Indeed, if the specialty distributions of the prepaid group practices were extended to the population at large there would be a glut of surgeons, which would get worse as more poured out of their existing training posts. At the same time there would be acute shortages of generalists and of physicians in various other fields, most notably otolaryngology and physical medicine.

Specialism and Maldistribution Encouraged

These shortages probably now exist. They are, however, camouflaged in the complex tangles of the present health care system, and in the assumption that free choice of specialty is part of the baggage of professionalism. The fresh graduate has the privilege of choosing a specialist internship and residency in virtually any field he/she chooses, for there are far more approved training positions in hospitals available each year than are filled. As a result, the structure of training posts represents two influences: the desire of a hospital to offer training in a particular specialty (the hospital's perception of need) and the desire of the student for that kind of training (the student's perception of interest). These two are joined by a third influence: the unwillingness of the AMA and its residency review committees to use the process of accrediting training posts deliberately as a means of influencing future manpower distributions. As a result, there are no barriers to entering the specialties such as exist, for example, at the level of entering medical school.

Such relative freedom continues. Once trained, the specialist may take examinations by the appropriate specialty certifying board. In the past some of the boards have had apparently exclusionary policies, in order to keep standards and prestige at a high level. But the boards—which have themselves had a major influence on the structure of residency training through the specification of educational requirements—have never acknowledged a composite manpower planning function. Again, moreover, certification is not necessary for specialist practice, although it is desirable for gaining the privilege of a hospital staff appointment.

As the next step, the physician may still move where he or she wishes and set up practice without permission (except for a general medical license) from any planning agency. Nor does the physician, unlike many less fortunate persons in other professions, have to seek a job opportunity. An increasing number of physicians are now taking salaried positions in hospitals (30,000, or as many as 11 percent of trained physicians were in such posts in 1968).[17] Over and above this, however, hospitals have not—at least overtly—used their own considerable power of granting or withholding staff privileges to develop balanced community staffing patterns.

Finally, the physician is not constrained by formal patterns of patient referral and consultation that forbid all physicians except general practitioners to accept walk-in patients from the street, and limit the specialist role to one of secondary consultation to the generalist. The specialist may openly compete with general practitioners, or may begin with general practice and abandon it as his specialist practice rises. Thus general practice has been in a relatively weak position; the professional structures themselves have encouraged specialism over generalism. This lack of a formally recognized primary and secondary function for general practitioners and specialists has been a major reason for the general practitioners' much more rapid decline in the United States than in countries such as Britain or Canada where traditional professional practice patterns have fortified the role of the generalist as the focus for primary care. It goes without saying that the reinvention of primary practice as a pivot of medical care in this country also rests on the establishment of recognized primary and referral functions.

There is no evidence to suggest that reliance on established professional structures alone will lead to modified specialty distributions in the future, at least in the absence of major changes in the health delivery system. The professional trends are toward the further decline of generalism (even allowing for the approval of a specialty certifying board for family practitioners in 1969), and continuing maldistributions among other specialties.

Prospects for the Future

These trends give rise to serious questions about specialist manpower production and policies. This country seems destined to have a health service system or "industry" that is increasingly financed through public funds, fed by a professional educational structure that is producing an inappropriate supply of physicians. Specialist manpower policies raise future, if not present, issues of public and professional accountability.

It is true that the health care system could impose its own controls over the desired number and distribution of physicians through, for example, the widespread development of health maintenance organizations, each of which would have its own planned complement of physicians. In this event, evidence of shortages in some specialties would appear through expressed demand—for example, through substantially higher incomes for physiatrists or family physicians than general surgeons, and through extensive advertising for physicians in certain specialties to join communities, partnerships, groups, or hospital staffs. Alternatively there might be a physician excess in some specialties, represented in insufficient income, the impossibility of securing a hospital appointment, denial of specialist certification, or an excess of applicants over specialist training posts. Physicians would thereby be obliged to change their specialty, to move, or even to emigrate, much as is now the case in university and high school teaching in some areas. But such organizational controls are as yet in the future.

Meanwhile, as has been remarked, the structure of health services in this country does not yet allow for effective market regulation of the supply of specialists. The diffuse, private system of medical care is sufficiently elastic to support increased numbers of physicians (and indeed other health professionals), even in specialties already reasonably staffed by the standards of closed-staff delivery systems. Despite the relatively large proportion of surgeons in the United States, surgical incomes remain so high that they may well be a decisive factor in encouraging new graduates into surgical specialties. A national health insurance scheme could seek to change the balance of incomes through control of fees for services; general practitioners could, for example, be given much larger office fees than, say, ophthalmologists. In Britain, the National Health Service performed the major feat of paying at least all specialists at a standard scale; but it may be noted that this was only one measure of control over the balance of specialties. Such an approach in the United States is, however, politically unlikely.

Specialist Manpower Planning

If redistributions of specialists—specialist manpower planning—are to be seriously contemplated, other routes will prove more realistic. The effect of a widespread development of health maintenance organizations has been mentioned. But specialist distributions could also be regulated through limiting the number of available positions offered for training in each specialty (and, indeed, in each geographical region); through a system of financial and other inducements for training in needed specialty areas; through certification or licensing up to a specified numerical ceiling in each specialty; and through other measures. It may be noted in passing that some of these suggestions are modifications of controls over the number of physicians that have been exerted with marked effect by organized medicine in the past at the level of entry of students into the medical profession; so far, however, they have not been used to regulate the specialties.

This distinction between entry into medical school and entry into a specialty should be stressed. It is one of the oddities of the continuing attitude that medicine is one discipline as well as one profession that inordinate attention has been paid to the overall number of physicians but very little to their subsequent distribution. The shortage of physicians has become a familiar byword, and there is a recognized policy of medical student expansion, stimulated by federal funding. Through the Health Manpower Act of 1968 and through active encouragement from the major professional organizations of medicine—notably the AMA and the Association of American Medical Colleges—the number of medical students is being rapidly increased.[18] There is little indication, however, that the additional recruits will of themselves choose different career patterns from their predecessors. Is the policy really meant to be one of producing more researchers, surgeons, and super-specialists?

In two specialties, psychiatry and clinical anesthesiology, limited federal funds have been made available for scholarships or grants for training. There are now also persuasive proposals for federal grants to encourage physicians to choose family practice. And resolutions have come up regularly (but unsuccessfully) to the AMA House of Delegates that all physicians should have a period in general practice before being allowed specialist recognition. But such moves are as yet embryonic. In terms of control over medical specialty distributions, there is a chicken and the egg situation. Which will come first—major changes in the organization of medical practice, or increased pressures from Washington to modify the specialist training system, if only to justify substantial federal support of medical schools for teaching at the undergraduate level? The first is possible given a scheme of national health insurance directed toward comprehensive local health care systems. In the absence of such national health insurance, the second is more likely.

To spell out what patterns of medical specialization will be in ten or twenty years requires a crystal ball rather than an analysis of trends; for the physician manpower situation, like other aspects of medical care, is volatile. Relatively little change may be observed in the next two decades. Alternatively, there could be rapid transition from a system that is now largely professionally regulated and diffuse, to one that has considerable governmental influence and is much more highly organized. And there are many other intervening possibilities.

Potential Readjustments

Some readjustment of existing specialty trends does, however, seem inevitable. Moreover, in the future, trends in medical specialization will depend increasingly on deliberate actions taken from outside rather than inside the medical profession. Taking the long view, there is a relatively limited selection of ways in which adjustments may be made.

First, it seems likely that closed-staff health service systems will develop in the United States, replacing the present, largely individualized practice system. These systems could take a variety of forms. They could be groups or networks of physicians who agree to contract for services with a third party payer; more highly-organized group practices or partnerships working as an integral part of a self-sustaining health service system; or hospital medical staffs with an expanded role in the community, with joint medical staffs of area hospitals acting as a medical staff planning unit. Even without national health insurance, the development of such networks would be accelerated through the incorporation of the idea of health maintenance organizations into Medicare and into any reforms or expansion of Medicaid.

Within these closed-staff networks there will be specialty distributions with some significant differences from existing national patterns. In particular one would expect a greater concentration of physicians in preventive medicine—in-

cluding physiatry, pediatrics, internal medicine, obstetrics, family medicine—
and relatively fewer surgeons. In networks that build medical care patterns
around the primary physician, or the primary care team, primary physicians
may represent as much as 50 percent of all physicians. This latter prospect is
not as unrealistic as it may appear, for to some unknown extent, the primary
care function may be mandated. For example, should a national health insurance
program require each person to have a personal physician, with specialist care
only to be given on the advice of that physician, there would undoubtedly be
many physicians who now label themselves specialists who would accept an
increased primary function. Whether their training is appropriate for such a
function is another question, and one that stresses the importance of the current
residency training systems.

Any general appearance of closed-staff medical systems would have certain other effects. The range of incomes among specialists would be narrowed
(and perhaps even reversed), with incentives for physicians to choose certain
specialties over others. At the same time the number of career opportunities
available to physicians would be drastically reduced, particularly in the more
popular specialties. This factor would have some geographical implications.
As in England, for example, the trained neurological surgeon might find no
available opening in a system or on a hospital staff in his preferred practice
area, and would thus gravitate toward another area. There would also be obvious implications for specialty choice, in terms of both income and geography.
A candidate might, for example, choose family medicine rather than a pediatric subspecialty knowing that career chances in the former were much more
promising than in the latter.

Incentives in the Specialist Training System

Either parallel with or independent of the growth of closed-staff health care
systems, direct efforts will be made to provide incentives in the specialist training system. The following are suggested.

Federal or third-party subsidies for graduate medical education may be
made available. This would be logical in a national insurance scheme that
separated training costs from patient care reimbursement methods. Hospitals
with residency programs would be expected to justify their training programs
to a national or regional medical planning unit, which would decide which
types of residencies to support. Training costs would not be reimbursed in
unapproved institutions.

Subsidies could apply to all types of graduate medical education. Alternatively, they could be limited to defined "needy" specialties such as family
practice in an effort to attract additional applicants. The most probable course
of events is for the latter to develop first. In the long run, however, government
subsidy of all approved training at the graduate level is foreseen as the logical
extension of government support at the undergraduate level, and of university

responsibility for graduate education. The subsidies themselves could be in the form of direct fellowships to students, to be paid with respect to education in approved teaching programs.

Concurrently or alternatively, direct federal grants may be made to medical schools to develop centers of excellence in certain specialties (and geographical areas) through a network of affiliated hospitals, with the universities responsible for house staff stipends. The grants mechanism would merely accelerate the existing trend toward concentrating graduate medical education in university-affiliated hospitals, and would extend the accepted use of federal grants. Under this system each university would be expected to justify for reimbursement its educational policies and specialist distributions. Some university networks might wish to limit or at least focus their contribution to training in selected areas. Under either system, scholarships, grants, or loans might be made to individual students for an eight- or nine-year training period, from the beginning of medical school to the end of specialist training, perhaps contingent on choice of specialist area. But in any event, there will need to be increased advisory services on specialty choice for undergraduate medical students in the light of alternative career expectations.

None of these suggestions would negate the important role of professional accreditation of training posts and specification by professional groups of appropriate patterns and standards of specialist education. Indeed the number and location of residencies could be regulated through exercise of the professions' accrediting machinery of residency approval. At its most draconian, this could drastically reduce training opportunities in some specialties, or reallocate the opportunity for training in well-filled and less-filled specialties, and in different types of institutions. Such a policy may be the ultimate outcome of a professional Commission on Medical Education, such as that being proposed by the AMA, the Association of American Medical Colleges, and related professional groups. It is suggested here, however, in light of past developments in undergraduate medical education, that the most appropriate (and most needed) role for professional organizations relates to questions of education and competence rather than of numerical production; and that qualitative and quantitative considerations are best divorced.

In brief, and on the basis of the developing characteristics of American medicine, logic suggests: specification of the number of specialists demanded at any one time as the sum of recruitment patterns by a network of local health systems or organizations; translation of these specifications into action through a national physician manpower committee responsible for federal funding of specialist training positions; increased responsibility for specialist training (and increased specialization of educational function in this area) by medical schools; and increasing the importance of professional standards of certification in defining (and probably also relicensing) specialists, and in guaranteeing the highest degree of competence to the public.

Practical Realities

The magnitude of administrative, professional, and even legal changes implicit in the logic should not, however, be underrated. All of these possibilities beg the question of whether accurate specialist predictions can be made in a technological environment that is changing so quickly, and in a sociopolitical environment whose norms are also subject to radical change. Accurate long-range predictions of the demand for medical specialists will probably always be impossible. Nor is this the sum of expected difficulties. If specialist educational policies are developed independently of hospital service expectations, hospitals will be forced to explore alternative means of staffing for the substantial services that are now given by interns and residents. Detailed research still needs to be done on career choice, attitudes, and expectations among student physicians, on the roles and workloads of hospital residents, and on the effect of specialist-mix in different practice situations. Above all is the attitudinal jump necessary in the medical profession to reconcile the gap between an educational structure geared to produce technological excellence with much that is humble in community health needs and irrelevant to the scientific situation—problems of poverty, nutrition, housing, behavior.

In all of these respects, however, difficulties can be overcome. Specialty manpower decisions can be made, on the basis of defined service needs, however inaccurate or crude the actual projections; and can, to a greater or lesser extent, be implemented. Hospital staffing patterns will be adjusted. More will be learned about specialist roles and functions, and this knowledge will be utilized in developing specialty manpower projections at national, regional, and local levels. Professional attitudes to patterns of physician supply and education have changed rapidly and radically in the past, when the situation has demanded: most notably in the revolution made in undergraduate medical education between 1905 and 1910, and again in the development of specialist education and certification in the 1930s. In both cases there were social as well as professional pressures for change: in the earlier period, economic incentives to reduce the large number of physicians; in the second, the equally compelling pressures of the Great Depression. A third period of radical education and manpower reform may be foreseen in the 1970s or 1980s in response to organizational and economic pressures, whether through national health insurance or government financing of medical education.

In terms of the broad framework of specialization with which this paper started, the issues are clear. If goals of reasonable access to health services are to be achieved in the United States, expressed through appropriate legislation, the trends of specialization within the medical profession will be changed. In the future trends in medical specialization will depend on the initiative of planning groups and service organizations, including physicians and non-physicians, rather than on the scattered decisions of 300,000 individuals.

This chapter was presented at the sixty-fifth annual meeting of the American Sociological Association, Washington, D.C., September 3, 1970, and was published as "Trends in Medical Specialization in the United States," *Inquiry*, 1971, VIII, 1: 9-19. It formed part of a research series on the development of specialization in medicine, supported by Grant # HS 00374 from the National Center for Health Services Research and Development, and developed in my book, *American Medicine and the Public Interest* (New Haven: Yale University Press, 1971).

Notes

1. Henry D. Noyes, "Specialties in Medicine." Read before the American Ophthalmological Society, New York, June 1865 (privately printed). The specialties were nervous diseases, eye and ear diseases, diseases of the throat, diseases of the skin, chest diseases, venereal diseases, midwifery.
2. Henry J. Bigelow, *Medical Education in America* (Cambridge: 1871): 6.
3. Michael M. Davis, Jr. "Organization of Medical Service." *American Labor Legislation Review* 6 (1916): 16-20.
4. Louis B. Wilson, "Report of Committee on Graduate Medical Education." *American Medical Association Bulletin* 14 (1920): 58-67.
5. Barbara S. Cooper and Mary F. McGee, "Health Care Outlays for the Young, Intermediate, and Older Age Groups." *Research and Statistics Note* (Social Security Administration, October 23, 1970).
6. Dorothy P. Rice and Mary F. McGee, "Projections of National Health Expenditures, 1975 and 1980." Ibid., October 30, 1970.
7. J. N. Haug, G. A. Roback, C. N. Theodore, and B. E. Balfe, *Distribution of Physicians, Hospitals and Hospital Beds in the U.S., 1968* (Chicago: American Medical Association, 1970): 13.
8. There were 91,932 physicians active in the surgical specialties (including anesthesiology) in 1968, out of a total pool of physicians in active practice of 298,401. Ibid.: 39.
9. Of 8,573 graduates of U.S. and Canadian medical schools who were in approved first-year residencies in American hospitals in 1968—that is, virtually one complete cohort of American physicians—3,684 were being trained in surgical specialties. See John D. Nunemaker, Willard V. Thompson, George Mixter, Ike Mayeda, and Rose Tracy, "Annual Report on Graduate Medical Education in the United States." *Journal of the American Medical Association* 210 (1969): 1-30, Table 11A.
10. Haug et al., op. cit.: 39.
11. See J. H. Knowles, "The Quantity and Quality of Medical Manpower: A Review of Medicine's Current Efforts." *Journal of Medical Education* 44 (1969): 81-118.
12. *The Graduate Education of Physicians*. Report of the Citizens Commission on Graduate Medical Education commissioned by the American Medical Association, Chicago, 1966.
13. *Meeting the Challenge of Family Practice*. Report of the Ad Hoc Committee on Education for Family Practice of the Council on Medical Education, American Medical Association, Chicago, 1966.
14. For example, the Griffiths bill for national health insurance (H.R. 15779, 91st Congress) specifies both primary and specialist physician services. The Health Security proposals sponsored by Senator Edward Kennedy (S. 4297, 91st Congress) also assume the establishment of qualifications for specialists in defined fields, and

the provision of appropriate patterns of referral between primary and specialist consultative care. A recent report of the staff of the Senate Finance Committee has also recommended that all Medicaid recipients be required to designate a primary physician to end "doctor shopping" by recipients. *Medicare and Medicaid, Problems, Issues and Alternatives.* Committee Print, 91st Congress, 1st session, February 9, 1970: 23.

15. See John P. Bunker, "Surgical Manpower, A Comparison of Operations and Surgeons in the United States and England and Wales." *New England Journal of Medicine* 282 (1970): 135.

16. A survey of six prepaid medical groups in 1967 indicated that for general surgery and its subspecialties alone between six or seven physicians were sufficient for an enrolled population of 100,000; in the same year for the country at large (excluding interns and residents) there were over thirteen physicians in general surgery and its subspecialties (neurological, plastic and thoracic surgery) for a population of 100,000. See *Health Manpower, Perspective: 1967.* U.S. Department of Health, Education, and Welfare, PHS publication #1667, 1967, Appendix Table 6: 75; and J. N. Haug and G. A. Roback, *Distribution of Physicians, Hospitals, and Hospital Beds in the United States, 1967* (American Medical Association, 1968): Table 1.

17. Haug et al., op. cit. 1970: 39.

18. The first-year enrollment in medical schools included 8,512 students in the academic year 1959-60; the number rose to 9,043 in 1964-65 and to 10,514 in 1969-70. Projected figures are for a first-year enrollment of 13,622 in 1974-75. "Medical Education in the United States." *Journal of the American Medical Association* 214 (1970): 1512-13.

13

The Future of the Medical Profession (1986)

Everywhere there are signs of constriction on traditional professional prerogatives: in high malpractice insurance rates, derived from huge settlements in the
courts, which reflect, in turn, a reservoir of public skepticism about the standards
and motives of medical professionals; in the frenetic growth of health care organizations, in which physicians are subordinate to highly-paid executives; in
the willingness of government to force change on medical practice and medical
education through Medicare and Medicaid; in the growth of consumer self-help
groups; and in the lay and business leadership of major disease intervention
programs for alcoholism, stress reduction, counseling, and weight control. The
physician's role seems, somehow, diminished. It is easy to sketch a scenario of
a profession in decline; to express concern about the quality, socioeconomic
mix, evolving attitudes, and motivations of students entering the pipeline in the
1980s; and to foresee a generation of disaffected medical cynics, carrying large
debts and unfulfilled expectations.

However, as in most of life, the picture is more complicated, ambivalent,
contingency-ridden, and subject to unexpected changes than any simple scenario
can suggest. There is not one future for the medical profession but a kaleidoscope
of possible developments. Even simple generalizations are difficult to make.
For example, the accepted notion of professional dominance—the physician's
autonomy in making clinical decisions, controlling medical resources, and
practicing as (and where) he or she thinks fit—is clearly weakened in the 1980s.[1]
Nevertheless, although the profession may lose power in one area, it may gain
power in another. Thus it is not enough to talk about the declining authority of
the medical profession without substantial qualification, including increased
opportunities for physicians to become managers and negotiators within health
care systems.

The theme of this chapter is that we are moving, awkwardly, but profoundly
and permanently, toward new definitions of the "medical profession" and
"professionalism" in the late twentieth century; toward fundamental shifts in
assumptions; and toward rearticulated roles for professional organizations.

Indeed, what is exciting about the next twenty years is the growing need—indeed, demand—for a new frame of reference in which to assess contemporary changes. The professional snake is shedding its skin. From the prospect of the late 1980s, the metamorphosis—the clean lines of the new order—is impossible to predict but there are hints, apparent in the pressures now being imposed upon professional behavior and roles, in the sociocultural environment of medicine, and in physicians' reactions to them. Here, I shall focus on three broad areas of change: (1) the trend toward organized and supervised practice of physicians; (2) the appearance of the articulate patient, in roles as diverse as a purchaser, a consumer of care, and a partner in medical treatment decisions; (3) challenges to the underlying cognitive and structural bases of medicine, as symbolized in the structure of medical specialties and in the educational milieu in which doctors are trained.

I do not intend to engage in detailed analysis of changes in different areas; rather, I seek to find patterns across these disparate areas that suggest specific changes in medicine as a profession. I will then return to the more general questions subsumed in my charge. What are the most likely futures for the medical profession and its institutions? How is the profession to view itself? And how will it be viewed? Since medicine has numerous possible futures, depending on decisions and events across an interdependent matrix of variables, it makes little sense to describe changes in a single, straightforward narrative. Thus, I will list my specific, illustrative observations as if each were, indeed, a cell within a larger matrix.

Supervised and Corporate Practice

1. Physicians in the 1980s are rushing toward practice in organizations: group medical practices, health maintenance organizations (HMOs), preferred provider organizations (PPOs), managed health care systems. Although opinions vary as to how much of the population will be served by HMOs within ten years (probably 20-40 percent of the population), most other individuals will also be served by physicians working in organized practice arrangements, including group practice and independent practice associations. Between 1980 and 1984 alone, there was a 44 percent increase in the number of identified group practices in the United States.[2]

The movement of physicians to organized arrangements will continue, pressured by the growth of organized payment arrangements (HMOs, PPOs) that require physician practice organizations of some sort; by the double economic whammy of declining visits to physician offices and hospitals and competition from an increasing pool of physicians; and by the convenience and emerging convention of a corporate environment as the appropriate place for practice. There is little future for physicians outside of practice systems, except perhaps on the fringes of medicine or in highly specialized activities. New definitions of the medical "profession," including codes of professional ethics, have to assume that the average physician's work and behavior are conditioned by organized, bureaucratic workplace arrangements.

2. The successful medical practice organization in the United States is business-oriented and highly sensitive to external organizational, economic, and political environments. A former president of the American Group Practice Association recently told an audience of group practice physicians that, "your success in the future will depend upon your ability to raise capital, the strength of your management, and your ability to do good, competent marketing. Growth will be a part of that capitalization and your ability to develop and market new services."[3] Traditional discussions within medicine, articulated most clearly in the 1930s, assumed that the notion of a "profession" is separate from and antagonistic to that of "commerce": The former is altruistic; the latter is driven purely by self-interest. This rhetoric has been useful in defining medicine as a profession with at least some public responsibilities, even though private, fee-for-service practice has long distinguished physicians as the proprietors of small service businesses. Present-day trends toward overt commercial practices within medicine demand an adjustment of the rhetoric, at least. Since the old rhetoric suggested that commerce corrupts ideals, it is important for professional organizations to articulate appropriate patterns of professional behavior that are free from the old dichotomous beliefs; in short, to replace or reinvent the rhetoric in terms that reflect today's practice pressures. If the notion of professionalism is to survive, it needs a new primer of etiquette. What are the acceptable and unacceptable modes of behavior that distinguish the term "professional" in the late twentieth century?

3. The trend toward more comprehensive patient care within organizations parallels a potentially widespread move to pay for physician services by capitation. Administration calls for capitation payments through Medicare,[4] which, if implemented, will have as profound an effect on physician practice patterns as DRGs have on hospital care. Notably, multi-specialist group practice will be encouraged and perhaps become the norm; physician groups or networks will have a direct incentive to evaluate the distribution of costs and resources across the specialty fields encompassed in the services they offer collectively; and the capitation fee system will provide a vehicle for external monitoring of performance and a need to justify practice-specific behavior by physicians. Under Medicare capitation, congressional committees would need to assure themselves that patients were not being shortchanged or given inferior care. Subscribers would benefit from information on comparative services given by different groups for the same capitation fee. Moreover, in a system dominated by organized groups, all physician groups in an area would have a collective interest in presenting a combined front to Medicare agencies or their agents in renegotiating the capitation fee. Thus, professional skills will increasingly require negotiating and public relations skills by the practice corporations as a whole and an awareness of individual physician behavior and external incentives

and controls by physicians within the groups. Resistance to external regulation will, in the long run, be self-defeating.

4. Medical group practices traditionally have not developed tight self-policing mechanisms over their own physicians.[5] However, peer review organizations as well as major hospitals have begun to monitor physician behavior in terms of costs and benefits, identifying the relative profitability of individual practice patterns to the institutions, and designating individual physicians as money-raisers or money-losers. For example, the University Hospital of Cleveland was featured in a recent cover story of a major health management journal for its "manufacturing style management organization similar to those used in automobile plants,"[6] based on productivity. General managers are expected to step in if a physician orders too many tests and to keep watch on physicians who attract a large number of lawsuits.

One organizational model for the future is balanced confrontation; that is, sharper physician/hospital or physician/health system conflicts, pitting managers against both individual physicians and physician organizations. However, hospitals have their own problems and they no longer form the single, natural, organizational center of the health care system. A more interesting possibility is the development of coalitions of interest between health care organizations and medical groups, with each side responsible for its own sphere of operations, held in tension by mutually reinforcing goals: the survival and prosperity of a health care system, challenged from without by competing systems, payer groups, and public and private regulation. This model requires the development of well-run physician practices (corporations) that are able to develop organizational policies and exert management authority over their physician members. It remains to be seen whether the medical profession will be able to see the benefits of self-organization and self-policing in corporate units—either as freestanding units with negotiated relationships with independent health care corporations, or as subsidiary units of health care systems.

5. I do not see the future health care system dominated by a few huge national corporations. Perhaps no more than 35 percent of all hospitals will be part of chains by 1990.[7] However, at the local level, for example, within a city, it seems increasingly likely that health care will be carved up among a relatively small number of organized systems, some of which will be part of larger chains. As the physician marketplace becomes, in effect, a closed system of competing units, the doctor's professional allegiance will be to a health care organization. The role of local medical societies may become either less or more important: less, if corporations meet physicians' needs; more, in climates of general physician dissatisfaction.

6. The physician of the future will be able to practice because he/she holds a "job." The job will be sought by advertisement, a recruitment firm, or the use of formal and informal networks (such as referral of residents by trusted evaluators in specific teaching programs). The individual will be recruited through competition. Significantly, he/she will be assessed not only on technical and

behavioral skills but on conformance to the prevailing corporate "style," corporate goals, and corporate ethos. Medical students and medical residents will need to be sophisticated readers of the job market and be aware of divergent corporate expectations.

7. Supervised medical practice by external agencies will continue: through government (through peer review organizations and other mechanisms), through health care organizations (via management information systems and other controlling mechanisms), through other insurance intermediaries, and through fourth parties, notably employers. Employers are already intervening in physician decision-making through requirements for hospital utilization reviews and second surgical opinions. In one study of 1,185 companies in 1984, 40 percent reported that they required retrospective hospital utilization review, 34 percent required concurrent review, 25 percent required preadmission review, and 28 percent mandated a second surgical opinion.[8]

Large physician groups may be able to counter some of the supervision and control by providing alternative self-policing mechanisms. Indeed, in the long run, attempts by outside agencies to establish detailed practice norms (and to enforce them) may become both economically meaningless and functionally self-defeating. Regulation assumes that practice can be standardized—hence DRGs. However, medicine is not infinitely reducible to standards of measurement. Indeed, in many chronic diseases we may see increased variety in practice style in different settings, rather than increased conformity. Where responsible physician organizations are recognized, regulation over practice may be delegated to these in the future—provided such organizations are in place—leaving, as external controls, cost limits and patient satisfaction measures. Large-scale organizations may thus imply a wider collective responsibility by professional groups for professional standards in the future.

8. Supervised and corporate practice represents a significant and lasting change in the American medical profession, bringing both problems and opportunities in its wake. It is easier to see the problems than the opportunities because: supervised and organized practice represents a shift in the traditional professional doctrines of American medicine, which have long emphasized individual autonomy in practice and distrust of the "corporate practice of medicine;" the shifts have been engineered by forces external to the medical profession, thus threatening the control of medicine by its own national professional organizations; and perhaps of most significance, these shifts coincide with other major challenges to medicine in the late twentieth century, creating a combined sense of powerlessness, onslaught, and doom within the medical profession. Such challenges include the increasing physician supply and changes in the formal social regulation of professions as trades, including the role of the Federal Trade Commission and antitrust regulation.[9]

Even more central to the future role of the medical profession are the overlapping changes in the behavioral and cognitive aspects of medicine, suggested in the next two sections; that is, in the doctor-patient relationship, and in the structure and meaning of medicine. These combined pressures mask the opportunities inherent in changing organizational forms; opportunities, that is, both for individual and for collective professional authority.

Public Distrust and Patient Power

9. The basic tenets of the medical profession have come under increasing criticism in the past decade inside, as well as outside, the medical profession. Medicine's most venerable icon, the Hippocratic Oath, is openly criticized at medical meetings in the 1980s as inappropriate and outdated: for example, by giving paternalistic power to physicians over patients, by excluding a social role for physicians, and by implying that interventionist treatment is always better than doing nothing.[10]

10. Concerns about physician incompetence and the ability of the profession to police itself—at least, as yet—are commonplace. Medical licensing boards are criticized as understaffed and as tending to work in isolation from each other. Fraudulent medical credentials are often accepted; hospital medical staffs have been reluctant to inform upon physicians known to be of inferior competence, even dangerous; most disciplinary actions, when they do exist, have not been publicized, and there continues to be enormous variation in the rate of disciplinary actions from state to state.[11] The phenomena themselves are not new. What is new is public interest and awareness through television reporting and the press, and acknowledgment by professional organizations that self-policing does not work effectively through the traditional licensing and credentialing system. There is much breast-beating.

Rather than blame the failures on the licensing boards, it may be better to ask how physician competence can be assured, in the future, within organized practice systems. Moreover, it should be observed that the licensing boards, as basic mechanisms of professional control, were developed in the late nineteenth and early twentieth century to create a strong, unified profession—and that they were very successful in achieving this goal. They are not necessarily appropriate to medicine in the late twentieth century. Thus, the criticism itself is perhaps misdirected.

11. Physicians are also criticized for not fulfilling patient expectations; that is, for failing to deliver on the promise of technological and scientific "progress" that was the main message of the reform of the medical profession at the beginning of the century (the so-called Flexner reforms in American medical education) and was carried further by formal specialization between the two world wars. The promise was to advance medicine as applied science. Yet ironically, in its most dramatic applications this movement, too, is questioned. The heralded era of organ transplantation from the mid-1950s, the increased technical potential of artificial organs and body parts, and the ability to sustain life on machines—each representing dramatic technological developments

in medicine—have also emphasized the limitations of technology in improving the quality of life, and hence the limitations of physicians. For example, widespread use of kidney dialysis—and the boast that the United States, unlike more "rationed" countries, makes this technique available to all in need—has been joined by a growing awareness of problems in the clinical area, including side effects, and in the moral and psychological spheres of patient care.[12] The definition of good medical care has gone far beyond the scientific and technical. Yet, at the same time, the physician has lost much of his/her mystique. The future physician is neither fully scientist nor shaman. The new role model (or myth) does not yet exist. It will.

12. The obvious difficulty in reconciling the heroic status of artificial heart transplant teams with the subsequent strokes and sufferings of the supposed beneficiaries has been managed, in part, by making the patient part of the treatment team. Thus the recipient, too, becomes a kind of hero. Indeed, the artificial heart recipient may be seen as an emblem of a wider set of shifts, in which the patient gains power vis-à-vis the physician; that is, where the old doctor-patient role of superior and dependent, or expert and passive recipient of expertise, is replaced by a doctor-client or partnership arrangement. The patient, in short, becomes an active participant in jointly made decisions.

The end of the era of the passive patient is most noticeable in decisions affecting the terminally ill. Such decisions have moved, in large part, from the private, informal domain of physician decision to the negotiated or bureaucratic domain. Physicians have been indicted for murder in cases where life-sustaining equipment was withdrawn from a comatose patient, even where family approval was assumed. Patients' wishes about life or death may be codified in "living wills." Indeed, the very definitions of life and death, originally the exclusive province of physicians, have become a matter for legal guidelines and national debate.[13]

13. If patients are seen as consumers as well as partners in the healing process, a major shift in power relationships between the public and the profession can be observed. Insuring organizations have become agents of consumers rather than of providers, able to exert control through the power of the pocketbook. At the same time, the increased role of non-physicians in areas of great importance to health maintenance has challenged the central role of physicians in the medical arena. Much of the work now being done in the United States to control obesity, alcoholism, anorexia, stress, and individual behavior is being done under the aegis of lay organizations such as Weight Watchers or through the health programs of major business corporations. Moreover, much of this work has been defined as education and behavior modification rather than as "medicine." The cumulative impact of the increased role of patients in clinical decision-making, of public criticism of medical organizations and of medicine itself, and of developments of health services outside medicine, could suggest a more limited role for the medical profession in the future. However, these

changes can be seen, equally, as part of the larger readjustments in medicine. Direct comparison of the present with the recent past is less important—certainly less fruitful—than reassessment of the full range of physician activities in the present.

Physicians appear to have accepted, even to have welcomed, the new emphasis on the role of the patient in decision-making and the patient's right to refuse treatment. However, there is also concern lest the pendulum sway too far in the other direction: toward abdication of responsibility by physicians, unsound medical judgment by patients, and unwilling collusion by physicians and patients, leading to decisions against the patient's own better judgment.[14] This tension reflects the (as yet) uncompleted shift to a new kind of medicine that seeks to involve the patient through adequate understanding of the patient's approach to life, health, and disease, through a doctor-patient encounter that explores the psychodynamics of the illness in each and every specific case. How can physicians, collectively, manage a positive readjustment of their role to allow for major changes in doctor-patient relationships? What are the incentives and opportunities for the profession that are inherent in this change?

In terms of previous attitudes and ideologies of medical practice the emphasis on "talking medicine" has three profound—indeed revolutionary—implications. First, it puts psychosocial skills and joint planning at the forefront of the medical encounter, forcing the physician to think of health and disease in terms of subjectively defined notions like suffering, hope, and pain, rather than in terms purely, or even predominantly, of the external, concrete evidence of disease. Various attempts to define the approach and skills necessary to undertake this complex task have been grouped under calls for a new "humanism" in medicine.[15] Second, this type of encounter takes time: to talk, to listen, and where necessary to educate and to persuade—thus potentially lengthening the physician encounter at a time when fees are being controlled and shorter encounters appear more "cost-effective." Third, it assumes a potentially wide variability in the nature of individual treatment decisions, rather than the repetition of standard treatment measures in all cases that present similar "medical" symptoms.

15. The new humanism thus runs counter to pressures imposed on physicians via Medicare reimbursement. Indeed, there is a worrying dissonance between perceptions of medical practice that suggest increasing variation in individual patient care, based on effective patient-physician encounters, and a reimbursement system based on standardization and reproducibility across medical care incidents. Not only do DRGs assume the systematization of medicine around standard forms of practice, but interest in small-area variations in practice patterns assumes that there is, somewhere, some arbitrary, if not ideal mean for defined categories of care. Excessive standardization of medical practice through the reimbursement system will lead to profound moral questions about individual patient care and individual (patient) freedom of choice of care. One major task for the medical profession is to map and justify the type, range, and

nature of practice in the era of the "active patient," and suggest how it should be assessed and monitored—and by whom.

16. Just as the notion of the patient's role is shifting from the legitimated dependency of the "sick role" to more active involvement in clinical decision-making, physicians are seeking to develop roles and skills that allow for complexity and uncertainty, rather than assuming that scientific expertise lays down "one best way" of proceeding in most cases. In turn, redrawing the doctor-patient relationship implies new definitions of medicine, diagnosis, and disease. The medical profession has ridden triumphantly through most of the twentieth century along a road paved with assumptions and structures about disease that are based on the infectious diseases. Today's major medical problems encompass chronic diseases—conditions that are often long-term and messy, and are not usually susceptible to a single diagnosis, intervention, and cure. Neither doctors nor patients have yet developed an appropriate set of behaviors or an ethos for a medicine based on chronic disease. These are major activities for the future.

Medicine and Its Institutions

17. As Anselm Strauss and others have pointed out, there is a curious inappropriateness in today's prevalence of chronic illness amid the profession's images and practices of acute care. In hospitals, personnel still tend to think of themselves as treating patients who are acutely ill and of cure as the only successful outcome of disease. Nevertheless, the work of physicians, nurses, and technicians has been radically altered by the prevalence of chronic illness and the technologies to manage such diseases. Chronic disease patients, playing an active rather than a passive role in the management of a chronic condition, also engage in substantial work in the course of the illness. The patient's role in hooking up and monitoring kidney dialysis equipment is a notable case. The increased diffusion of technology from hospitals to patients' homes also involves patients in active work with machines. However, the patients' own effort, or work, has usually been ignored in the hospitals where most nurses and physicians are trained.[16] The two sets of perceptions are potentially (and dangerously) at cross-purposes.

18. The shift from an infectious to a chronic disease mode of thinking within the profession—and from a single diagnosis to a complex of problems—is not new; it has been developing for at least fifty years. The effect is cumulative and can no longer be ignored.

19. Major professional institutions are out-of-date in both their structure and assumptions. There is an acknowledged gap between medical education and major health problems such as asthma, arthritis, or chemical dependence.[17] There have been few studies of the effect of health care programs on individual health. Indeed, the general lack of outcome measures for chronic diseases—and a serious lack of interest in outcome studies—has created a major gap in

knowledge about the relative effects of different forms of medical intervention on patients' health and well-being.[18] Clinical studies performed in health facilities may have little relevance for assessing the health status of the majority of individuals in any one year who are sick outside of institutions. There are few measures of the effectiveness of home care. Of perhaps most importance, the professional "culture" of medical schools has given little importance to such questions—at least, as yet.

20. The infectious disease era was based squarely on medical research. Identifying bacteria and viruses in the laboratory was translated, at least in theory, into scientific interventions—"magic bullets"—against specific diseases. In contrast, research on chronic diseases is enormously varied, drawing on a wide range of biomedical and applied sciences, focused on underlying biological mechanisms. Basic research into disease mechanisms and processes, which may have long-term payoffs in understanding and treating diseases such as cancer, is undertaken in large part by research specialists who are not physicians. Epidemiological research on chronic diseases is a peripheral activity in most medical schools. The odd position has been reached where American medicine is distinguished, in part, by its emphasis on research and technological development, but medicine as a profession in the late twentieth century lacks a discrete, focused, formal body of knowledge for application in the field.

21. In the early years of the twentieth century, the reform of the American medical profession, with medical education based at universities, was justified by centering medical education around research, in laboratories and on the hospital wards. The second major professional movement, the growth of specialization, was predicated on technological advances in research and practice. In an era of chronic disease, the medical profession cannot define itself and its institutions so sharply around scientific research and/or technology, as they are presently understood. A new defining focus is needed. What this will be is not yet clear.

22. Marked differences of medical opinion about treatment have appeared in recent years, in cases ranging from breast cancer to coronary bypass surgery. A current example is the debate on whether psychosocial variables can affect the course of cancer. Different research draws diverse conclusions about the relationship between the patient's emotional state and the outcome of disease.[19]

Such debates, however invigorating and good for the advancement of medical knowledge, have important structural effects. First, they further weaken the traditional authority of the physician as the "expert with the answer"—a matter of concern only if one believes that this traditional authority should be maintained. Second, such debates lead to the involvement of the patient in discussions of alternative forms of care and relative risks. Indeed, they require that the patient be sufficiently sophisticated to understand that physicians may have an individual style of practice and beliefs about particular diseases. One physician may be more interventionist than another; a second may lean towards surgical intervention; a third towards chemotherapy; a fourth may favor psychotherapy; and so on.

There is, in short, a climate of medical uncertainty, for both patients and physicians.

23. In this environment of uncertainty and risk, doctor and patient are, ideally, bonded as allies, working jointly to achieve the optimal effect. It follows that they may need mutual reassurance that each did all they could, when medical intervention fails to arrest the course of disease. For example, a recent contribution to the *New England Journal of Medicine* urged physicians to be present at the patient's funeral.[20] By doing so, the physician may reassure family members and help with their guilt after a patient's death, and demonstrate his/her caring about the patient as an individual, particularly when the last days have been dominated by machines. In turn, the funeral provides the physician with a ritualized "ending" to a course of treatment in which there were no single or obvious decisions. The typical physician has not been trained to cope with notions of disease that transcend his/her actual "medical attendance," nor to share any sense of defeat with patients or their relatives. The opportunity here is for the physician to become more "human" and, perhaps, more trusted as an individual. The fear is lack of authority and lack of distance. Enormous psychological shifts are required of individual physicians during this period of transition, at a time when morale is already low. Such an observation suggests aggressive efforts by professional, corporate, and other groups to encourage or establish discussion and intervention programs, designed to develop perceptual change.

24. The structures of medical education still largely follow the pattern set up at the time of the Flexner Report (1910), designed to streamline and standardize medical curricula to produce a well-trained medical journeyman, educated in the basic and clinical sciences within a university setting. Graduate medical education (residency training in the specialties) follows the patterns set up in the 1920s and 1930s: training based on acute care in hospitals, within subdivisions of medicine or "specialties," based on technologies, diseases, organs, systems, or age groups. Neither pattern of education is ideally designed for, or easily adjustable to today's practice, which applies a wide range of technologies to a wide range of chronic diseases.

Both undergraduate and graduate medical education are therefore under stress. Medical school curricula are criticized in blue-ribbon reports for requiring the memorization of facts, rather than the acquisition of skills, values and attitudes, and the development of knowledge through self-critical, independent learning.[21] Meanwhile, under the onslaught of numerous crosscutting specialized fields, the structure of specialty certification is becoming complicated and unwieldy. There are now twenty-four approved medical specialties, with forty-two subspecialty areas. However, many of these new areas are attempts to reinvent generalized practice or to link established technologies across traditional specialties. For example, both internal medicine and family practice have an interest in geriatric medicine, while six specialties (anesthesiology, internal medicine, obstetrics and gynecology, pediatrics, psychiatry and neurology, and surgery) have endorsed a subfield of critical care.

Continuing appraisal of medical education by professional groups is expected in the next decade, culminating (perhaps) in major changes. Possibilities for change include new national specifications about undergraduate medical education, enforced through accreditation, external funding, or consensus; more flexible specialty board requirements; alternative forms of specialist education offered by universities and/or health care systems, outside the board system. One possibility is for major service organizations to train their own physicians at the graduate level, or to contract for training in different fields with selected universities. In any event, the large health care systems (via their medical groups or otherwise) will have an increasing voice in specifying the nature of the specialties.

25. External influences on academic health centers and on the financing of graduate medical education, even in the 1980s, attenuate the traditional authority of medical organizations to dictate the form and structure of professional education. Notably, the reform of medical schools in the early twentieth century was accomplished under the strong medical leadership of the Council on Medical Education of the American Medical Association, in a climate of public compliance and/or approval. Likewise, the specialty boards were generated from preexisting specialist associations and interests within medicine. The present crisis in medical education forms a major, third phase of professional development in the twentieth century. In this phase, the game will be played by different rules, in which the power of professional organizations has to be justified and negotiated anew. Strong, effective leaders could build confidence within the profession and create confidence in the profession from outside. Weak or disorganized leadership may lead to a steady erosion of professional self-governance and prestige.

26. Changes affecting the medical profession are easiest to see where they take place in the external political arena rather than within; for example, in debates over reimbursement policy, physician supply, or the number of residencies. It is also easiest for any group to rally its forces to cope with outside threats, rather than to rethink its basic assumptions and its internal order. Nevertheless, the assumptions built up in the old era of educational reform and infectious diseases conflict, in numerous ways, with the demands of consumerism, cost-control, and chronic disease. The educational system has produced an abundance of physicians practicing in the subspecialties; relatively few with knowledge ranging over the technology of home care, the management of large physician organizations, and the development of comprehensive services, including social services for long-term care. Hospitals may no longer be the best or only place to train all specialists. Yet, inertia in the system has inhibited major change. How the institutions of medicine will change in response to the rapidly changing environment is still, alas, unclear.

27. Fundamental assumptions built into professional priorities and ranking systems demand reexamination. For example, the assumption that a specialty field is defined, in large part, by its claim to technique or to a focused body of research breaks down in fields such as family practice and general internal medicine: fields that define themselves functionally—as managers or gatekeepers of comprehensive care. Nevertheless, a national study of heads of departments of medicine, reporting in 1985, criticized programs in general internal medicine for their inability to conform to the focused research programs and NIH funding that distinguish other nonsurgical specialties. Development of a research program in general internal medicine was said to be the most significant reported problem in the field, as perceived by the departmental chairman.[22] However, there was no specification as to what this research might be, and no discussion of the possible value of a field whose research interest might be wide-ranging, across a variety of disciplines—or even, of a field with relatively little focus on scientific (laboratory) investigation. Research has become a Pavlovian reflex.

There are, in short, changes both in the external environment and within the profession of medicine. These changes are interlinked. They include pressures on both the structures, and underlying ideology and assumptions of the profession. The future success of the medical profession rides on the ability of its leaders and organizations to manage change in both the external and internal spheres.

The Medical Profession: Possible Futures

One possible future for the medical profession is to hold on to the old ideas and assumptions of medical authority, developed through the earlier successful periods of medical reform (1890-1917) and of specialization (1920-1970), and to resist further changes for as long as feasible. But this stance is self-defeating. Indeed, the American medical profession is already embarked, willy-nilly, upon a new period of major change.

For students of the professions, the present period is of enormous intellectual interest. I expect a flowering of good sociological analysis of concepts such as professional dominance and authority, the patient's role, the doctor-patient relationship, and the social construction of disease. The very nature of a "profession" is under reappraisal. Such a prospect may seem a hollow comfort to physicians struggling with the impact of present-day changes. Nevertheless, I think that a better understanding of the magnitude and multifactorial character of present shifts will allow the profession to escape the dangers of unthinking opposition. The opportunities need also to be created. In earlier periods of professional change in the twentieth century, professional leaders and groups developed new, even radical institutions and movements, based on clearly stated missions: Upgrade the medical schools, control standards in surgery, provide an orderly subdivision of medicine into specialties. Today, there is ambivalence about the appropriate role of a profession at all—ambivalence that calls for clearer statements by those major organizations. Otherwise, action will be frozen.

Charles Bosk recently reviewed assumptions about professions in terms of two competing traditions in sociology,[23] and these serve well here. First, there is the "classical myth": that the professions are essentially different from other occupations, that they deserve a high degree of autonomy in the workplace, and that they can be trusted by society to operate in the public interest through a rigorous code of ethics and through governance by their own associations. Second, there is the "anti-myth": that professions are merely devices created out of the self-interest of an occupational group, in order to further its goals in the marketplace. Hence, in Bosk's phrase, discussions of the profession oscillate between idealism and cynicism, depending on the author's point of view. Arnold Relman's plea for a "return" to a medical profession infused by idealism and moral principle is the clearest example of the tendency to choose one of these views.[24] By choosing the "myth" as a basis for argument, physicians can be seen as swept into a period of commerce and greed, and as losing some of the attributes that make them a "profession." Alternatively, all medical actions can be couched as self-serving exercises of power, a jockeying of interests in which rhetoric services economic interest. Both these points of view are useful. Alone, neither is an ideal mindset for viewing the present, complex picture of professional change in medicine, with a view to prediction or prescription.

I think that we are now in a remarkably exciting, fluid period, which may last for many years, of constant debate, negotiations, organizational and ideological adjustments, out of which a new consensus about the nature of the medical profession will emerge. It is too soon to see what this consensus will be. However, it is fruitless to see present changes as having only deleterious effects upon the profession. The future profession may well be different, but it may be equally powerful and equally successful. The key is the ability to shift from outmoded expectations and perceptions.

Perceptual shifts are difficult, in part, because the potential pluses and minuses of professional change do not always fall within the same category of analysis. Thus, an apparent economic or organizational constriction might have unexpected cognitive or clinical benefits—or vice versa. Even among the changes I have sketched out here—and many others could be delineated—positive elements of change have to be set against the more obvious negatives. For example, for individual physicians, practice in large-scale medical organizations may be much more interesting and relevant to clinical work, in an era of chronic illness, than practice in a relatively narrow specialty setting. The identification, within the corporate setting, of a large group of patients also provides the element of what the British call a "practice," that is, the opportunity for a group of physicians to accept collective responsibility for a community of care and to review the progress of patients through their careers of health and disease. Large organizations also centralize information systems, providing physicians with a potentially better means of self-examination, clinical and epidemiological research than is available to government through peer review organizations (PROs), or to organized payers.

The fee-for-service private practice system has long made physicians mini-business executives. Translation to an organized setting may make such skills more sophisticated, specialized, and useful. At the same time, organized systems may allow for increased physician-participation in resource allocation across the spectrum of medical care, and perhaps for the exercise of more clinical initiative within the sheltering arms of a corporation, than in more exposed forms of practice. Large corporations can also extend their grasp much more readily than small group practices to encompass social services, home care, and other necessary adjunct services for the effective management of chronic disease.

Positive as well as negative outcomes can also be suggested in other areas. In the future, physicians will undoubtedly earn less, in real terms, than they have in the period of enormous physician incomes in the past forty years. However, they may also have more time to spend with patients—a necessary aspect of doctor-patient cooperation—and they may also find that practice is more intellectually engaging and satisfying as a result. The number of malpractice suits might even decline in number. Debates within medicine about the nature of disease, appropriate forms of treatment, and the role of patient attitudes and behavior promise a fertile, open, exciting arena for debate about fundamental questions within medicine. We do not yet know what the various results will be. My point is that change is not necessarily all in one direction.

The development of the medical profession in the late twentieth century may be seen by future historians as the third major period of professional change in the twentieth century—at least as important as the changes that led to a reformed medical educational system by 1917 (and to a national medical profession), and to a structure for specialization by World War II. Today, as in the earlier periods, basic ideas about medicine demand as much attention as the structure of professional organizations, controls, and incentives. How far—and how—the organizations of medicine will respond to the complex changes in medicine's environment remains to be seen. Meanwhile, the system itself is implementing change, just as it did at earlier periods of professional reform.

If professional organizations and individuals see today's changes as necessary, manageable, and negotiable, and as having potentially positive effects, the present generation of medical students may feel privileged to be entering medicine, despite its various uncertainties—and the profession may have a stronger voice in its own destiny. Medical schools may become more varied in the future than they have in the past; the structure of specialty certification may become a less controlling system; the role of practitioners within physician organizations may produce new forms of practice. All such developments, and others, carry with them the opportunity for creating a new, more appropriate, more interesting profession.

This chapter was originally given at the Cornell University Medical College Second Conference on Health Policy, New York City, February 1986, and published as Rosemary A. Stevens, "The Future of the Medical Profession," in Eli Ginzberg, ed., *From Physician Shortage to Patient Shortage: The Uncertain Future of Medical Practice* (Boulder: Westview Press, 1986): 75-93.

Notes

1. See Eliot Freidson, *Professional Dominance: The Social Structure of Medical Care* (New York: Harper and Row, 1970); and Paul Starr, *The Social Transformation of American Medicine* (New York: Basic Books, 1983).
2. Carol Brierly Golin, "Remodeling the House of Medicine," *American Medical News*, 17 May 1985.
3. David J. Ottensmeyer, President of the Lovelace Medical Foundation, cited in Golin, "Remodeling the House."
4. "Changes Sought in Doctors' Pay under Medicare," *New York Times*, 7 December 1985, 1-8.
5. See Eliot Freidson, *Doctoring Together* (New York: Elsevier, 1975).
6. Kathy A. Fackelman, "Cleveland Hospital on the Road to Product-Line Management," *Modern Health Care*, 22 November 1985, 70-77.
7. Editorial, "Hospital Chain Expansion Over?" *Modern Health Care*, 22 November 1985, 5.
8. Hewitt Associates, "Comparing Practices in Health Care Cost Management, 1984," reported by Jeff Charles Goldsmith in Eli Ginzberg, ed., *The U.S. Health Care System: A Look to the 1990s* (Totowa, N.J.: Rowman & Allanheld, 1985): 53.
9. See, for instance, Clark C. Havighurst, "Doctors and Hospitals: An Antitrust Perspective on Traditional Relationships." *Duke Law Journal* (1984): 1071-1162; Leigh C. Dolin, "Antitrust Law versus Peer Review." *New England Journal of Medicine* 313 (1985): 1156-57.
10. For example, Thomas Swick, "At ACP Session, an Ancient Code is Scrutinized," *American College of Physicians Observer*, December 1984, 20, 22.
11. For example, a CBS "60 Minutes" program featuring fraudulent credentials, 1 September 1985, and a series of articles on physician incompetence in the *New York Times*, 2-3 September 1985.
12. See Renée C. Fox, Judith P. Swazey, and Elizabeth M. Cameron, "Social and Ethical Problems in the Treatment of End-Stage Renal Disease Patients," in Robert O. Narins, ed., *Controversies in Nephrology and Hypertension* (New York: Churchill Livingstone, 1984): 45-70.
13. President's Commission for the Study of Ethical Problems in Medicine and Biomedical and Behavioral Research, *Deciding to Forego Life-Sustaining Treatment* (Washington, D.C.: GPO, 1983); and Barbara Mishkin, "Decisions Concerning the Terminally Ill: How to Protect Patients, Staff and the Hospital," *HealthSpan*, the Report of Health Business and Law, 2 (March 1985): 17-21.
14. Peter M. Marzuk, "The Right Kind of Paternalism." *New England Journal of Medicine* 313 (1985): 1474-76.
15. See, for instance, Richard Gorlin and Howard Zucker, "Physicians' Reactions to Patients: A Key to Teaching Humanistic Medicine." *New England Journal of Medicine* 308 (1983): 1959-63; and American Board of Internal Medicine, "A Guide to Awareness and Evaluation of Humanistic Qualities in the Internist," June 1985.
16. Anselm Strauss et al., *Social Organization of Medical Work* (Chicago: University of Chicago Press, 1985).

17. For example, see D. Shine and P. Demas, "Knowledge of Medical Students, Residents, and Attending Physicians about Opiate Abuse." *Journal of Medical Education* 59 (1984): 501-07; Health and Public Policy Committee, American College of Physicians, "Chemical Dependence." *Annals of Internal Medicine* 102 (1985): 405-8.

18. Barbara Starfield, "Motherhood and Apple Pie: The Effectiveness of Medical Care for Children." *Milbank Memorial Fund Quarterly/Health and Society* 63 (1985): 523-46.

19. B. R. Cassileth et al., "Psychosocial Correlates of Survival in Advanced Malignant Disease?" *New England Journal of Medicine* 312 (1985): 1551-5 and correspondence, ibid. 313 (1985): 1354-59; "Strong Emotional Response to Disease May Bolster Patient's Immune System," *New York Times*, 22 October 1985, C-1.

20. Patrick Irvine, "The Attending at the Funeral." *New England Journal of Medicine* 312 (1985): 1704-5.

21. A notable recent example is "Physicians for the Twenty-First Century." *Journal of Medical Education 59* (1984), Part 2.

22. Robert H. Friedman and Janet T. Pozen, "The Academic Viability of General Internal Medicine." *Annals of Internal Medicine* 103 (1985): 439-44.

23. Charles L. Bosk, "Social Controls and Physicians: The Oscillation of Cynicism and Idealism in Sociological Theory," in Judith P. Swazey and Stephen R. Scher, eds., *Social Controls and the Medical Profession* (Boston: Oelgeschlager, Gunn and Hann, 1985): 31-51.

24. Arnold S. Relman, "The New Medical-Industrial Complex." *New England Journal of Medicine* 303 (1980): 963-70.

14

Professional Competence and Specialty Board Certification (1999)

It is a great pleasure to be here in two roles: as a historian who has long been interested in specialty certification, and as a new public member of the American Board of Medical Specialties.

In my "public" role, I will ask the obvious questions. Have not the boards always been interested in competence? If not, what is the purpose of their existence? The historian in me asks more complex questions. How have the boards defined and redefined themselves over the years? And how does this history explain where we are at present? What, for example, does "competence" mean to this group, in this room, in 1999? Does it have a clear set of meanings, or is it perhaps some form of code? A vehicle for action, perhaps. Or a resounding cry for redefining the boards' structure and public purpose. I'd like to suggest that "competence" means all of these things. "Competence" includes defining what physicians ought to do and measuring the necessary traits; but it is also a rallying cry for defining and measuring the boards' own professional capabilities.

This is a particularly good time to look at the role of the medical certification system in relation to that of other professions. Comparisons are useful in at least three areas: performance measurement itself; how other professions are defining competence in relation to the jobs their members do; and the social or public functions of certification as an exercise of professional responsibility.

The specialty certifying boards, like the examining processes of other professions, are also distinctly *American* institutions, forged by a distinctively American history. Unlike the basic pattern set for the British Royal College system, for example, the specialty certifying boards are twentieth-century institutions. Their independent, sometimes idiosyncratic foundations reflect the patterns of specialization writ large, and a willingness to engage with the realities of changing markets. Ophthalmology, the first board (1917), was a response in part to the successful, competitive campaigning of optometry; Otolaryngology (1924) was founded in the midst of enthusiasm for hospital-based tonsillectomies;

Obstetrics and Gynecology (1930) achieved success as middle-class women sought hospital-based deliveries; and so on up to the present. In many ways, as part of American social, scientific, and technological history, the boards may have more in common with other American professions than with medical organizations in other countries.

Status of the Boards Today

During the twentieth century the medical specialty boards have become august, successful American social institutions—part of what the British call the Establishment. This is a good time to review the avowed purpose of competence assessment, if only to overcome the inertia of prestige. Nineteen of the present twenty-four primary boards are now more than fifty years old. Even the American Board of Medical Specialties, which was formed after the appearance of four independent boards, has exceeded the age of Medicare eligibility (sixty-five years of age). Longevity can be seen as a mark of maturity, but may also burden the recipient with the accretions of the years, making it difficult to take risks and make bold changes. There may, after all, be more at stake.

A question that has been raised more than once at ABMS conferences is whether twenty-four independent boards, working with and through the ABMS, and with locations in different states, can agree on a common agenda for competence and move with sufficient speed to implement it. I am optimistic for three reasons. First, the information age in which we live makes geographical location and administrative structures far less relevant than they used to be. We are now all enmeshed in webs and networks, and communicate across the world with the same facility that we converse electronically with our neighbors. Second, there is nothing like a common set of external pressures to mobilize groups to unify and change; and those pressures are certainly here today. Third, the nature and function of the Boards have actually changed significantly over the past few years through common certification and recertification processes—setting the stage for further changes to come.

a) Changes Achieved

As a system—and the boards *are* a system, as was evident when ABMS was founded in 1933—the medical specialty boards have successfully added new fields over the years, and solidified their collective authority in medicine. As a historian I last looked carefully at the role of the board system in 1970, when fewer than half of all practicing physicians were diplomates of [i.e., certified by] approved specialty boards—only yesterday in historical terms, but it now seems another era.

Think of some of the significant changes since then. Perhaps most significantly, the implementation of certification and recertification in Family Practice [now Family Medicine] in 1969 completed the historical shift in the role of the boards as elites certifying the few, to examiners over the full span of medicine. Among other major changes: the establishment of new primary boards in Emergency Medicine, Nuclear Medicine, and Medical Genetics; the proliferation of approved subspecialties; and a major extension of function in accepting the role of recertification. Recertification brought the boards, together with other specialty organizations, into the domain of practice evaluation. Not least, there has been a flowering of psychometrics, and continuing questioning of the value and validity of the oral examination (which fifteen of the boards now require, as well as a written exam and specified training).

What is most striking to me, looking at the boards in 1999, is the degree of cooperation among different boards that has accompanied these and other changes—even though independence is cherished and defended, and the different boards have strikingly different organizational cultures. Some of this cooperation may have been limited, even perhaps grudging, for example where two, three, or four boards have negotiated some of the joint subspecialties. Nevertheless, there is a much greater level of cooperation and a shared sense of purpose than there used to be—signified in this conference on competence as a fundamental, overarching theme.

b) Functional Shifts: Market Definition

Two shifts in functions seem to me particularly critical to discussion of professional competence today, and I want to take these in turn. The first is how the boards collectively define a "specialty" or "subspecialty"; that is, under what categories recertification will be administered in the future—and why. The second is the role of the specialty board system as arbiter of competence over the whole span of clinical medicine; that is, what is the desired role of certification in the health care system.

First, what is a specialty? In the early history of the boards—say up until the 1970s—specialty elites carved up medicine's domain into specialties as if medicine were a pie that could be sliced into sections; the subspecialties represented smaller pieces within the sections. Once a section was "taken," the only way for a new field to be established was by taking another piece of the pie or organizing as a subspecialty. For many years this model of specialization, largely laid out in the 1930s and 1940s, contained the number of specialties and ordered the structure of specialty medicine in the United States. But by 1970 this model was breaking down. Family practice had clear overlaps with other established specialty fields. New fields were developing that cut across established lines: emergency medicine, geriatrics, sports medicine, critical care, and many more. Over the years since 1970 the model of medicine as an ordered domain of discrete specialties has largely broken down. Many of today's subspecialties are arguably cross-specialties. The model of specialization has shifted from that of a divisible pie to an expansionary network of cross-cutting fields.

The exuberance of this process is remarkable. It has become impossible to diagram the entire specialty structure in a way that makes any sense of the whole to the outsider—such as a member of the public. You can start by listing the primary boards as the basic elements of a hierarchy, and then list each board's subspecialties as a second tier. However, drawing links across subspecialty fields and allowing for double-boarding (for example, through defined programs in internal medicine and pediatrics) creates an extraordinarily messy, ultimately incomprehensible diagram. How to link together subspecialties where more than one board is involved: hand surgery, for example, or dermatopathology, or critical care medicine? At my last count there were thirty-seven primary areas of specialization, and seventy-five areas of subspecialization, with many more on the way.

Of course, drawing a diagram is at one level a trivial pursuit—it may even reveal an over-rigid desire for rationality. But organizational charts do say something about the way an organization perceives itself, and this in turn has a bearing on the boards' collective mission as self-appointed guardian of professional competence.

On the face of it, this set of organizations has been moving rapidly to meet the demands of a multiplicity of specialty groups. One definition of "specialty" or "subspecialty" is that it is whatever is plausible at the moment and able to rally appropriate professional adherents. There is nothing new in such an observation; this is how the older primary boards were created. The question is how far this definition of fields is to go in the future. Are we to congratulate the boards for consumer (or constituent) awareness of the potential of new fields in the medical marketplace—the consumers in this case being sufficiently powerful professional groups seeking new credentials? Are the boards to be compared, for example, with the pharmaceutical industry, where new products suggest a constant search for improvement?

Why not forty or fifty primary specialty certificates and a couple of hundred subspecialty certificates? This organizational model could be described as a supermarket for specialty credentials. Physicians, health care organizations, and licensing authorities could select from the shelves whatever combination of certificates met their needs.

The supermarket model suggests that the boards might (or should) develop as service agencies, marketing sophisticated measurement techniques. Under this model, specialties and/or subspecialties might be defined by buyers as a mix-and-match collection of multiple competencies. For the board system the focus would be on measurement expertise. In a break with the past, the definition of a specialty or subspecialty might be left to the marketplace. Some would say this is already taking place.

An alternative model is to extend the boards' role, collectively, as an instrument to improve quality in the health care system. This would require the boards to grapple more overtly than in the past with wider, collective professional responsibilities.

There is an irony in recent changes in certification. While engaged in enthusiastic fragmentation of credentialing to such an extent that the very notion of a "specialty" seems to be in jeopardy—the new terminology is "primary care" plus "subspecialty"—the board system has acquired, in parallel, de facto responsibility for naming or labeling the *entire* medical profession. Are the twenty-four boards capable of acting as a collective force for this single purpose? Alternatively, is the public (whoever this is) willing to accept that medicine is reasonably divisible into the present twenty-four medical segments? These are looming policy questions.

The ABMS estimates that 87 percent of American physicians are certified by ABMS-approved boards. In essence, virtually all clinicians seek certification. As a result, the boards as a collective have become the most important national arbiter of clinical competence in American medicine. The boards' sheer scope of responsibility—certifying almost all American physicians—would provide a wake-up call, should one be needed, for looking ruthlessly and dispassionately at what physician competence should mean, generically, as a core value of the American health care system.

Arguably, the board system is now also the most important professional institution for American doctors as a whole. In the future, for example, far more doctors will be regularly involved in recertification than belong to the AMA or any other single professional association. It is a good time—I think it is essential—to reexamine the potential and the limits of the two roles, *arbiter of competence* and *professional entity*, recognizing that they are not necessarily the same.

The supermarket model limits itself to the former, offering a technical array of tests. The role of the boards as professional entity—as a national force for guarding and improving health care on behalf of the medical profession and the public—is an idea that has long been built into the credo of the board system, and is present in today's discussions about "competence." However, as an idea it is as yet far from fully articulated. What does it mean to be a national professional guardian of competence?

Other professions seem to offer little guidance on this issue. The professional responsibility for assessing competence is far greater for the certifying system in medicine than, for example, in law, where responsibility for specialty certification rests at the state level and there are far fewer lawyers than physicians currently certified as specialists. There are certainly other fields where safety and fiduciary issues are as important as in medicine, as we will hear about [in the conference] today.

But in some ways medicine presents special problems. This is not only because of the boards' scope of influence over the profession as a whole. It is also because of the long and eager identification of the medical profession with the competence of the entire health system. Think, for example, of the responsibilities assumed by the profession in the twentieth century, notably by the AMA and the American College of Surgeons in the early years of the twentieth century, and of the lofty phrases long associated with board development. There has long been an implicit social pact between the medical profession and the public. Traditionally the profession has claimed independence by virtue of producing a competent profession based on the best possible medical science—this was indeed the central message of the Flexner Report. The quality of health services was equated with the competence of the individual physician.

Unless they are on strike, airline pilots are not blamed if an airline drops scheduled flights, or strands passengers in planes on the runway for nine hours. Doctors are much more likely to be blamed for high medical costs or deficiencies in hospitals, managed care, and Medicaid. In some sense, the medical profession has stood as the symbol of excellence in the health system as a whole. And the specialty boards have been part of that process; a great deal is expected of them.

Quite apart from such historical considerations, recertification has placed the question of professional competence squarely within the health care system. Where initial certification, like licensing, certifies education completed, knowledge, and basic skills, procedures for recertification in any occupation bring the idea of competence firmly into the practice environment: into the individual's workplace. This is a huge jump in role for the board certification system. It requires a perceptual shift in goals that breaks with the past, and it conflicts with the supermarket model as a model for the future. With general acceptance of recertification and growing commitment to continuous (or at least periodic) measurement, the boards have crossed a historic line.

Engagement with the health system enlarges the cast of characters involved in physician competence and expands the traditional network on which the boards have long relied, to include employers as well as members of the public. In the past, board leadership could be characterized as an extension of leadership in specialty departments of medical schools and specialty associations, with strong links to residency education in the specialties. Each element of this network reinforced the other. The existence of specialty residency programs helped justify the creation of a board; and the existence of a board validated specialty identification for departments and divisions in medical schools. For each defined field there was in effect a web of influence.

However, this web focused on undergraduate and graduate medical education (and indirectly on the strengthening of the specialty's research base in the medical schools), rather than on the health care system. It was assumed that well-educated specialists would be competent, and would continue to be so throughout their careers. The practical advantage of this approach was that it was reasonably clearly focused. It was the justification for the system of specialty boards we have today.

Recertification, requiring engagement with the world of practice and with health services research, has extended the boards' gaze from the educational to the health care system. Remember, too, that we are talking about a process that affects virtually all physicians practicing in that system. Done well, the definition of competence for recertification may influence the health care system, just as board requirements have influenced the educational system for medicine in the past. By articulating, ostensibly for the public, what is important to the health care system's major profession, the boards inevitably make major statements about professional responsibility on behalf of the entire profession. How far other professions attempt to do this—or whether they do it at all—is a matter of some interest for this conference.

All of these actual or potential board responsibilities—defining specialties, assuming professional responsibility for competence measures, and assuming public roles in quality of care in the health care system—infuse debates about professional competence today. I want now to look briefly at the external threats that make action of some urgency, and conclude with some more specific questions for the future.

External Threats

All of us here are only too aware of the environmental pressures that have called the roles of certification into question:

- calls for professions to justify their social value on the grounds that professional institutions are self-interested monopolies;
- the parallel upheavals of managed care and the incentives of the marketplace;
- the rapid fragmentation of medicine, not only into subspecialties but also into new roles—gatekeeper, hospitalist, interventionist, rationer of managed care;
- major changes in the science base of medicine;
- strides made in the ability to measure what physicians know and do;
- the rise of competing credentialing processes; and, not least,
- increased public and industry attention to qualitative measures as a means of standardizing practice, regulating costs, and improving patient care.

The recent report from the Pew Health Professions Commission stated baldly that the goal of certification should be continuous self-assessment, that there should be a move toward national standards (a long time internalized agenda for the boards), and that accreditation or certification should be reconceived as a "facilitator for improvement."[1] Improvement in this context means improvement in the actual services delivered (or not delivered) to patients, not merely the demonstration of an isolated competence by any given individual. The focus is on the competence of a health care team, and how well the individual physician works within a given health care system.

As a result of these and other clarion calls, the "professional" part of professional competence has often seemed under siege. Books, articles, and speeches have sounded the alarm that the professions have had their day. "Fall of a Giant" was the way one recent author described the American medical profession in a book on the history of professions[2]—a message I believe to be at the very least premature, as Dr. Samuel Johnson said on hearing rumors of his death.

My message is not one of gloom and doom. Rather, I am struck by the sense of urgency and opportunity generated by various boards and by the ABMS. Today's opportunities to advance the public influence of the boards as guardians for competence in American medicine may be unparalleled—and may wane. There may be countervailing arguments in favor of reticence; that is, to define professional competence narrowly, field by field, and claiming that the boards should have minimal national, collective influence in the health care system. But, if so, these views, too, need to be fully articulated. For better or worse, certification is in the limelight.

Can the boards as a system provide creative professional leadership in defining and measuring competence as a professional responsibility, rather than as a function of the market, government, or other professional groups? And if so, in what terms? Will the boards lose out to the more rapid actions of other groups? Who *owns* competence in all of its regulatory dimensions? Do practicing doctors and the systems that contract with them really want all these certificates? Are the boards obsolete? Alternatively, in what demonstrable ways is certification associated with improvement in care? Such questions are not new. What is new is that the messages of urgency in the current environment dislocate us usefully from complacency. It becomes easier to recognize that there is nothing inevitable about present goals, activities, or structures.

Futures

As scientists, we should ask why we need national standards for competence at all, and for whom; and what advantages there may still be in the claims the boards have traditionally made of providing the "gold standard" for qualifications for defined specialties and subspecialties, and only in medicine, and not in other health professions. Other professions may be instructive here. The American Bar Association accredits private certification groups. Theoretically, at least, the ABMS could extend its reach to accredit other organizations.

The ABMS lists well over a hundred non-accredited specialty certification bodies, but has little or no information about them. Should the ABMS provide a public clearing house of information on all forms of certification, and rate them, as one element of the boards' responsibility to the public? If interdisciplinary cooperation is to be tested as one of the measures of competence for physicians (as the Pew Commission suggests), why should there not be much more cooperation between specialty areas in medicine and related specialties in other health professions?

Other questions follow. If the approved boards are able to set a reasonable standard for "competence" of virtually all practicing physicians, through certification and recertification, will this be an exclusive definition? That is, will it be assumed that physicians without board credentials are incompetent? Or still on the way to becoming competent? And if so, will this be legally valid and/or politically acceptable to state licensing agencies, physician employers, and contractors? Again, the use of competence measures by other professions may be instructive.

In my view, the structure of the board system is far less important than strategic mobilization around a common set of purposes. Nevertheless, as scientists, we should ask whether recertification should apply to organizations (i.e., the boards themselves), as well as to individuals. It is not clear that the present boards represent the requirements imposed on new entrants; that is, that they represent major concepts of medical science, and justify one board per specialty, each a "distinct and well-defined field of medical practice." Given that most of the boards were established in the environment of medical science and practice of fifty or more years ago, there is no particular reason why they should. But it is always useful to pursue self-examination.

It is also urgent. A larger notion of "professional competence" is implicit in the title of this conference; that is, the organizational competence of the boards as a system. The Pew Commission urges that future health workers have the "skills as professionals to move organizational systems and policies toward strategies that can change the reality"; and surely that should apply to the certifiers too. If the competence of physicians (and other professionals) can and should be measured on a periodic or continuing basis, it is fair to ask what the organizational competence of the specialty certifying boards is as a whole. What is the job description and how well do the boards, collectively, fulfill it?

This is not a trivial question. Without competent institutions—and that means a demonstrably effective specialty certification system designed for the environment and public expectations of the future—the testing of physician competence is an exercise in measurement techniques that could probably be performed by other expert groups, outside of professional leadership.

The virtue of continuing the present system unchanged as a supermarket for credentials is its flexibility in the face of changing patterns of specialization, and in the range of choice offered to physicians, health care organizations, and thus ultimately to patients—assuming the choices reflect the competencies they seek. Even if the range becomes even more byzantine than it is today, the ubiquity of information technology could help employers and patients more creatively than it does at present, where information is still largely organized by certifying board rather than by area of public interest. It is now possible to have an organizational system designed along one set of principles, with a virtual system announcing to the world another set of specialty configurations.

For example, the boards might perform a public service by listing the collective professional competence that a reasonable person or health system might draw on for cancer care, heart disease, depression, chronic back pain, or other major health conditions, signified by an array of specialty and subspecialty certificates across the boards, irrespective of primary board. This might indeed be an interesting exercise to do for its own sake: one way of assessing how "competence" as defined by certification relates to the health service needs of today's population.

In today's fragmentation of medicine there is much to be said for unifying principles, based on the core values of competence and professionalism. If anyone can do it, it is this distinguished, creative, and dedicated group. But to this neophyte, at least, it seems that if competence is to be seen as a common denominator, a unifying activity across all components of the board system, then the actual measures will have to be limited to what is relevant across a diversity of fields, encompassing areas as different from each other as geriatric psychiatry, blood banking transfusion, reproductive endocrinology, neuropathology, undersea medicine, and pediatric surgery—to take just a few current subspecialties.

It is difficult to reconcile unifying measures of competence with the fragmentation of the examining and organizational structure of the boards and the diverse practice environments in which physicians work today. I know that many of you have been grappling with these questions for some time, so I speak with some hesitation on these points. But it seems to me that another form of generalism and specialism will have to be invented. In some areas general measurement may make sense (such as interpersonal or informational skills). For others, packages will be designed for specialized knowledge and techniques, some parts of which may be common to more than one field, and perhaps even to more than one profession.

A couple of final observations. First, competence testing has a potentially important role to play in forming specialty and subspecialty fields as liberal professional occupations, with wide knowledge and wide-ranging views of medicine; in improving quality in the practice of medicine; and in shaping the boards as a unified professional force working in the interest of patients and the public.

Second, there is no magic formula for the future. We may learn from what other professions are doing in the face of similar opportunities and pressures. But it is also useful to think through the implications of the information revolution as a true revolution, changing *both* the way we can think about issues, *and* the way change can be implemented. The old board structure as a pie or set of hierarchies was a form of linear thinking. We are now more likely to think in patterns and are much more comfortable with complexity. To some extent the health care system has itself become a vast information system.

I am honored to be part of the medical profession's national credentialing system at what is, I believe, a unique historical period. The underlying questions are perhaps quite simple. How far will this formidable credentialing system focus its role on measuring "competence" as primarily a technical undertaking (that is, developing the best possible, and most appropriate, measures of individual capabilities)? How far will the boards extend their professional and public responsibilities beyond this to improve the quality of clinical services? Will board certification become a supermarket for tests, to be purchased in the market? Will the boards, represented by and through the ABMS, be a leader in defining what American medicine ought to do?

This chapter was originally given, under the title "Professional Competence and Board Certification," as the keynote address to the American Board of Medical Specialties Conference on Professional Competence and Board Certification, March 18, 1999. Unpublished except by www.abms.org.

Notes

1. E. H. O'Neill and the Pew Health Professions Commission, *Recreating Health Professional Practice for a New Century* (San Francisco: Pew Health Professions Commission, December 1998).
2. E. A. Krause, *Death of the Guilds: Professions, States, and the Advance of Capitalism, 1930 to the Present* (New Haven: Yale University Press, 1996).

15

Public Roles for the Medical Profession in the United States: Beyond Theories of Decline and Fall (2001)

What is the future of medicine in the public sphere, as expressed through its professional organizations? Will the profession continue to be just one of many competing interest groups, whose influence will continue to wane? Or is there a basis on which the professional organizations of medicine might assume a new position of moral leadership in American health care? This paper sets out to examine this largely neglected question by considering alternative explanations for that role in the past, assumptions in the present, and possibilities for the future.

Is there potential for the professional organizations of medicine to serve a positive policy role? Doubt attends upon the answer to this question. First, strong competition has developed over the issue of quality, a topic long monopolized by medical organizations through their control of education, training, and credentialing of physicians. Quality is now seen as a legitimate concern for purchasers, managed care plans, provider organizations, politicians, and consumers and is the subject of serious measurement and reporting efforts under a variety of auspices. Quality improvement of patient care requires effective management of complex systems (Kohn, Corrigan, and Donaldson 2000; Committee on Quality of Health Care in America 2001).

Second, organized medicine has fragmented structurally. These days, physicians see their specialty societies as their primary professional representatives, and the medical profession has splintered into hundreds of diverse organizations. The American Medical Association (AMA) represents a minority of all physicians. A recent article in the AMA's *American Medical News* put the question succinctly: "Is it time for the end of organized medicine as we know it?" (Booth 2000) For those who see medicine's public role only in terms of its efforts to enhance the well-being of its members, such a prospect would not be regretted (or perhaps dismissed as inconsequential). However, this is hardly the most intellectually creative or socially helpful stance one can take when considering what medicine's national voice and organizational roles in American health care might be in the future.

On the positive side, scholars are redefining the multifaceted meanings of "professionalism" for our time (Freidson 1994; Wynia et al. 1999; Rothman 2000; Mechanic 2000), and professionalism is being widely discussed in medical meetings, in medical schools, and as part of bioethics programs throughout the United States—though it is only beginning to be developed as a rationale and strategy for the profession's collective, organizational, public roles. Beyond new definitions, there is an incipient movement toward finding new concepts and language through which change might take place. Historical narratives dominated by the story of organized medicine's rise and fall, suggesting a defeated profession, have sustained its weakened political status. Nevertheless, an alternative history, which stresses the value of organized medicine's public activities, could be recounted in a way that allows the profession to play a role that does in fact further public interest. These tasks represent a challenging undertaking for scholars and other commentators on medicine in the United States.

Plausible arguments can be made for strengthening the profession's public roles, on grounds of practicality, effectiveness, timeliness, and common sense. Attacks on the imagined role of medicine as an entity, as well as major changes in purchasing arrangements and the power of payers since the 1990s, have caused demoralization, confusion, and cynicism within the profession, which affect, in turn, those people who wish to negotiate with it. Physicians now feel marginalized and under siege, not only because of the constrictions and regulations of health insurance contracts but also by their symbolic understanding of where the profession stands today. Historical theories of a profession in decline have lost their utility for explaining the present; that is, as grounded policy assumptions on which to build high-quality health services for the next twenty or so years. In theory, at least, a revived, socially confident medical profession, exerting moral leadership at the national level, might help create reform coalitions and build practical consensus among otherwise competing groups. In any event, the profession's public roles are overdue for updating to meet today's scientific, economic, and political conditions. Despite recent negative critiques, the American medical profession actually has a long history of public service, though that history has been submerged in recent years. There is thus an alternative (or secondary) history of the profession on which to build.

Basic Questions

Policy groups and medical leaders throughout the world are tackling the restructuring of professional roles, responsibilities, and organizations in the first decade of the twenty-first century. In most countries, the role and authority of the medical profession have been strongly influenced by the extension of national government health policy over the past fifty years. For example, in the

Canadian provinces, which have a single-payer insurance system under government auspices, medical organizations carry substantial delegated authority. In Europe, medical organizations may constantly find themselves renegotiating and contesting for power with government, but they at least have a national role to renegotiate and contest (Freeman 2000; Moran 1999). In the United States, there has been no similar concentration of responsibility for universal health insurance at national, state, or local levels, and no single government agency responsible for delegating formal power to medical organizations in relation to organized payment and service systems.

The growth of managed care in the 1990s, though in some ways as revolutionary in its effects on doctors as universal governmental health insurance might have been, was a dispersed rather than national experience, with substantial variations from place to place. With the typical physician having contracts with multiple insurers rather than with a single payer, the financial power of insurance corporations is disseminated—and so, therefore, is the negotiating power of physicians. Thus, even at the local level, there have been no overarching authorities, public or private, to empower (or restrict) the medical profession on behalf of the wider health care system in the United States. The profession lacks clear-cut policy roles in the health care system.

Compared with the situation in countries with established policy roles for medical organizations in national health services or insurance systems, the medical voice also lacks political definition in the United States. The long-term social values and social costs inherent in delegating responsibility to the profession are at this time barely discussed in the United States—in terms of incorporating medical authority in the power structure of major health care corporations, or of the profession's public accountability for the standards and scope of services in major tax-supported programs, most notably Medicare.

Without a formal public-private partnership role to serve as a model, and without designated help from outside groups (at least as yet), the leaders of medical organizations, ranging from the AMA through a battery of specialty organizations, have been left to invent and negotiate new public roles on their own, insofar as they can, pulling their constituencies along with them. This is an enormously difficult task, because of the profession's status as an independent private enterprise that must struggle for public influence in an arena crowded with other players. Would-be professional reformers at all levels also have to work within a context of "negativity among their colleagues" (Mechanic 2000). An obvious first challenge for the profession is to be able to convince the public that it has different, perhaps loftier goals than other players. What does the medical profession stand for, over and above the actions of its individual members and self-interested actions by its associations? What does it wish to stand for? Can membership organizations, sensitive to the immediate problems of their constituents, ever represent the public's interest, or even appear to do so? What can the profession or others do (if anything), to build socially responsible organizations?

Asking such questions in the abstract may engender vigorous philosophical debate and even generate consensus, but talk will not necessarily lead to action. For that, three practical issues are crucial. First, is the medical profession willing and able to work as a partner with managers, policymakers, and insurers—public and private? The jury is still out on this question. The current health care system has been going through so many changes that it is not even clear which partners are the ones to work with on a long-term basis. Second, does the profession have the organizational capability to act as a unified whole? And third, will influential critics be prepared to entertain the idea, even hypothetically, that professional organizations could be more than self-serving?

The enthusiastic specialization, subspecialization, and sub-subspecialization in American medicine over the past three decades, endorsed by multiple constituencies, has fractured the profession into multiple associations, leaving the core organization—the AMA—vulnerable. This process has been accelerated by the organization and funding of the health care system. The organizational parallel to pluralistic (rather than single-payer) insurance arrangements in the United States has been representative structures for the medical profession that are fragmented and opportunistic, based on specialty interests rather than on the profession as a whole. Moreover there is a long history of tension and mutual distrust between the medical profession and health care management (Stevens 1989). Even if we were to believe that valuable social goals could be furthered in the future through a strong, self-regulating medical profession with a mandate to act on behalf of the public, could the profession rebuild itself though robust alliances, both across specialties and with outside groups? And how could outsiders help?

Historical Reflections on Ideas and Agendas

The history of medical organizations is not much help in addressing these questions, except in underlining the cultural contingency of professional authority and emphasizing persistent themes of dominance and conflict. Much of the most interesting historical literature on medical organizations published since the 1960s focuses on battles won and lost—chiefly by the AMA and its associated societies at the state and local levels, and by the medical schools (e.g., Harris 1966; Rayack 1967; Hirshfield 1970; Marmor 1973; Burrow 1977; Numbers 1978; Poen 1979; Starr 1982; Ludmerer 1985; Ameringer 1999). Though it has long been clear that some AMA policies—notably its opposition to government-sponsored health insurance for most of the last century—have not served the profession well in the long run, the impression remains that organized medicine has always fought government on a single agenda of professional self-interest.

Well into the 1990s, the AMA was portrayed as the change-resistant agent of a narrowly self-serving profession. A book about the AMA published by two knowledgeable Chicago journalists in 1994 included such chapter headings as

"Looking after Medicine's Special Interests," "Stopping National Health Insurance at All Costs," "Playing Politics with Tobacco and the Public's Health," and "Bungling Health Policy on the AIDS Epidemic" (Wolinsky and Brune 1994). Self-interest and ideals can, of course, coexist. However, there is not yet an authoritative history that takes seriously the possibility that idealism played any role in the profession's political decisions.

Involvement in a national health insurance system might have strengthened the role of medicine's professional organizations (though it might also, of course, have polarized the issues further). Theoretically, stronger central health care organizations would have forced professional leaders to reconceive the ideals and roles of medical organizations through years of rapid changes in bioscience and technology, social expectations of what medicine can do, complexity in the provision of care, rises in the costs of services, the information and consumer revolutions, and, not least, the increasing burden of chronic illness (Fox 1986; 1993). Such involvement also probably would have led to different scholarly appraisals of the profession's larger social roles than the ones we now have—perhaps more critical, perhaps less.

As it was, the American medical profession was shockingly unprepared to face the question of its public role in the late twentieth century. There was no national system to provide a concrete framework for negotiation about the profession's new public place, or even a few monopolistic health care corporations that might have served a similar purpose. At the same time, the inherited ideology of organized medicine rested on outdated precepts—specifically, on patterns and policies that were developed in the first half of the twentieth century, when doctors were primarily general practitioners, health care costs were relatively low, and there was little health insurance, or even a health care "system" as we think of it today.

A century ago, it was not unreasonable to assume that providing a well-trained, science-oriented, increasingly specialized cadre of experts, working within the dictates of a professionally defined code of ethics, was a good and sufficient guarantee of the profession's obligation to serve the public. This ideological stance was represented by standardized educational programs in medical schools with a strong scientific base, support of biomedical research, a national network of licensing laws, standardized specialist training and certification programs, and national accreditation of hospitals. From today's perspective, the profession's public service agenda could be described as enhancing the quality of the doctor-patient relationship, improving scientific standards, and intervening at the national policy level where standards of patient safety were threatened. Thus the AMA supported food and drug legislation, which formed the basis of subsequent procedures for the regulation of new drugs and devices up through the present. In all of these respects, the profession seemed clearly to be serving public roles, and to be doing so remarkably effectively: unifying the medical profession, standardizing medical education, building the science base, and upgrading the competence of the average practitioner.

There were thus two distinct threads to the profession's public service agenda in the twentieth century, one representing an individual orientation and the other a collective orientation. While the AMA, then embodying organized medicine, supported funds for public health and clinics for the very poor, and promised the public that any person seeking an individual doctor should find him or her to be reasonably well-trained in a defined field, to act in a principled way, and to give charity care where necessary, there were no similar promises about the quality of the health care system as a whole. As the effective organization, accessibility, and delivery of health services rested increasingly on multiple occupations and institutions, the medical profession isolated itself from other aspects of the system.

Organized Medicine and the Scholarly Critique

By the 1960s, when concern about access to care and inequalities in services came dramatically to the forefront of policy debates in health care, society at large took for granted the profession's primary public agenda—promoting high standards of entry and education for individual physicians and encouraging biomedical research. Its second public agenda—opposing organized, collectivist health policies—appeared rampantly antisocial. Eliot Freidson noted in his landmark book, *Profession of Medicine* (1970), that despite claims that the medical profession was dedicated to high-quality services, no reliable information indicated that a service orientation was in fact widespread. A medical system based on professional autonomy had increased scientific knowledge, he wrote, but had also "impeded the improvement of the social modes of applying that knowledge," and encouraged the profession to be blind to its own shortcomings (Freidson 1970, 82, 371). It was but a short step from that position to the claim that professional authority seemed destructive of the public interest, at least in the United States.

A series of well-known critiques described the "autonomous" or culturally "dominant" roles of professions not only as outmoded but also as socially counterproductive (see Wolinsky 1988; Light 1988; Light and Levine 1988). Inside and outside the United States, scholars were observing that the conditions that gave rise to the institutions of professionalism were no longer the norm in industrialized societies (Johnson 1972), and that politics was not best served by the exercise of private interests, such as a powerful medical lobby. American political institutions, wrote Grant McConnell, "have in many ways been designed more to gain the acquiescence of power holding groups than to achieve a balance of public and private values" (McConnell 1966, 367). The professions were being socially reclassified, moving down a moral continuum away from the role of benevolent agents of the public and toward that of self-interested players in the economic marketplace, as if they could not be both at once. Magali Sarfatti Larson set out to examine "how the occupations we call professions organized themselves to attain market power" (Larson 1977, xvi). Like other professions, medicine was relabeled as a social institution in the 1970s and 1980s. No longer seen as working quietly for the public good by producing well-trained experts, the American medical profession took on sinister, even antisocial characteristics in its role in the culture at large. Some influential critics and participants also revised its history from a glorious narrative of success to a more ominous tale of hubris.

Whatever the scholarly debates, the language of battles, rise, loss, decline, and defeat—associated with the ideas of dominance, autonomy, and authority—became part of more general, typically negative critiques of the medical profession. Historians created, and physicians (and others) accepted, an explanatory history of organized medicine in the United States based on the familiar cultural myths of paradise lost and vanquished heroes. Paul Starr's widely cited book of the early 1980s was perhaps the most compelling, and the most expropriated among medical groups, of the rise-and-decline interpretations. Starr (1982) depicted the rise of a "sovereign profession," imbued with cultural authority, which lost its legitimacy in the 1970s, and was then challenged by the "coming of the corporation." Concurrently, John Burnham (1982) described the 1950s and early 1960s—those years in which the profession could apparently do no wrong—as the profession's "golden age," and this phrase was appropriated into the myth. Eventually, it seemed, the forces of corporate America vanquished a heroic profession.

The language of decline and fall has been pervasive, as illustrated by two (of many) recent examples. "Fall of a giant" is how Elliott Krause (1996) summed up the American experience for medicine in his historical study of four professions in five countries since 1930. Kenneth Ludmerer (1999) depicted today's medical schools as "vassals of the marketplace," and used the creation and breaking of a "social contract" as a powerful organizing theme for the recent history of American medical education.

Criticisms of the profession's lack of a tradition of service in the 1970s and 1980s came at a time when service issues were urgent in the public eye, forced by the new conditions of rising health care costs, the failure of governmental health planning, the emergence of antitrust regulation for professions, new Medicare policies and procedures, and later managed care. In theory, at least, the passage of the Medicare and Medicaid legislation in 1965 abolished the need for charity care by doctors and hospitals for the largest, most vulnerable social groups: the elderly and poverty-stricken. The profession's lack of service orientation in the 1970s can be attributed at least in part to the impact of these huge governmental financing programs, which removed charity care from the expected repertoire of medical practice. As an anonymous reviewer of this paper pointed out, this ubiquitous aspect of medical practice in the 1950s and 1960s (and in the rhetoric of ideal practice) was not replaced by another social good.

In the absence of effective governmental, nonprofit, or market-driven health care strategies (or a working combination of some or all of these), the medical profession became a convenient villain for failures elsewhere in health care policymaking. Its villainy was enhanced by the powerful narratives of failure that were built into conceptual explanations of the profession's larger social role: the decline in professional authority, with the medical profession overcome by the power of public disillusion and then by the more potent power of insurers. From the 1970s through the 1990s, as cost concerns marked U.S. national policy and the quality of care was seriously questioned, the idea of professional dominance as a negative social force merged neatly into contemporary (pro-market) policy critiques and helped to justify those critiques. The Clinton health plan deliberations of 1993-94 included little input from medical organizations, directly acknowledging their lack of political power and relevant social agenda as well as, perhaps, deficiencies in that policymaking process. The scenario was simple: Doctors were players in the economic marketplace who had gained inappropriate control of their workplace for their own financial ends.

At the same time that governmental efforts to provide health services for all people largely failed, professional organizations of all kinds lost credibility. In the process, the medical profession lost an opportunity to become a champion of modern, efficient health services through organizational innovation, and lost the government as a potential ally. Instead of the profession receiving a responsible delegation of authority from the government, doctors became conspicuous as adversaries, first of the government (notably in opposing Medicare in the 1960s) and later of managed care. The government, the corporations (the market), and the professions could be seen as three competing forces (see, e.g., Krause 1996). James Robinson described the recent history succinctly: The antitrust critique of professional institutions from the 1970s on "ultimately contributed to the breaking up of the guild" and led directly to the "creative chaos of the moment" (Robinson 1999, xii, 29).

Reinventing the Public Mission

Critiques of medicine over the past thirty years appear at first to rule out a public mission for the medical profession in the future. However, since the mid-1990s, both the health system and the policy context have radically changed, making this a useful time for reevaluation. Managed care is not the panacea it once seemed to be. Medical groups are working with Congress and with state legislatures to regulate insurance practices and to protect the interests of both doctors and patients through patients' rights legislation. While organized medicine may have declined to press for a role as a delegated public agent under a governmental system for financing care in the past (as they declined to fight for private group practices such as HMOs), this option is not precluded for the future. Today, it is easier to see than it was ten years ago that public interest and professional self-interest are not necessarily, or even usefully, antagonistic.

It is in this context that the profession's strong, if one-sided public service agenda for the last 100 years should be stressed. The forms of public service that predominated in the early years of the last century did not vanish; they have remained as subordinate purposes through the years and are available for expansion and updating.

Challenging the Myths

The medical profession and its critics need not continue their negative, perhaps self-fulfilling critique of the profession. Indeed, only by revising old ideas can there be a liberating language for this decade. Scholarly work on the utility and functions of language, narrative, and myth as part of the received history and ideology of the medical profession might usefully concentrate on the continuing mythological themes of strife and heroes, and on the long historical juxtaposition of "ideals" and "business" as rival descriptions (or mirror images) of America. The first theme provides the profession with a scenario for failure in the present; the second suggests conflict rather than cooperation with insurance and health care corporations.

Health insurers have come to symbolize business, in the sense that a necessary antagonism is assumed to exist between them and the "ideal" medical profession (Stevens 1998; Stone 1998), rather than a sense of shared mission, constructive mutual criticism, and even shared success, in the long run. Here, again, ideas from the first quarter of the twentieth century linger, when the concept that commerce and ideals were antithetical social spheres (however counterfactual) was useful rhetoric for the rise of professions in the United States (e.g., see Haskell 1984). This set of beliefs informed the AMA's long opposition to "corporate" or "contract" medicine in the twentieth century, through sanctioning the role of the medical profession as a source of idealism set against the market, on the assumption that the two were mutually exclusive. This notion lingers today in the belief that insurers and other large health care corporations will inevitably destroy the hallowed, selfless properties of "true" professionalism. Such instrumental, but largely unexamined, assumptions continue to structure behavior. For health care managers and researchers, as well as members of the health professions, thinking in terms of winners and losers, or victims and antagonists, may block the potential for confident, proactive, and innovative leadership in the future.

Identifying Partners

Reinventing professional idealism in the market, rather than in opposition to it, would require medical organizations to have available and willing partners. Visionary leaders within the profession may find themselves in a double bind. They are challenged to develop forward-looking public policies that move beyond divisive rhetoric, but they may be thwarted in the search for national allies because of the decentralized, competitive power structures of the health care system and the inertia of federal policymaking (and at least some suspicion of their goals). Their policies, whether or not upheld by the membership at large, or seen merely as idealistic statements, drop into an implementation vacuum.

In the process, efforts by some organizations to create real change in health care go unrecognized within medicine as a whole, and ignored by the health services research and policy communities. For example, the American College of Physicians (ACP) developed and published a major policy paper in 1990, calling for a uniform minimum package of insurance benefits for all, irrespective of residence or employment, and for financing mechanisms adequate to eliminate barriers to care (American College of Physicians 1990). In 2000, the Board of Regents of the combined ACP-ASIM (the ACP and American Society of Internal Medicine), representing 115,000 physicians, approved an extended policy statement, calling for a sequential, planned strategy for health policy in the United States. This would include the explicit public goal of having all Americans covered by an adequate insurance plan by a specified date; a "uniform, evidence-based package of benefits that would be available to all Americans"; the use of federal budget surpluses to expand health insurance to the uninsured; progressive financing; efforts to eliminate disparities in health care for those living in the inner cities; and programs of accountability to reduce medical errors. In this process, the medical profession should "embrace its responsibility to participate in the development of reforms to improve the U.S. health care system" through partnering with government, business, and other stakeholders (ACP-ASIM 2000).

Other medical organizations have developed public policy statements, and have sometimes signed joint statements, such as the one calling for health insurance for all Americans that was signed in 1999 by representatives of family physicians, pediatricians, emergency physicians, obstetricians and gynecologists, internists, surgeons, and the AMA (All Americans Must Have Health Insurance 1999). However, it is not yet clear how national medical organizations can move beyond divisive rhetoric and rally their members to effective action without strong external partners.

In the short run, national charitable foundations and other nonprofit, policy-oriented organizations might fill part of the gap in national policy structures. Programs such as the Commonwealth Fund's Task Force on Academic Health Centers, the Open Society Institute's Medicine as a Profession Program (MAPP), the Robert Wood Johnson Foundation's Investigator Awards in Health Policy Research and other programs, the Institute of Medicine's Committee on Quality Health Care in America, and the National Quality Forum, among others, provide organizational bases for discussion both of health care policy and of the role of professional organizations. While these not-for-profit institutions rely primarily on their claims to objectivity and moral leadership, and on their ability to foster consensus, sway public opinion, and mold expert judgment as levers for change (rather than the direct exercise of power in the health care system), these and similar efforts could prove vital to supporting and defining medical leadership in the United States for the foreseeable future.

Changing the Rhetoric

The medical profession itself is, of course, a diverse army of individuals with a wide range of skills, interests, and agendas. In the short run, a unifying body of rhetoric may be important in giving this army a sense of identity and purpose as members of one profession, and it is reasonable to expect that the major organizations will vie with each other to develop resounding phrases. Vilifying managed care has played this unifying function to some extent, and there have indeed been egregious problems and destructive controls on doctors and patients that needed to be fixed in the interests of both the public and professionals.

Medical organizations have used this tactic quite successfully. "Don't Let Big Insurance Ambush Patients' Rights," trumpeted an AMA advertisement in the *New Orleans Times Picayune* in April 2001, citing the "abuses" of managed care (American Medical Association 2001). Passage of patients' rights legislation in more than thirty states represents political success and may even restore some of the lost privileges and "autonomy" of the old fee-for-service medicine (Kesselheim 2001), although this might be seen as a retrograde step. However, this accomplishment may prove short-lived as managed care shifts to new forms, and battle statements do not mesh easily with the measured calls for public policy just discussed. Making managed care the "fall guy" for necessary (and overdue) rationalization of the medical marketplace seems misguided, even counterproductive, as a long-range strategy for any actual or would-be policy group.

What organizing rhetoric might be useful? Addressing this question offers an intriguing policy task (and intellectual challenge) not just for the medical profession but for any individual or group studying, working with, or attempting reforms of the major health professions. Available social science theories seem to sustain a conflict model for interorganizational relations. David Frankford and others have pointed out that the language of power is structured into health care debates and scholarly analyses to such an extent that each type of power is thought to have a challenging or countervailing power (Frankford 1997; Schlesinger 1997; Light 1993). Under this model, the power of professional self-regulation is countered by increasing regulation of doctors by outside agencies. Buying into the concept of countervailing power is likely to structure expectations by suggesting (or rationalizing) an attack/defense agenda, thus narrowing the possible outcomes to winning or losing, and excluding the possibility of a win-win scenario. However, assumptions are not immutable, and when images and stereotypes change, so may politics and policies (Morone 1997). The old rhetoric is tired and, in some ways, meaningless. For example, as other commentators have noted, the term "professional autonomy" in medicine seems to have shrunk and become a proxy for concerns about physician job security and income maintenance, while attacks on professional self-regulation as self-interest have left the term "self-regulation" without any coherent meaning or moral value (Wynia et al. 1999).

A recent article in the nursing literature reviewed models of positive identity developed for oppressed groups as relevant for the profession of nursing, so as to break negative stereotypes inherited from the past and liberate the profession from the "oppressor within" (Roberts 2000). Physicians, many of whom, like nurses, feel under siege from increased workloads and staff cutbacks, might be reluctant to declare themselves organizationally or individually "oppressed," despite their manifold complaints about the health care system. Nevertheless, the invention of new terms and the creation of new understandings of old terms are likely to be important elements in the process of change, whatever one's view about the future of professions.

There is renewed recognition in the scholarly disciplines of the importance of reappraising unexamined ideas that provide the conceptual framework in which we live: those words, ideas, and concepts that are "large in potential but not programmed," as the historian Thomas Bender put it (Bender 1997). New language can express cooperation rather than conflict, and act as an important bridge between participants with otherwise conflicting views. Working separately or together, policy analysts, consumer groups, medical leaders, and action-oriented researchers might address three tasks: to describe complex events in new ways, by drawing from common mythological understandings in ways that are helpful to the present; to reinterpret recent history in the light of the major organizational changes of the past decades; and to develop new organizing language and new story lines to spur innovation.

Imagining the Future

A movement to reimagine the present, past, and future is already evident in a scattered body of work, largely outside the formal structures of the medical profession. In his study of the science and politics of drug regulation, for example, historian Harry Marks (1997) has reconceived the first half of the twentieth century as the "era of organizational reform," and the second half as the "triumph of statistics." A rhetorical shift toward the value of statistical evidence in medicine, tailor-made for our present information age, provides one good way of conceptualizing organized medicine's role in the light of positive changes in the science base, and of opening up new possibilities for physicians in assessing and improving the health of communities. Discounting, for the purpose of argument, the very real difficulties of incorporating population health as an intrinsic part of medical education and clinical practice, such concepts could be more strongly framed by building on the medical profession's long tradition of support of biomedical science and public health.

In another example, Robinson (1999) has usefully ascribed "normality" to the turmoil in medical practice in the 1990s, by drawing analogies between health care reorganization and the deregulation of other sectors of the economy. He starts with the assumption that the old days are gone, that there is no going back to "unregulated professionalism," and that current upheavals are signs of "creative chaos," providing opportunities for innovation. In this scenario, the role of the medical profession is dynamic, not yet fixed, in terms of managing clinical practice in the future. To seize the challenge, medical groups, including professional associations, would have to work together across specialty boundaries, develop collective goals, buy into the culture of innovation, and (perhaps most difficult) cede management authority to effective leaders. The tone is one of moving forward, rather than of conflict or defeat.

Other scholars and reformers, too, are suggesting specific conceptual changes. Frankford argues for dropping the label "countervailing power" in favor of "participatory power," thus encouraging, at least at the symbolic level, different groups to work together more constructively in local communities (Frankford 1997; Frankford and Konrad 1998). Jordan Cohen (1999) has been using the term "collaborative care" as a rallying cry for change in medical education. Marc Rodwin (1993; 1995) has stressed the nature and importance of the doctor's fiduciary role, a term that extends readily to the profession's wider social roles. Gregg Bloche (1999) has focused on the nature of clinical loyalties, raising the issue of wider organizational loyalties among physicians and to the public, as well as the traditional loyalty to individual patients. David Mechanic (1996; 1998) has chosen trust as an organizing concept for thinking about professionalism, including the importance of "social trust" in the broader roles and institutions of medicine. The concept of trust also weaves into the management literature and thus provides a potentially useful bridge between physician organizations and health care management. *Trust Matters* is the title of a book for managers trying to rebuild shattered organizational relationships (Annison and Wilford 1998). In a related vein, Norman Daniels (1998) has stressed the importance of building ethical health care organizations (including health plans), as well as ethical professions. Language is not difficult to change. We live in a world of sound bites and buzzwords, with virtually instant communication.

The idea of a public service role is not difficult to grasp, either. Unarguably, no one in the United States, rich or poor, would be well served in the future by a disorganized, if not demoralized, medical profession. Why? Because individual doctors make life-and-death decisions for (and with) individual patients; because medical organizations have years of experience and expertise in educating and evaluating doctors, and this experience should be judiciously used; because there is a tradition of public service ready to be revived; and because no one outside the profession is capable of regulating the profession as well as the profession itself, though it may need help to change in ways that will enhance medical performance, confidence, creativity, and public trust.

Beyond Decline and Fall: Toward a New Public Service Ethos

What might a new public service role for the medical profession actually consist of? Any specific agenda would be context-dependent. Major changes in legislation, massive shifts in the structure and behavior of health corporations (perhaps stimulated by government regulation or by fiscal incentives), or some combination of the two might generate new collective professional roles quite quickly, by incorporating the professional voice inside insurance arrangements, program policies, and organizational practices. Absent such changes, consideration of a new public service role would require continuous, subtle engagement by medical leaders and many others, including consumers. Models are needed—and here the health services research community could provide a major service. We need good scenarios for constructive empowerment, different forms of empowerment—and, for that matter, disempowerment—of professional organizations under different policy models in the United States, including alternative forms of universal health insurance. Other models might assume enhanced roles for organized medicine in the present system (e.g., greater involvement in clinical policies within, and as part of, managed care networks), in specific areas (e.g., quality improvement and assessment, or privacy of medical records), or in alternative scenarios for services in the future (e.g., the profession's role in crafting rules for managed care that are workable, innovative, and acceptable to all parties).

Potential roles for the medical profession depend on the competence of professional organizations to take a public leadership role, the relative willingness of the public (however defined) to recognize the value of a strong profession in furthering social goals, the existence of willing organizational partners (public and private), and the development of concepts and new language to build policy consensus. This promises to be an active time for professional organizations, and for the action-oriented researchers who work with them. Among today's questions are: what doctors can and should do for patients in health plans; how to establish common goals for high-quality clinical services; how to measure and improve those services; and how to ensure that all members of the population actually receive appropriate care. Theoretically, all of these questions flow directly from the profession's traditional, "individualist" agenda: ensuring to the public a trusting, ethical relationship between one doctor and one patient; making a commitment to provide care to those who need it; furthering public health activities; establishing national standards for education and training; and supporting biomedical science and technology policy. These historical agendas remain, to be adapted to meet new conditions.

The doctor-patient relationship, a core value of professionalism, is at the heart of current medical critiques of physician relations with managed care corporations. This essential commitment could be extended in many different directions, however. Since teams of health professionals rather than one doctor often care for individual patients now, the doctor-patient relationship could simply be expanded to encompass the performance and behavior of the whole health team—a logical updating to take account of changes in the way medicine is delivered. The policy implications of such a shift range from joint training and evaluation of the team to increased cooperation between doctors and other health care workers (including those involved with quality evaluation). Looking at patient care from a systems perspective is critical for error reduction as well. Similarly, the term "patient" might be extended to encompass the local health system or groups of patients with similar conditions. In either case, the spirit of self-criticism (and learning from mistakes) that has long been a hallmark of medicine might be extended to the evaluation of specific health care systems, policies, or procedures—not as an attack on the power of the "system" or as a backhanded swipe at clinical practice, but as a natural extension of medical professionalism. The goal would be to learn from and improve care, rather than to punish or over-regulate practitioners—a noncontroversial goal that is clearly in the public interest.

Even the profession's long-standing charity tradition, however archaic in its original practice of giving services to the poor without expectation of a fee, might be revived to serve the original goal of ensuring needed care to every member of the population, through whatever means available. In today's context, that would logically lead to strong political positions on universal health insurance coverage, or some other means of providing reasonable access to services for the whole population. This goal might also encompass policies for expanded administrative and planning roles for doctors in insurance and service organizations to ensure that services are being given and that they are of high quality. Similarly, the profession's traditional commitment to public health suggests an increased medical voice for better health at the community and national levels.

Since the term "health" has long since widened to include coping well with chronic conditions, medical organizations might also pay more attention to how well patients are actually coping with such conditions, irrespective of their income level, ethnicity, or place of residence. Organized medicine could do more to encourage doctors to rate themselves and their teams by the health indices of the communities in which they work. Where those indices appear to be associated with factors extrinsic to the traditionally defined health system (such as improving education), the organizations might extend their collective moral reach in the interests of better community health.

The profession's traditional commitment to scientific standards also demands an adjustment in public roles, since major medical organizations are having to accept that other players have entered the standards business—including independent accrediting and credentialing agencies, such as the National Commission for Quality Assurance (NCQA) for health plans, and specialist credentialing groups outside the profession's nationally approved structure for physicians (see Millenson 1997). The development of patient-outcomes measures, clinical guidelines, and novel ways of testing for competence in the practice setting has shifted concern about medical competence away from educational and credentialing alone to involve a host of experts outside (as well as inside) the medical profession. State licensing boards are flexing their muscles as alternative vehicles for private, professional regulation. The rise of bioethics involves a further group of professionals with a legitimate role in medical decision-making. Medical organizations are trying to take account of these various shifts without defining them narrowly as power grabs by other players—not an easy transition to make. Again, the challenge is partly conceptual: to redefine "science" as a positive joint effort of numerous organizations and interests.

Medical organizations are becoming increasingly involved in defining and measuring medical service in the United States through specialty recertification and proposals for extension into the continuous evaluation of practice performance (see, e.g., Wasserman, Kimball, and Duffy 2000). Almost 90 percent of all practicing doctors (post-residency) are now board-certified specialists. In the future, evaluation might include appraising doctors' prescription patterns, appropriately early diagnosis, outcome measurements of patient care, effectiveness of the therapeutic team, and statistical analysis of the practice as a whole and of the larger group to which the doctor belongs. These action and others, if fully implemented, would bring American doctors firmly into the information age under private auspices. Logically, such actions would also generate demands by medical organizations (with or without cooperative efforts with insurers) for much better, more available data than exist at present.

Mark Schlesinger (1999) has suggested that it would be useful conceptually to explore the role of competing social institutions in dealing with issues that might otherwise be delegated to the profession. But if we stopped here in the analysis, we might buy into the downhill, post-professional-dominance conceptual model of the medical profession—that is, that a once-authoritative profession has lost much of its traditional cultural authority. Today's environment requires collaborative planning, management, and policymaking rather than conflicts; concerns about the health of populations as well as of individuals; and moral leadership in the allocation of scarce resources. Quality evaluation, a key aspect of professionalism, requires links between medical groups and nonmedical evaluators—in universities, consulting firms, government agencies, corporate health plans, and (where relevant) the information industry. All these considerations of professional roles and actions have a direct bearing on social policy relating to the health of the public; for, taken together, they might realign public and professional agendas in ways that would be constructive for both.

No organization has yet taken the high ground of defining a consensus position of what, ideally, the American medical enterprise should be in the early twenty-first century. While this task may properly lie in the public policy realm—with legislators, consumers, entrepreneurs, and economists at the forefront—stronger involvement of the medical profession is not necessarily contra-indicated. As caregivers in the most fundamental sense, literally and culturally, doctors are in a unique position. It is not unreasonable to expect the medical profession to work with other groups, including congressional committees, to help establish basic principles for health care for all and invent a workable social contract from which innovation could take place; that is, to re-empower the medical profession organizationally, recognizing that both power and its exercise would have different meanings than in the past.

The medical profession is only one potential source of leadership, of course. But there are strong reasons why the role of medical organizations as moral leaders makes considerable practical sense. The profession has long had an authoritative voice in American culture. Indeed, the very narrative of rise and fall was based on medicine as an American success story. Despite the gloom and doom expressed over managed care from the early 1990s to the present, doctors have not lost their normative roles in American society. They embody a huge reservoir of goodwill, inherited from the past. This is derived in various parts: from long respect of the doctor as healer; from the ideology of medicine as a public service and the doctor as hero; from the huge advances of scientific medicine in the twentieth century, continuing through promises for the future; from claims for scientific objectivity; from the symbolic value of medicine as culturally suited to other American values (such as ingenuity, technology, and international superiority); and, not least, from the sheer visibility of national medical organizations, even in the absence of a unified governmental health policy. At a practical level, the medical profession might also be easier to mobilize as an influential force in American culture than newer, less visible organizations.

Can medical organizations in the United States rally with sufficient speed to claim a new public agenda? This may depend on if they have external help (or effective external goading) to do so. Organized medicine could continue to be stigmatized (and stigmatize itself) by the myth of a profession in decline, if not defeat. At this point, no one knows. By raising and commenting on these themes, I hope to stimulate debate and research on medicine's future public roles among scholars, managers, and policy analysts, to raise consciousness within the medical profession, and to encourage cooperation across these groups.

This chapter is a slightly modified (slightly shortened and clarified) version of my article, "Public Roles for the Medical Profession in the United States: Beyond Theories of Decline and Fall," *Milbank Quarterly*, 2001, 79 (3): 327-53.

References

All Americans Must Have Health Insurance. 1999. (Joint Statement of the American Academy of Family Physicians, American Academy of Pediatrics, American College of Emergency Physicians, American College of Obstetricians and Gynecologists,

American College of Physicians American Society of Internal Medicine, American College of Surgeons, and the American Medical Association.) Philadelphia: American College of Physicians American Society of Internal Medicine.

American College of Physicians. 1990. "Access to Health Care." *Annals of Internal Medicine* 112: 641-6.

American College of Physicians-American Society of Internal Medicine. 2000. "Providing Access to Care for All Americans: A Statement of Core Policy Principles." Approved by the Board of Regents, October 29. www.acp-asim.org. Accessed April 23, 2001.

American Medical Association. 2001. "Don't Let Big Insurance Ambush Patients' Rights." www.ama-assn.org. Accessed April 24.

Ameringer, C. F. 1999. *State Medical Boards and the Politics of Public Protection.* Baltimore: Johns Hopkins University Press.

Annison, M. H., and Wilford, D. S. 1998. *Trust Matters: New Directions in Health Care Leadership.* San Francisco: Jossey-Bass.

Bender, T. 1997. "Intellectual and Cultural History." In *The New American History*, rev. ed., eds. S. P. Benson, S. Brier, and R. Rosenzwieg. Philadelphia: Temple University Press.

Bloche, M. G. 1999. "Clinical Loyalties and the Social Purposes of Medicine." *Journal of the American Medical Association* 281: 268–74.

Booth, B. 2000. "Fractured Federation." *American Medical News* (October 9): 14.

Burnham, J. C. 1982. "American Medicine's Golden Age: What Happened to It?" *Science* 215: 1474–9.

Burrow, J. G. 1977. *Organized Medicine in the Progressive Era: The Move Toward Monopoly.* Baltimore: Johns Hopkins University Press.

Cohen, J. J. 1999. "Collaborative Care: A New Model for a New Century." Address given at AAMC Annual Meeting, Washington, D.C.

Committee on Quality of Health Care in America. 2001. *Crossing the Quality Chasm: A New Health System for the 21st Century.* Washington, D.C.: National Academy Press.

Daniels, N. 1998. "Professional Values and Their Institutional Context." New York: Open Society Institute, Program on Professions. (Manuscript.)

Fox, D. M. 1986. *Health Policies, Health Politics: The British and American Experience, 1911–1965.* Princeton, N.J.: Princeton University Press.

———. 1993. *Power and Illness: The Failure and Future of American Health Policy.* Berkeley: University of California Press.

Frankford, D. M. 1997. "The Normative Constitution of Professional Power." *Journal of Health Politics, Policy and Law* 22: 185-221.

———, and T. R. Konrad. 1998. "Responsive Medical Professionalism: Integrating Education, Practice and Community in a Market-Driven Era." *Academic Medicine* 73: 138-45.

Freeman, R. 2000. *The Politics of Health in Europe.* Manchester: Manchester University Press.

Freidson, E. 1970. *Profession of Medicine: A Study of the Sociology of Applied Knowledge.* New York: Dodd Mead.

———. 1994. *Professionalism Reborn: Theory, Prophecy and Policy.* Chicago: University of Chicago Press.

Harris, R. 1966. *A Sacred Trust.* New York: New American Library.

Haskell, T. L. 1984. "Professionalism versus Capitalism: R. H. Tawney, Emile Durkheim and C. S. Peirce on the Disinterestedness of Professional Communities." In *The Authority of Experts: Studies in History and Theory*, ed. T. L. Haskell. Bloomington: Indiana University Press.

Hirshfield, D. S. 1970. *The Lost Reform: The Campaign for Compulsory Health Insurance in the United States from 1932 to 1943*. Cambridge, Mass.: Harvard University Press.

Johnson, T. J. 1972. *Professions and Power*. London: Macmillan.

Kesselheim, A. S. 2001. "What's the Appeal? Trying to Control Managed Care: Medical Necessity Decisionmaking through a System of External Appeals." *University of Pennsylvania Law Review* 149: 873-920.

Kohn, L. T., Corrigan, J. M., and Donaldson, M. S., eds. 2000. *To Err Is Human: Building a Safer Health System*. Washington, D.C.: National Academy Press.

Krause, E. A. 1996. *Death of the Guilds: Professions, States, and the Advance of Capitalism, 1930 to the Present*. New Haven: Yale University Press.

Larson, M. S. 1977. *The Rise of Professionalism: A Sociological Analysis*. Berkeley: University of California Press.

Light, D. W. 1988. "Turf Battles and the Theory of Professional Dominance." *Research in the Sociology of Health Care* 7: 203-25.

————. 1993. "Countervailing Power: The Changing Character of the Medical Profession in the United States." In *The Changing Character of the Medical Profession: An International Perspective*, eds. F. Hafferty and J. McKinley. New York: Oxford University Press.

————, and Levine, S. 1988. "The Changing Character of the Medical Profession." *Milbank Quarterly* 66 (suppl. 2): 10–32.

Ludmerer, K. M. 1985. *Learning to Heal: The Development of American Medical Education*. New York: Basic Books.

————. 1999. *Time to Heal: American Medical Education from the Turn of the Century to the Era of Managed Care*. New York: Oxford University Press.

Marks, H. M. 1997. *The Progress of Experiment: Science and Therapeutic Reform in the United States, 1900-1990*. Cambridge: Cambridge University Press.

Marmor, T. R., with the assistance of J. S. Marmor. 1973. *The Politics of Medicare*. Chicago: Aldine. (See also Marmor, T. R. 2000. *The Politics of Medicare*, 2nd ed. New York: Aldine de Gruyter.)

McConnell, G. M. 1966. *Private Power and American Democracy*. New York: Alfred A. Knopf.

Mechanic, D. 1996. "Changing Medical Organization and the Erosion of Trust." *Milbank Quarterly* 74: 171-89.

————. 1998. "Public Trust and Initiatives for New Health Partnerships." *Milbank Quarterly* 76: 281–302.

————. 2000. "Managed Care and the Imperative for a New Professional Ethic." *Health Affairs* 19: 100-11.

Millenson, M. L. 1997. *Demanding Medical Excellence: Doctors and Accountability in the Information Age*. Chicago: University of Chicago Press.

Moran, M. 1999. *Governing the Health Care State: A Comparative Study of the United Kingdom, the United States and Germany*. Manchester: Manchester University Press.

Morone, J. A. 1997. "Enemies of the People: The Moral Dimensions of Public Health." *Journal of Health Politics, Policy and Law* 22: 993-1020.

Numbers, R. L. 1978. *Almost Persuaded: American Physicians and Compulsory Health Insurance, 1912-1920*. Baltimore: Johns Hopkins University Press.

Poen, M. M. 1979. *Harry Truman versus the Medical Lobby: The Genesis of Medicare*. Columbia: University of Missouri Press.

Rayack, E. 1967. *Professional Power and American Medicine: The Economics of the American Medical Association*. Cleveland: World.

Roberts, S. J. 2000. "Developing a Positive Identity: Liberating One-self from the Oppressor Within." *Advances in Nursing Science* 22: 71-82.

Robinson, J. C. 1999. *The Corporate Practice of Medicine: Competition and Innovation in Health Care*. Berkeley: University of California Press.

Rodwin, M. A. 1993. *Medicine, Money and Morals: Physicians' Conflicts of Interest*. New York: Oxford University Press.

———. 1995. "Strains in the Fiduciary Metaphor: Divided Physician Loyalties and Obligations in a Changing Health Care System." *American Journal of Law and Medicine* 20: 147-67.

Rothman, D. J. 2000. "Medical Professionalism—Focusing on the Real Issues." *New England Journal of Medicine* 342: 1283-6.

Schlesinger, M. 1997. "Countervailing Agency: A Strategy of Principled Regulation under Managed Competition." *Milbank Quarterly* 75: 35-87.

———. 1999. Personal communication.

Starr, P. 1982. *The Social Transformation of American Medicine: The Rise of a Sovereign Profession and the Making of a Vast Industry*. New York: Basic Books.

Stevens, R. 1989. *In Sickness and in Wealth: American Hospitals in the Twentieth Century*. New York: Basic Books. Reissued 1999, with a new introduction (Baltimore: Johns Hopkins University Press).

———. 1998. "Old, New, and Déjà Vu: The Social Roles of the Medical Profession." New York: Open Society Institute, Program on Professions. (Manuscript.)

Stone, D. A. 1998. "The Doctor as Businessman: The Changing Politics of a Cultural Icon." In *Healthy Markets? The New Competition in Medical Care*, ed. M. A. Peterson. Durham, N.C.: Duke University Press.

Wasserman, S. I., Kimball, H. R., and Duffy, F. D. 2000. "Recertification in Internal Medicine: A Program of Continuous Professional Development." *Annals of Internal Medicine* 133: 202-8.

Wolinsky, F. D. 1988. "The Professional Dominance Perspective, Revisited." *Milbank Quarterly* 66 (suppl. 2): 33-47.

Wolinsky, H., and Brune, T. 1994. *The Serpent on the Staff: The Unhealthy Politics of the American Medical Association*. New York: G.P. Putnam's Sons.

Wynia, M. K., Latham, S. R., Kao, A. C., Berg, J. W., and Emanuel, L. L. 1999. "Medical Professionalism in Society." *New England Journal of Medicine* 341: 1612-6.

V. The American Health Care State

Introduction to Section V

What does history teach us? Humility, for sure. The two chapters in this section focus on the very rapid, largely unpredictable changes that assailed American hospitals from the late 1980s through the 1990s. But the messages are larger than for hospitals alone. Together with the concurrent uncertainties and changes in other parts of health care, including the medical profession, described in Section IV, the stage was set for organizational uncertainty, hand-wringing, and blame-calling across the American health care state in the first decade of the twenty-first century.

Chapters 16 and 17 explore themes that continue to engage us today. For example, are hospitals (or, for that matter, doctors or other health organizations and professions) expected to demonstrate responsibility for the health needs of their local communities; and if so, how much responsibility, and how should this be achieved, measured, or enforced? Is it reasonable to expect a hospital to cater to the needs of individuals or social groups whose members cannot play a full role as paying consumers in a market-oriented health care system? And if hospitals (or doctors or anyone else) should take on a larger community role, where are they to find the funds to do it?

For those who have read chapter 1 of this volume—on hospitals seeking state funds for "charity" in Pennsylvania more than a century ago—these questions may sound uncannily familiar. The reason is, of course, that the question of community has been a continuing theme in policy debates through many different sociopolitical and economic contexts. Charity and community responsibility have been interlocking themes. With Medicare and Medicaid, the federal government claimed responsibility for important aspects of charity by paying for hospital services for individuals who were elderly, disabled, and/or indigent, according to specific eligibility and payment rules. However, as in the earlier history of Pennsylvania, the implementation of government responsibility for charity, through policies thought to benefit all participants, soon collided with the exigencies of governmental budgets.

I wrote chapter 16, "The American Hospital as a Social Institution: Past is Prologue," for a 1986 book of essays edited by sociologists Linda Aiken and David Mechanic on the applications of the social sciences to clinical medicine and health policy. A modified version appeared in *Society*, also in 1986. Writing the essay gave me the opportunity to address "community" as a concept that had woven its way through hospital history. I discuss the wide array of meanings it has held—to the point of becoming functionally meaningless by the late 1980s. Nevertheless, it was still symbolically important in the 1980s, and one can make a similar observation in our present. Hospital managers and boards see themselves as being more than a commercial venture. Though being selected to a hospital board is taken much more seriously today in terms of fiduciary responsibility than in the 1980s, it is still regarded as a social honor, and still evokes some sense of community service.

The word "community," like many other descriptive words in health policy, brought feel-good emotions to the fore in the 1980s—representing, perhaps, as potent a social aspiration as at the beginning of the twentieth century. But like many other values and buzzwords in health care, much of its utility lay in its ambiguous meaning when translated to the real, money-driven world. Then, as later, health care providers were happy to receive government subsidy but reluctant to strengthen government's role as regulator as well as payer. Quite apart from this, community agendas could vary considerably; aiming for example, to improve access for all members of the population, or use available resources more efficiently, or strengthen private organizations (thus ensuring their success and avoiding direct government intervention), or solidify social class divisions, or ratify the local entrepreneurship of community power structures. Hospital advocates in Pennsylvania in 1910 had recognized community value in a hospital enterprise that was segmented into religious and ethnic hospital ownership. This value was strongly supported by the state through subsidy in response to the community claims of powerful, self-selected local leaders. At the end of the century ownership seemed less important as a marker of a specific community than social stratification of hospitals by clientele.

Medicare, Medicaid, and private insurance, including managed care, responded to hospitals in an owner-neutral way, buying services in for-profit, not-for-profit, and government hospitals on a similar basis. In the 1980s each type of hospital struggled to survive and prosper where they could. Communities other than the local community or the state—communities of interest, largely but not wholly in the private sector—had become powerful players by the 1980s, including consultants, lawyers, and monetary advisors. Federal control, exercised through Medicare regulation, represented the national fiscal interests of a community of taxpayers. In the 1980s, as earlier (or later), community in the American context was inevitably defined in terms of influence, power, and money.

My book on the history of American hospitals, *In Sickness and in Wealth*, was published in 1989. Chapter 17 was written to reintroduce the book when it was reprinted in 1999. The introduction was only too necessary for new readers, given the strains and stresses that faced hospitals in the 1990s, particularly the greatly enhanced influence of insurers over providers of care. The so-called managed care revolution was in full force. The introduction also gave me a second chance to survey the twentieth century by bringing the history forward another ten years. Timing alone made the attempt irresistible, in anticipation of the coming of the much-touted, new "millennium."

Apart from generic concerns about "community," what *were* the themes that marked the century? The policy surge toward "market solutions" to health care organization and financing suggested that older organizational assumptions might be irrelevant or dead. Medical science and technology bore little comparison with that of the early twentieth century, when hospitals became recognized as quintessential, quasi-public American institutions. Was it merely quaint and outmoded to think that hospitals embodied symbolic social aspirations as emblems of civic pride and scientific medicine? Were hospitals more usefully categorized as competitive supermarkets for services; or as focused factories, using Regina Herzlinger's term in her book, *Market-Driven Health Care* (1997); or as cogs in giant, investor-owned health care corporations, nimbly responding to the combined 3-Ms of public and private revenue streams—Medicare, Medicaid, managed care?

The central theme of *In Sickness and in Wealth* was that twentieth-century American hospitals were both charities and businesses, leaning toward one depiction or the other as circumstances changed. Hospitals were organizational chameleons, revealing themselves as more business-oriented (for example in the 1920s or 1980s) or more charitable (as in the 1930s) as economic and political contexts changed. They were also intensely and pragmatically political. As shown in this volume, as well as in the book, hospital representatives and their organizations have long been attuned to political advantage, particularly where money is concerned.

Compared with a hundred years ago, organized charity is *not* how we would describe the role of twenty-first-century for-profit or even not-for-profit hospitals—competing, as they must do, in a tumult-driven, public-private marketplace in which organizational goals are constantly renegotiated. Nevertheless, whatever words define them, hospitals remain culturally powerful institutions in the United States, whatever the type of ownership. While not-for-profits have become more savvy about finance and operational balance sheets in the past decades, for-profit hospitals have been seeking community approbation, if only for marketing purposes and to advance their brand name. Advertising, from billboards to glossy magazines, became ubiquitous in the 1990s, irrespective of type of hospital ownership; and hospitals trumpet their relative rankings (usually where these are high, of course) in local and national ratings of hospital and service "excellence."

I concluded in 1999 (chapter 17) that a mix of ownership, for-profit, not-for-profit, and governmental, is on balance a good thing. Arguably, it still is. Since each type of institution must constantly watch and adjust to the relative advantages of the others, the hospital industry works in an environment of continuing tension, uncertainty, and interdependence that spurs each on to greater efforts, and allows for future policy changes. In our present as in earlier decades, it is not clear what the future will bring: whether hospitals will (or should) play a role in American popular and political culture simply as profit-driven factories for bodily treatment (or shopping malls for boutique medical specialties) to be sold to customers (caveat emptor), or whether they also speak to higher cultural aspirations; demonstrating, for example, American ideals of caring and professionalism, providing an assist to the goals of individual opportunity, or spreading American technology thrillingly to all.

Other larger themes of this collection include the ambiguity inherent in not-for-profit status; the larger, societal implications for services when they are contingent on buyer-seller contracts; the continuing, often lively, sometimes desperate interdependence among for-profit, not-for-profit, and governmental maneuverings; and the successes and failures of the market (and of government) as social engineer.

Perhaps most evidently, the United States has lacked a consistent set of policies for health care over the decades. But it is also evident that, despite energetic, largely quixotic efforts to invent them, there have never been simple "solutions" to providing health care. Indeed there has never been agreement on what "health care" is. American health care policy is typically expressed as multiple streams of money flowing from government and other money-collecting organizations (such as employment-sponsored or other private insurance) to organizations and professions in the business of providing care. Not surprisingly, much policy discussion in health care focuses on huge expenses by the federal government as a single payer, such as in Medicare, NIH, and federal grants to states for Medicaid. Discussions over Medicaid as a fiscal burden in state budgets in the early twenty-first century echo similar concerns in Pennsylvania in 1910 (chapter1).

The reasons for the money flows vary, as illustrated in these essays. There has been considerable ingenuity in justifying funds for different purposes. In the process government funds have transformed private institutions, but not necessarily in ways that could have been predicted. The implementation of Medicaid in the late 1960s and early 1970s (chapter 5) provides a good example of the continuing, intense, and mutual relationship between the political, economic, and organizational spheres of health care. The cycle repeats: Legislation is passed, but then implementation changes the landscape (and sometimes the players), and politics comes to the fore again. Public and private realms are interdependent and sometimes intermixed. As I write this, the federal government is providing millions of dollars to private employers as an incentive for them to continue to provide benefits for prescription drugs to their own retirees, so that those individuals will not participate in the federal program for prescription drugs offered as Medicare part D. In the light of history this is not as illogical as it may seem; but, rather, part of a long tradition of public subsidy of private institutions.

For much of the twentieth century health care provision in the United States could be contrasted, favorably to its supporters, as the antithesis of the "socialist" approaches in Western Europe. With the end of the Cold War the capitalist vs. socialist rhetoric lost its edge—we are all democratic capitalists now. Nevertheless, important distinctions remain in what is meant by the health care state. If the National Health Service in Great Britain still reflects, to its critics, the excessive fussiness, rigid rules, and suffocating virtues of the "nanny state," the United States might be described as the "pocket money state." Here money, not rules, is the apocryphal child's (i.e., society's) incentive for proper behavior—whatever "proper" might mean in either nation. In the United States, monetary opportunities suggest liberating the child to go in new directions, wherever those directions may lead.

Not surprisingly, each system has recently been attempting some correction. Changes in the National Health Service are designed to encourage managerial innovation and entrepreneurship and to increase scientific information about outcomes and processes of care, in order to make the service more flexible and base rules on established evidence. The United States has begun a process of reining in. The American problem is conceived not as one of hyperactivity or bad behavior, but of expense and lack of assigned responsibility. Policies favoring consumer responsibility express the desire to improve health care in two ways: through informed consumer choice of services, which would in theory allocate available resources more rationally; and through encouraging individuals to manage their own medical care more forcefully. Hence come proposals for financial incentives to encourage individuals to be more prudent in spending health care dollars and more rational in their purchase decisions, aided by knowledge gained from individually owned, portable patient records. Policies favoring audits and inspections, which have become ubiquitous, establish and enforce organizational and behavioral rules on providers.

At first glance, the most surprising aspect of the U.S. system is the lack—so far, at least—of standardized, transportable, electronic health care information, including patient history, clinical information, outcomes, and use of services. Why this is so is a historical question. The answers lie in part in the self-conscious independence and aloofness of hospitals one from another; in part in the traditional hostility of hospitals and doctors to the imposition of standards by external organizations, especially government; in the natural American urge to celebrate the vitality (and supposed superiority) of independent private organizations over government—as reflected in the clause in the original Medicare legislation (1965) that proscribed changes in the health care system even as it poured a golden river of money into that system; in no one being particularly interested until recently; and in the reluctance to favor one information system (or company or product) over another. The search now is for software to create a seamless compatibility across disparate information systems. Given its very different history, the British system may perhaps move more quickly.

I hope it has become abundantly evident in these essays that the American public-private health care state is about much more than health care. The health care industry has no clear boundaries. It involves, among other things, the interests of biotechnology, pharmaceutical, and medical devices corporations, the banking and insurance industries, large legal firms devoted to health care, an army of consultants and accountants, and political lobbies of manifold persuasions. "You see a financial opportunity and it sets off a gold rush," reported a banking lobbyist in 2006, in response to President George W. Bush's program for establishing individual Health Savings Accounts (Eric Dash, "Savings Accounts for Health Costs Attract Wall Street," *New York Times*, January 27, 2006, A16). Banks were contemplating a windfall of $2.3 billion over five years for payment processing costs on the new accounts. The health care state is not primarily about the health of American citizens but about the multiple roles played by the health care enterprise in the dynamic American economy. This is an exciting process to be involved with, to watch, and—not least—to try to influence so that health services are better as a result.

16

The American Hospital as a Social Institution: Past is Prologue (1986)

Because American hospitals developed as modern institutions at the time they did—largely between 1870 and 1914—they assumed an unusually important function as the embodiment of cultural aspirations. The hospital served both as a modern and an ideal institution, symbolizing the wealth of the new and expanding American cities, the order and glamour of science, the happy conjunction between humanitarianism and expertise in a society rife with money making. It is not coincidental that American hospitals have been among the most luxurious and costly structures ever built. An observer writing about the New York Hospital for *Harpers Magazine* in 1878 described its elevator, which was larger than those of a fashionable hotel, as so smooth in motion that it was like "a mechanical means of getting to heaven."[1]

Demonstration or show, even conspicuous waste, became a lasting aspect of the American hospital as a symbol—one that has as yet received too little attention by social scientists, and one cause of increasing costs. That the modern American hospital is a monument, symbolizing in its architecture and equipment more than its basic function, is apparent not only in the historical literature, but in the lavish style of buildings erected even in time of depression (including those built by the WPA in the 1930s). Another example can be drawn from the early

1960s, when there was enormous public concern about the poor hospital care available in run-down hospitals in inner-city areas. The solutions sought were for rebuilding and major renovating, rather than for the kind of making-do in draughty basements that has been a continuing characteristic of British hospital care. Today's hospitals, despite concern about the massive costs of hospital care, are among the most modern, high technology, costly structures being built in modern America. They continue to speak, subtly, to an implied link between cost and expertise.

The hospital was also to symbolize medicine as a vehicle of precision and control. Mastery of diagnosis (understanding the causes and progression of disease) gives a comforting illusion of control to both doctors and patients, even when little effective treatment is available—and for most nonsurgical conditions there was little effective treatment except good nursing techniques, until the advent of sulfa drugs in the 1930s and antibiotics after World War II. The promise of surgery and of specific remedies against infectious diseases, inherent in major discoveries before World War I, consolidated the image of the doctor as a hero fighting disease with twentieth-century tools. The increasing subdivision of medicine into specialties after World War I carried forward this image by placing the greatest emphasis, in terms of prestige and income, on the most heroic interventions. Thus neurosurgery carried greater prestige than psychiatry; radiotherapy than pediatrics.

As a projection of a profession whose archetypes were control, daring, and entrepreneurship, the twentieth-century American hospital (along with the medical schools) was always ill-suited to deal with chronic diseases—of which causes were mutifactorial and for which medical success was often problematic—and with the collective realms of public health. Even before World War I, hospitals could be criticized for a tendency to view the hospital merely from the inside; that is, from the self-generated perceptions of its board of trustees and its physicians. It followed, as S. Goldstein wrote in the 1907 *Charities and the Commons*, that the hospital did "not feel itself an intimate part of the social order; it stands forbiddingly isolated and aloof."[2] The fact that the potential existed, in theory at least, for the hospital to provide health services to the whole population in a defined service district, to compile epidemiological statistics, offer public health education and maternal and child welfare clinics, and to deal with the patient's family as well as with the patient, was to be a source of irritation to generations of disappointed critics.

The success and visibility of the hospital in providing acute, specialized care obscured its relatively limited role in the overall picture of health and disease. Nevertheless, the hospital could be described by the 1920s, as later, as an expression of pessimism, a "negative instrument of evolution," somewhat akin to refuse and sewage disposal, in that it dealt with problems of society rather than with positive solutions.[3] Departments of social work were started in leading hospitals, following the example at the Massachusetts General Hospital in 1905, with the belief that such facilities would help to eradicate the widely-held notion that the hospital was an impersonal institution and would help to elucidate the social causes of disease. Social service failed to become the core of community health care efforts for at least three reasons: the concentration of social service work on the poor, who attended outpatient departments with socially unappealing conditions—including venereal diseases, unwed motherhood, and tuberculosis; the lack of fees for social work, making it dependent on charity and on cost shifting from the hospital's paying patients; and the lack of power and the desire by the social workers themselves to become a clinical profession on the medical model, dealing with the psychosocial symptoms of individual patients rather than with community service needs.

American hospitals became successful at marketing acute services to paying patents. Public relations became an acceptable aspect of hospital management in the 1920s, with hospital fairs, radio spots, and even movies extolling the virtues of hospital care. Even in the depths of the Great Depression of the 1930s—with enormous pressures put on local government hospitals, as the unemployed sought free medical care, together with the closings of hundreds of small institutions—most of the income to the hospital industry came from patient fees. In not-for-profit hospitals, the standard bearers for hospital quality in the United States, 71 percent of hospital income came from patients in 1935.[4] The development of Blue Cross insurance plans in the 1930s, commercial hospital insurance in the 1940s, and Medicare in the mid-1960s buttressed the idea of hospital care as acute services, while increasing hospital income. None of these schemes typically included out-of-hospital diagnosis, preventive services, health education, or social services, whereby hospitals could reach out to the community as comprehensive health care centers. There were no financial incentives to override the heroic, specialized medical model for hospital care.

Community Ties

Besides the emerging character of the American hospital as an acute care facility, thriving in a market for paying patients and oriented and a money-value nexus, the hospital acquired values whose properties were largely mythological—and no less powerful for that. One of the most potent of these values was (and is) the idea of community.

Nonfederal acute care hospitals are termed "community hospitals" by the American Hospital Association, irrespective of their location, size, or level of care. The term appears to be idiosyncratically American.

Two initial points can readily be made about the notion of the community hospital. First, since hospitals are not community heath centers, the term has an ironic ambiguity. Second, the word "community," like the world "voluntary" (long applied to not-for-profit hospitals) has emotive power in a much larger social and political context than the hospital field. Community flexibility stands in contrast to state or national standard-setting; voluntary activity against the implied rigidity of government intervention. Communities suggest creative, local, private activities in America, such as volunteer fire departments, school boards, or the PTA; they are part of American cultural tradition. Part of the attachment of the word "community" to hospitals reflects vague assumptions about the public good. Yet, in three specific ways American hospitals have traditionally had strong community affiliations. First, hospitals have traditionally served communities of interest within local power structures. Second, hospitals have been an important part of the hierarchical organization of the medical profession. Third, hospitals have provided centers for training, employment, and voluntary work for community residents. The combined effect of these patters has been to define, further, the American hospital as "American."

As major expressions of charitable, social, and economic interests, the hospitals that developed in the late nineteenth and into the twentieth-century reflected the segmentation of American society into diverse ethnic, religious, and occupational groups and into defined social classes. Hospitals were both a concrete expression of solidarity and a means of providing training for nurses and doctors in groups likely to be excluded from other institutions (notably, Jewish and black physicians and black nurses). They represented both community successes and community failures. By 1920 America was dotted with hospitals run by hundreds of different private associations, including Roman Catholics, Lutherans, Methodists, Episcopalians, Southern Baptists, Jews, blacks, Swedes, and Germans, depending on the power structures of local populations. Philadelphia, for example, had seventy-one hospitals in 1923, general and specialized; it now [1986] has seventy-two. Most were run by not-for-profit associations Their varied social origins were apparent in names such as Hospital of the University of Pennsylvania (for teaching), Jewish Hospital of Philadelphia, St. Mary's (Roman Catholic), Methodist Episcopal, Frederick Douglass (founded by the black community), and Lankenau (originally a German hospital, the name being changed because of the German role in World War I).

In many areas local governments developed hospitals out of their poorhouses for the indigent. These hospitals, like hospitals under not-for-profit auspices, ranged from tiny units of twenty-five or fewer beds to enormous barracks-like institutions (Philadelphia General Hospital, run by the city, reported 2,000 beds in the early 1920s). Railroads, lumber companies, and occasionally other corporations built hospitals for their employees. For example, in the first decade of the century, the Santa Fe Railroad, which ranged from Chicago to Houston and Galveston and from Santa Fe to San Francisco, would report emergency hospitals for accidents at all its major maintenance shops.[5] These were supported by monthly contributions from employees.

The federal government operated a string of hospitals in seaports and on the major rivers, to care for sick and injured merchant seamen, and developed veterans hospitals after World War I; army hospitals served U.S. camps and forts. An uncounted army of physicians opened their own small hospitals to serve their paying patients, technically on a profit-making basis. In short, American hospitals arose concurrently as diverse and multipurpose institutions, serving different clienteles, with different communities of interest, and with a distinctive set of social meanings.

Reflecting patterns of social stratification and discrimination in their local communities, the new hospitals of the early twentieth century were rarely community hospitals in the sense of serving the entire population on an equal basis, even for inpatient care. The city and county hospitals that developed from the old poorhouses, such as Philadelphia General, Bellevue and Kings County in

New York, Cook County in Chicago, or San Francisco General, remained institutions primarily for the very poor. When governmental or voluntary hospitals accepted private patients, they were typically housed in separate buildings, in well-furnished private rooms rather than wards, with better food cooked in separate kitchens, and with less restricted visiting hours. Indigence continued to carry the heavy weight of social stigma, even as hospitals were medicalized around progressive scientific ideas.

Until well after World War II, major differences in the patterns of disease treated by public and not-for-profit city hospitals added to the sense of social distinctions. Cleveland City Hospital (with 785 beds) was excluded from a major survey of hospitals in Cleveland in the early 1920s because it treated large groups of patents with tuberculosis, alcoholism, venereal diseases, and contagious diseases that did not appear (because patients with them were not accepted) at any other hospital in the area.[6] Cook County was criticized in the late 1930s, as it has been since, for its poor physical surroundings, overcrowded waiting rooms, patients lying on stretchers in corridors, machinery that does not work, and shortages of even common equipment.[7] In short, American hospitals have never, as a group, served as egalitarian forces in the culture as a whole.

Mirroring the diversity of community structure across the United States, there have also continued to be enormous variations in the relative roles of tax-supported, voluntary, and profit-making hospitals from place to place. In a settled city such as Philadelphia, class differences could be seen even among the poor patients admitted to the Pennsylvania Hospital ("respectable," "deserving" poor) and the city hospital, dumping ground for all the rest. However small, governmental hospitals in counties with only one hospital probably always behaved similarly to not-for-profit or profit-making institutions in the same circumstances—taking in all social classes, with income from paying patients representing the great majority of their budgets. Such an observation suggests that control of the hospital may be less important as a distinguishing factor of American institutions than segmentation of hospital services across diverse social groups. The important variable, for social policy purposes, is not stratification by ownership but stratification by clientele, a direct reflection of "community" organization. Relatively homogeneous communities (as in rural areas or suburbs) are likely to produce more homogeneous institutions, with less social distance between patients and between staff and patients than, for example, in a major city teaching hospital, which may attract two kinds of patients—the relatively rich (on its boards and committees and as private patients of leading physicians) and the very poor, the traditional recipients of charity care.

Such differences shape differing institutional personalities for different hospitals and add to the diversity across hospitals in the United States. The differences have also been sharpened recently, at least in perception, by the location of investor-owned hospitals in relatively homogeneous middle-class areas—suggesting that ownership and social class are necessarily correlated—and by the lack of funding for indigent patients.

The passage of Medicare (for the elderly and disabled) and Medicaid (for the indigent) in 1965, in a brief period of egalitarianism, was to indicate that, at least for a short time, everyone—rich, poor, young, and old—were to be given similar if not identical hospital treatment. The power of community patterns, as well as cutbacks in Medicaid, were to prove such optimism unrealistic and short-lived. In retrospect, the egalitarian expectations for Medicaid appear as an aberration in a long history of class discrimination in hospital care in the United States. Financially tottering city and county hospitals remain the dumping grounds for patients no one else will take.

The focus on competition and managerialism of the 1970s-80s has added a new dimension to the diversity of hospital care across different communities and classes by sanctioning, on business grounds, the refusal by hospitals to serve patients who cannot pay (either directly or through insurance, Medicare, or Medicaid). For example, in Pensacola, Florida, the city turned over the management of its hospital to a profit-making organization in the 1970s, closed its emergency room, and opened a fee-paying ambulatory center instead. Hospitals can indeed be seen as community institutions, in the broadest sense, reflecting the patterns and priorities of the societies in which they are based—both at the local and national levels.

At the same time, the community of reference for many hospital purposes has expanded beyond the local area, to national and state programs and national consensus-building. Physicians, through the American College of Surgeons, launched a major movement to standardize hospitals around national norms and expectations in 1917-18: the beginnings of hospital accreditation. As Blue Cross plans developed after the 1930s into statewide programs, the definition of hospital care for reimbursement purposes was extended beyond the town or city. Statewide planning of hospital care was initiated at the time of the Hill-Burton Act in 1946, stimulated by federal construction monies provided to the states under that program and further developed through the federal health planning programs in the 1960s and 1970s, and through state certificate-of-need legislation. Medicare provided the force of national regulation and national expectations, while allowing for substantial local service variations. The diagnosis related group (DRG) program can be seen as an extension of national standard-setting through attempts to define and standardize courses of hospital treatment across the United States, for Medicare patients at least.

The courts have also had a role to play in defining national community norms, whether through asserting hospitals' responsibility for the quality of their medical care, requiring racial desegregation, or providing definitions of life and death. In these examples, the term "community" can be seen as divisible into questions of community service, community control, and community consensus. Community still remains a vague concept at best, a cherished aim with ambiguous meanings, constantly to be sought but never to be fully achieved. Its strength may lie in its idea that something should be done at the local level. In this sense the present development of local health care coalitions (of businesses, other groups, or some combination) can be seen as a continuation of a traditional theme.

The development of competing hospital systems sets up new forms of segmentation of hospital service at the local level, threatening the idea of the hospital as part of its local community power structure, or structures. The visibility of groups other than boards of trustees, physicians, and administrators is changing the broader power structure of hospital care. Stockbrokers, fringe benefit managers, business leaders, self-help groups, and unions also have legitimate, often powerful roles to play in hospital development. A forty-seven-day strike against thirty hospitals and fifteen nursing homes in New York City in the summer of 1984 affected 18,000 patients and 52,000 workers. A single bond issue can lock a hospital into a pattern of fiscal operation for thirty years, whatever its pattern of ownership may be. The activity of major purchasers of stocks and bonds, including pension funds and insurance companies, affects the availability of capital for hospital development.

In these and other examples, there is a growing array of new communities—vested interests, with diverse purposes, in constant conflict. The idea of a hospital as the embodiment of medical expertise has given way to the exercise of monopoly power by numerous groups. Hospital management and planning become the outcome of a continuing process of bargaining, negotiation, and consensus-building among differing points of view, both inside and outside the institution.

The relationship of the community of doctors to hospitals has also been marked by ambiguity. In comparison with hospitals in most other countries, American physicians have had, and still largely have, a peculiar relationship to medicine's major institution. The typical American physician remains in private, fee-for-service practice, working independently or as a member of a physician group. When the modern hospital developed in the United States, local fee-for-service practitioners volunteered their services in the hospitals, serving charity patients without charging them a fee. The medical profession became, in effect, a volunteer attending staff, since the doctors who admitted patients (and were thus crucial to the financial viability of the hospital with respect to admitting private paying patients) were not employees of the institution. From the hospital's point of view the physician could be seen as a guest of the institution. To the physician, the hospital was an extension of his or her private practice of medicine.

American hospitals have also developed in large part as open staff institutions—that is, with the expectation that all qualified physicians in a given field ought to have appointments on the attending staff of local institutions. The great majority of all physicians had some kind of hospital attachment by the late

1920s, a pattern that has continued since then. Hospital affiliations have been necessary for many of the most specialized fields. The relationship between physicians and hospitals in America is sharply distinguished, for example, from the system in Great Britain where only salaried specialists typically have hospital affiliations. Although there has been a rapid increase in the number of salaried hospital physicians in American hospitals in the last decade, the formal separation of doctors and hospitals largely continues, requiring new readjustments as hospitals become part of competing systems.

Past and Present

What emerges out of a review of American hospital history is a set of culture-specific characteristics that mark the hospitals as American institutions. These include the segmentation and diversity of ownership of hospitals, the division between hospitals and the medical profession (a division echoed in the separate development of hospital insurance and medical insurance in the United States), the acceptance of social stratification of the patient population both among hospitals and within different institutions, the pervasiveness of the pay or commodity ethos in American medicine, and the general expectation that the role of government is necessary but should be limited to filling in gaps in medical care (through programs such as Medicare or Medicaid) and in providing an atmosphere conducive to the development of services in the private sector.

More generally, the fundamental values attached to the hospital industry and its power structures—its communities of interest—are marked by ambiguity. Strauss and his colleagues observed, of a single hospital in the 1950s, that because its overall goals were unclear, goals were constantly being negotiated within the established order of the institution.[8] It is useful, in the 1980s, to think of this process of goal negotiation as an intrinsic, continuing element of the national hospital system.

Over and above these general observations, three specific themes mark the continuation of hospital history from past to present. First, American hospitals remain segmented in their interests, communities, and control. Second, decision-making continues to be diversified; that is, diffused over communities of interest, ranging from the health professions to individual hospital boards, corporate headquarters, government programs, and major purchasers of hospital insurance. Third, American hospitals are expert at adapting very rapidly to explicit external incentives, usually financial incentives.

Where social needs are made explicit (for example, in civil rights legislation or with the passage of Medicare) American hospitals are socially responsive institutions. Where there is ambivalence or apathy (for example, in providing medical care to the homeless, uninsured, or indigent) hospitals· look to other institutions—notably to government—to meet such needs, disclaiming the responsibility of being public institutions. In this respect, too, hospitals can be seen as socially responsive; that is, as reflecting the messages from the broader culture in which they are based. Lacking a unified hospital or health system, and lacking consensus about the appropriate philosophy for an American welfare state, American health policy is marked by skittishness and change.

In the absence of consensus, decisions about hospital policy have been left to the jockeying of influence among communities of interest. Part of the uneasiness about high costs and increased profit-making in hospital care derives from a perceived need to develop national consensus about hospital policy without resorting either to a government-dominated health care system or one dominated by a few massive corporations. A high-cost system is the tradeoff for avoiding either of these two extremes. The present system allows for organizational experimentation and diversity, for avoidance of draconian management decisions (the specter of rationing) and overt limitations of care for middle-class Americans, and for accommodation of conflict among reasonable but opposing points of view. In this sense the hospital system can be described in terms of constructive ambiguity. To those struggling with their implications, rapid changes cry out for simple theories of explanation and simple solutions. DRGs became the solution to the rising cost of hospital care in the 1980s, just as Medicaid was the apparent answer, in the late 1960s, to bringing the poor into the "mainstream of medicine."

The hospital system can be seen as analogous to the development of other industries; for example, consolidation of the manufacturing industry at the beginning of the twentieth century, which again followed the consolidation of the railroads. Under this model, hospitals are small firms that will inevitably move toward industrial consolidation (and that may have been held back by the monopoly interests of the medical profession). Such analogies beg the question of whether hospitals are legitimately businesses, and if so, what this means. How far hospital service may be appropriately compared to manufacturing is another question that demands elucidation; indeed, whether any service industry can be appropriately compared to any manufacturing industry is an important question. The urge for simple explanations remains. Meanwhile, there are those who claim that profit-making in health services is ethically wrong and socially dangerous, while others are more concerned that medicine is rapidly being dominated by a "medical-industrial complex" in which the traditional rights of doctors and patients will be swamped by the coming of the monolithic "corporation."[9]

The search for simple theories and the "one best way" of doing things ignores the fact that organizational life in the late twentieth century is messy and complex. Decisions have to be taken in a climate of conflict and negotiation, whether we are speaking of hospitals, factories, government, or schools. Hospitals, like other institutions, carry with them the burdens and potential of their history.

Chapter 16 was initially published in extended form as "The Changing Hospital," in Linda H. Aiken and David Mechanic, eds., *Applications of Social Science to*

Clinical Medicine and Health Policy (New Brunswick, NJ: Rutgers University Press, 1986): 80-99; and in similar form, as "Past is Prologue," in *Society* 1986, and reprinted for the Thirty-Fifth Anniversary edition of that journal, January/February 1998, 35, 2: 312-318.

Notes

1. "Hospital Life in New York," *Harper's New Monthly Magazine,* 1878, pp. 171-189.
2. S. Goldstein, "The Social Function of the Hospital." *Charities and the Commons* 18 (1907): 160-166; and see C. Rosenberg, "Inward Vision and Outward Glance: The Shaping of the American Hospital, 1880-1914." *Bulletin of the History of Medicine* 53 (1978): 346-395.
3. E. C. Meyer, "Relative Value of Hospitals and Dispensaries as Public-Health Agencies and as Fields of Activity for the Rockefeller Foundation" (New York: Rockefeller Foundation, International Health Board, 1919); and see I. Cannon, *Social Work in Hospitals: A Contribution to Progressive Medicine* (New York: Russell Sage Foundation, 1913).
4. E. H. Pennell, J. W. Mountin, and Kay Pearson, "Business Census of Hospitals, 1935: General Report Supplement No. 154 to *Public Health Reports.*" U.S. Public Health Service, 1939.
5. C. B. Going, "Methods of the Santa Fe: Efficiency in the Manufacture of Transportation." New York: Reprinted from *Engineering Magazine*, March-July 1909.
6. Cleveland Hospital Council, *Cleveland Hospital and Health Survey* (Cleveland: Cleveland Hospital Council, 1920).
7. H. F. Dowling, *City Hospitals: The Undercare of the Underprivileged* (Cambridge: Harvard University Press, 1982).
8. A. Strauss, L. Schatzman, D. Ehrlich, R. Bucher, and M. Sabshin, "The Hospital and its Negotiated Order." In E. Freidson, ed., *The Hospital in Modern Society* (London: Free Press, 1963): 147-169.
9. A. Relman, "The New Medical-Industrial Complex." *New England Journal of Medicine* 303 (1980): 963-970; P. Starr, *The Social Transformation of American Medicine* (New York: Basic Books, 1982).

17

Hospitals at the End of the
Twentieth Century (1999)

The 1990s engaged hospitals in a rip-roaring, anxiety-provoking, roller-coaster ride. It has become a commonplace that the health care system is in the midst of major transition, though the transition to *what* is murky and unclear. Do the 1990s signal the end of an era for American hospitals—one marked by relative autonomy, ambiguous goals, flexibility in the use and amount of hospital income, and a perceived social value in their predominantly private, not-for-profit ownership? Is this the beginning of a new, more rigid period, marked by stringent oversight by government and purchasers of services, by investor ownership, by a less central role for hospitals in the health care system, and by their reduced importance as nationally significant American institutions? Given the magnitude and speed of changes in the financing, structure, control, and role of hospitals in the 1990s, will American hospitals, long marked as organizational chameleons, be able to adapt to external forces in the future as successfully as in earlier decades? Are hospitals as we have come to know them even necessary?

It is easy to point to the degree of change in the American health care system as a sign that the great era for American hospitals is past.[1] It is certainly possible that historians looking back from the comfort of fifty years or so from now will mark our present and immediate future as a period in which the twentieth-century hospital disappeared; for hospitals are not inevitable institutions, and their role has often been contested. Much depends on what happens next in the tussles for money, authority, and power that are currently running through the health care system. For all their complaints in the 1990s, hospitals are by no means passive players in these games.

Power Shifts: From Producers to Purchasers

Many, if not most, of the changes to hospitals in the 1990s were evident in the late 1980s. The pressure on hospitals in the 1990s was not new and sudden, but cumulative and visible, tipping the balance of power in the health care system toward the organized purchasers of services. Health care analyst David Drake put it nicely: "It really was a quite modest change in employers' buying practice that broke producer dominance of the market and introduced price competition."[2]

By the late-1980s, the profit-oriented climate for hospitals had put stresses on all three sectors of the American hospital system, not-for-profit (the great majority of hospitals), investor-owned, and public. Medicare had attained strong influence as a major purchaser of hospital services for its elderly and disabled beneficiaries, buying its services in an undifferentiated hospital system; that is, as if type of hospital ownership were irrelevant. There was already a double threat to the longtime ability of not-for-profit hospitals to set their own fees: first, the implementation of prospective payment for hospital services based on pre-set prices per diagnosis (DRGs); and second, the increasing importance of health maintenance (or managed care) organizations. It was increasingly difficult for the not-for-profit (or voluntary) hospitals to transfer internal profits to non-revenue-producing activities such as charity care and medical research, activities that were embedded in their self-perceived, historical mission as not-for-profit, "voluntary" institutions.

The relationship between traditional, private, fee-for-service health insurance and providers remained virtually unchanged between the 1930s and the 1980s. Private fee-for-service insurance was an enabling mechanism rather than one with strong financial incentives to direct patients to particular hospitals or select the physicians they could see. The person insured could usually obtain services from any licensed hospital, doctor, or other covered provider, and any licensed provider could be included automatically as a participant. Managed care organizations, in contrast, contracted with a network of providers, typically on the basis of discounted prices. Both of these elements, selective contracting and negotiated payments, offered the potential for rationalizing services and for cost containment, *the* big theme of the early-1990s.

From the historical perspective, managed care represented a much fuller acceptance than ever before of long-existing principles for organizational rationalization that were laid out most vividly in the final report of the Committee on the Costs of Medical Care in the early-1930s; that is, the principles of group payment and group organization of health services. These principles were demonstrated in what were then called prepaid group practice systems, and later (after 1970) called health maintenance organizations (HMOs); the additional term, managed care, was coming into currency in 1989, and took off in the 1990s. Group purchase and group organization of services remain a rational approach for the coordination of fragmented, specialized services as these have developed in the American system. However, up until the late-1980s, a combination of organizational inertia (including hospital reluctance to upset hospital-doctor relations), and problems in raising capital or taking the necessary risks to establish what was still an unusual form of health insurance, made

HMOs the exception rather than the rule—though the number of enrollees was rising steadily. By the late-1980s and especially in the 1990s major employers were seeing managed care as a lever for controlling the rising costs of health care as an employee benefit. All of the ingredients were in place for a rapid move to managed care.

Managed care was heralded for its potential to reduce hospital admissions, redirect the focus of medicine from inpatient care of the sick to broader services outside the hospital, and save on expensive hospital costs by managing private insurance benefits. I was one among many observers at the time who did not envisage the rapid extension of managed care into the standard form of insurance for American workers and their families, and for a large minority of Medicaid beneficiaries in the states (with a relatively small extension, so far, into the Medicare population). The term, managed care, does not even appear in the index to my book *In Sickness and in Wealth*, published in 1989! If I were writing the book now, it clearly would.

The steady shift in balance toward managed care and away from traditional insurance in the 1990s was to change the dynamics of power for hospitals in critical ways. First, the monetary power shifted to the insuring (managed care) organizations, and thus to new contractual obligations between hospitals and insurers in which the latter had the upper hand. These insurers were not the creatures of hospitals as Blue Cross had been to some extent, nor were they not-for-profit organizations. Managed care firms were owned increasingly by insurance companies and other investor-owned corporations, with a primary fiscal duty to their communities of stockholders.[3] In 1996, 58 percent of the community hospitals in the United States reported at least one managed care contract with an HMO, and 68 percent with the more loosely organized form of managed care, the preferred provider organization (PPO).[4]

In the past both employers and insurers had been relatively passive "payers," collecting and passing through funds to those who actually provided the care. Now both saw their role as active "purchasers." Employers negotiated and contracted with managed care organizations as their insurers (or formed their own organizations to contract directly with providers). Managed care in turn contracted with providers, including hospitals. The *contract* became a central, instrumental element in organizational relations in American health care, as indeed was happening elsewhere.[5] On one side were the purchasers. On the other were hospitals, doctors, and other providers, but new relationships were being forged among these parties too.

Where managed care contracts specified payment of a relatively small capitation fee to cover hospital services as needed for a group of insured beneficiaries, hospitals accepted new, difficult to estimate, financial risks. These risks were hard to turn down in the 1990s urban marketplace, since if one hospital declined, another might well acquire the potential patients, and thus increase its market share. Teaching hospitals found themselves in a special bind. The traditional mark-up of teaching hospitals costs (averaging 20 percent above that of non-teaching hospitals in the mid-1990s[6]) had been justified by the extra expense of research and teaching, and extra benefits to patients were assumed in the more intensive teaching settings. Both of these justifications lost much of their plausibility in the 1990s. Insurers wanted to negotiate the lowest price for hospital services, irrespective of their teaching status. At the same time, the traditional monopoly on innovation by academic centers was being weakened: by the rapid rise of specialty services outside teaching hospitals, by uncertainty about government research funding, and by the increasing role of investor-owned companies in biomedical research. Teaching hospitals were also coming under fire for the costs and workforce implications of hospital-based medical education, represented in efforts to cut back payments for graduate medical education (i.e., salaries for resident physicians) under Medicare.[7] In 1989 the continuing centrality of the medical school as an influence on the hospital system could be assumed. Instead, academic health centers were pushed off their pedestal as the diffusing agent and organizing symbol for high-technology medicine. It is not at all clear what will happen next.

Most, if not all, hospitals felt financially squeezed in the 1990s. How far hospitals responded by cost-cutting measures that have affected the quality of patient care (for example, by delegating professional tasks inappropriately to less qualified personnel) is hard to say, although nurses, in particular, have expressed anxiety about this. Adding to the general worry has been the need for hospitals to work with doctors in new ways, as they have grouped and regrouped outside the hospital into single specialty, multi-specialty, and disease-oriented corporations. Some hospitals forged new relationships better than others. An illustrative article from 1996 described a "major western teaching hospital" that was inappropriately "stingy" in its efforts to affiliate formally with a 350-member medical group with which the hospital had long-standing referral relationships; the deal failed, the doctors sold their practice to a national practice management company, and thus they shifted their primary allegiance.[8] Being a hospital chief executive (or a board member) in the 1990s is one constant, difficult learning experience.

Rethinking the Hospital's Boundaries and Roles

As happens in complex systems, one set of changes set off other, interactive changes. With the increasing organizational efforts of purchasers came a counter-response and collaboration with the "hospital industry," as it was generally described. There was an acceleration of hospital mergers and acquisitions, expansion of services into out-of-hospital fields, and the organization of groups and networks of physicians—sometimes in competition with the hospitals that had long served them as "doctors' workshops." The capture of what were traditionally "hospital services" by non-hospital groups was nicely delineated by John D. Stoeckle, of the Massachusetts General Hospital, in 1995.

Among the elements were an abundant supply of medical specialists; recognition by doctors and the public of the speed, convenience, and marketability of diagnostic testing in smaller centers near to where people live; the routinization and growing prevalence of expensive technologies such as MRIs that could be provided in independent sites, staffed and serviced outside of the hospital; the relative safety and dissemination of minimally invasive surgical technologies (such as laparoscopic surgery); growing medical skepticism about the value of bed rest—a value central to the hospital's traditional core identity; and the availability of insurance coverage to pay for all of this.[9]

A second, related set of changes was stimulated by hospitals themselves. By 1989, virtually all hospitals were shifting their focus to outpatient services. This movement was to mushroom in the 1990s. By 1997, more than a third of hospital revenues derived from outpatient services. The trend was not only to expand the repertoire of hospital services but also to shift many procedures from an inpatient to an outpatient setting. In 1996, hospitals reported that almost 50 percent more of their *own* surgery was being done on outpatients than on inpatients: 53.6 compared with 36.5 surgeries for a population of 1000.[10] And many more surgeries were being done in free-standing ambulatory facilities; not just for laparoscopies, but for cataract surgery, plastic surgery, and other procedures that for most of the century had been performed on inpatients. Surgery was no longer the monopoly of the hospital, nor even necessarily its central defining theme. The ambulatory surgical center, whether independent or run by a hospital, was a service station to which patients took their bodies for renewal or repair, and then went home to sleep in their own beds.

If the hospital no longer had a monopoly of medical technology, and if the center of interest had shifted to outpatients who had not been, and did not expect to be, inpatients, what was the role of inpatient care? How far was the hospital to be categorized as a hospital in the future because of its commitment to overnight stay? By the late-1980s, the typical inpatient was someone suffering from an acute phase of a chronic illness, such as heart disease, cancer, stroke, or AIDS. The latest figures at the time of writing show a continuation and strengthening of the general trend. Almost 40 percent of admissions were sixty-five years of age or over in 1995. More than one-fifth of hospital admissions were at least seventy-five years of age. This latter group accounted for almost one-sixth of inpatient surgeries in 1995, most commonly for heart conditions and prostatectomies among men, and for improving mobility or treating the results of falls (reductions of fractures and hip replacements) among women. The seventy-five-plus age group used relatively more acute hospital services than any other age group. Compared with other age groups, children used inpatient hospital services least, admitted most commonly for pneumonia, injuries and poisoning, and asthma.[11] These patterns were a far cry from the use of hospitals in, say, the 1920s, when tonsillectomies, appendectomies, and deliveries characterized the American hospital as a center for the young. In the 1990s, younger, healthier patients tended to be seen as outpatients or in the doctor's office. One potential future for the hospital inpatient unit is as a center for geriatric and disabled patients—the role that public hospitals played at the beginning of the century. But hospitals also continue to serve as inpatient maternity centers, and to provide intensive care for the treatment of acute problems in all age groups.

In terms of the hospital's role and self-presentation in the 1990s, it is significant that obstetrics is a major exception to the shift to out-of-hospital care, for in this role, the hospital does indeed serve the whole community, retaining its emotionally charged role as the center for both birth and death. The great majority of births still take place on an inpatient basis in the United States. Neonatal intensive care units provide a potent image for hospitals as a center for life-saving technologies, even miracles. In contrast to the shift to outpatient surgeries, the fundamental issue for care at both the beginning and the end of life is not decentralization of technologies out of the hospital, but the high costs of an inpatient hospital stay. Home-based midwifery, local birthing centers, and hospice care remain the exception rather than the rule. How far these patterns will persist is a big, undetermined issue for the role of hospitals, as well as the costs and quality of care in the future. In obstetrics the national focus has centered on shortening the period of inpatient care, and on limits on the length of stay by managed care. The so-called practice of "drive-through-deliveries" became an emotional battle-cry for consumer advocates and a feel-good reform issue for hospitals and legislators in the mid-1990s. Between the spring of 1995 and early-1997, twenty-nine states adopted legislation or regulations requiring insurers to cover minimum postpartum days (typically a forty-eight-hour stay).[12]

Responses to the costs of dying are less clear. There continue to be concern about the high cost of dying in hospitals for the Medicare program, and for the moral as well as the economic value of the expensive, last-ditch efforts at prevention that often accompany death in an acute hospital. Economist Eli Ginzberg pointed out that almost 30 percent of all Medicare patients who were hospitalized in the early-1990s failed to survive for twelve months; the implicit question is whether the hospitalization was worth it, on any terms.[13] On the other hand, the restricted regulations for hospice payments under Medicare biased the use of hospices in favor of individuals only weeks away from death. The questions of how best to handle death, what choices to offer patients and their families, and what choices individuals actually prefer, will require continuing attention in the next few years; again the outcome is by no means clear. Nor is it clear what implications changing social attitudes to death might have on the social standing of the hospital. This is an institution that has been based historically, after all, on the image of heroic physicians intervening against the ravages of nature, rather than on acceptance of dying and death. Palliative care for dying patients in hospitals is a promising specialty, but one that is still in its infancy. Will the American hospital remain the accepted place for birth and death in the future? Should it?

Steadily shorter lengths of stay modified the hospital's internal environment in the 1990s. The average length of stay for inpatients in community hospitals was 6.2 days in 1996, a day less than in 1989, with the shortest average stay in investor-owned hospitals and the longest in state and local government hospitals, which remain the hospitals of last resort in many places.[14] There are great variations around the mean, within and across institutions, and by geographical area. To the staff, many patients are brief visions passing through. Nurses complain that they are spread too thin, partly because of the greater average intensity of care, partly because of increasing demands of management, insurance, and regulation. In large institutions, at least, nursing stations on hospital floors look like the command centers of a spaceship, twinkling with computers. Patients' families provide additional eyes, ears, and legs for individual patients, isolated as they often are in single rooms. Many hospitals now encourage family members to stay. Much more work needs to be done in the future on the patterns and conditions of work in hospitals, the experiences of patients and nurses in particular, and the work being done by family members, both during and after hospitalization.

The new term "hospitalist" appeared (and blossomed) in 1996, signifying a major conceptual change already underway in hospital inpatient staffing, and thus in the relationship of attending physicians to their hospitalized patients. The hospitalist is a physician, typically a specialist in internal medicine, perhaps with training as an intensivist (in critical care) who takes responsibility for the care of inpatients.[15] By the beginning of 1998 the new National Association for Inpatient Physicians estimated that there were 2500 hospitalists in the United States. "Insurers and hospitals like the idea," wrote a journalist describing the move toward hospitalists in both teaching and community hospitals.[16] The rationale was straightforward: Inpatient services have become geared toward the shortest possible stay and the most intensive treatment; the hospitalist is an expert trained to focus on hospital care and coordinate other specialists as necessary; and the attending physician might not be available to visit the patient on admission, thus losing valuable time and incurring additional costs to the hospital and/or insurer. Teaching hospitals, which had traditionally relied on residents in training for continuity in medical staffing, had a further incentive. Crackdowns on unsupervised services given by residents marked the 1990s, both via the courts of law and Medicare audits. Much of what residents now do has to be signed for by a responsible physician—and the hospitalist is the physician most likely to be present.

Hospital Systems

Despite all the changes in services and functions in the 1990s, the core of a hospital is still usually a recognizable building, or a hodgepodge of buildings representing accretions over the years. The building stock is often heavily mortgaged, as was evident in the 1980s; thus the hospital's survival depends on a steady stream of income to pay down debt. Protection of capital was one stimulus in the "urge to merge" of the 1980s and 1990s, paralleling merger activities in business. Other stimuli included jockeying for a stronger market position and a more concentrated power in contracting with purchasers. Some hospitals were undoubtedly motivated by ego and by the herd psychology of mergers. There was fear of being left out in the cold as competitive hospitals in a local market merged and/or sought affiliations with wider systems, based on prevailing beliefs about managerial and competitive advantage in the market and the destabilization of traditional ways of doing things. According to American Hospital Association data for 1996, over half of the community hospitals with 200 or more beds were members of a hospital system. The probability rose with hospital size: 33 percent of the smallest hospitals (fifty to ninety-nine beds) belonged to systems and 66 percent of the largest institutions (500 beds or more). In addition, more than a fourth of all community hospitals reported membership in networks.[17]

By 1996 there were at least 200 not-for-profit hospital systems in the United States, large and small, compared with thirteen in the for-profit sector. *Modern Healthcare* reported in its 1997 annual survey: "It looks as if not-for-profit systems are making a rush on smaller hospitals in rural areas and outlying cities. For-profits, meanwhile, are probably at a stage much like reorganization of closets that follows a shopping spree."[18] The historical diversity of hospital ownership is reflected in these systems. Among the ten largest systems reported in 1996 were five systems based on Roman Catholic hospitals. The public New York City Health and Hospitals Corporation was also on this list, despite its continuing attempts to streamline services and cut back costs, while the largest system was the for-profit Columbia/HCA, which then had 319 hospitals, 57,000 staffed beds, and net patient revenues of $19.9 billion. However, even this large system represented only 5 percent of total hospital revenues in the United States. There were interlocking relationships between for-profit and not-for-profit forms of organization, chiefly through subsidiaries and through contract management. "As usual, every measure of acute-care system size is up," reported *Modern Healthcare*.[19]

Not-for-profit systems have tried to sustain their reputation as the representatives of charitable or exemplary organizations as they pursue the equally traditional roles of money-making and outrunning the competition. The systems, like individual hospitals, were well aware of the easy slippage into failure in the 1990s. Illustrating the downward slide was Michael Reese Hospital in Chicago, formerly a hospital of stature in that city. Facing fiscal problems by the late-1980s, despite its attempts to lure well-heeled patients, Michael Reese's board sold out to an investor-owned corporation, Humana. "You can't run a $200 million operation on nostalgia," said the board's chairman.[20] This hospital was soon sold again, as Humana concentrated its business on managed care, this time to Columbia (later Columbia/HCA). Stringent efforts to cut costs through staff reductions generated considerable hostility, but soon (in 1997) Columbia/

HCA went through its own upheavals, following raids on its facilities in Texas by federal agents investigating Medicare fraud. The future of Michael Reese Hospital is unclear, including its very survival as a hospital.

The recent history of Michael Reese stands as a cautionary tale for individual hospitals with a historical mission to care for all social classes in major cities, and for hospital systems seeking to demonstrate their efficiency. At the other end of the scale are dangers for nonprofit systems when they appear *too* successful in business terms. A much-quoted example is the critique in 1998 in the *Wall Street Journal*, which referred to the leaders of one of the largest systems, the Daughters of Charity, as "Daughters of Currency." The *Journal* noted that the Daughters system had divested itself of money-losing or non-competitive hospitals in favor of suburban hospitals, served fewer Medicaid patients than the national average, and held "billions in cash and investments," a portfolio that had grown rapidly. Former system president Sister Irene Kraus put the problem succinctly, as she saw it, "No margin, no mission."[21]

Whether mergers made sense in terms of hospital efficiency and costs is a debatable point in the late-1990s. A study of hospital mergers in the cities of St. Louis and Philadelphia cast doubt on the extent to which hospitals have been willing (or able) to merge their corporate identities, integrate their cultures, consolidate clinical services, and close redundant or inefficient hospitals.[22] Those familiar with the history of hospitals might have predicted such an outcome. The oldest hospital in the eastern United States, the Pennsylvania Hospital, became part of the University of Pennsylvania Health System (based on the Hospital of the University of Pennsylvania and its associated practices) in the 1990s, following dramatic competitive negotiations with rival Thomas Jefferson University (and its hospital), but it remains the Pennsylvania Hospital in name and spirit—at least as yet.

There was relatively little acquisition of not-for-profits by for-profit systems in the 1990s, less than one might have expected looking forward from the 1980s. But the numbers were smaller than their impact might suggest, stimulating reactive reorganizations and consolidations among not-for-profits in local markets. Huge amounts of money changed hands in the 1990s, enriching individuals and creating new community foundations (representing, at sale to a for-profit organization, the assessed value of the not-for-profit's social benefits). What is striking in all of these moves is how in the 1990s, as in the past, not-for-profit, for-profit, and government roles intermingle and coexist.

Speed and Complexity of Recent Changes

Behind the speed of changes in the 1990s were the dual messages, "let the market rip," and "let's keep government out of this." Health care analyst Bradford Gray stressed in 1990 the steady move of the health system to contractual relationships. There was concomitant dissatisfaction with relationships built on the idea of trust (a core assumption for not-for-profit institutions), and what Gray calls the "near religious status" of belief in market forces.[23] The not-for-profits were once again lined up as card-carrying members of the "private sector." Observers and critics of the late-1990s use words like "revolution," as in the "purchaser revolution"; this is defined as the shift from a "producer-dominated" market, characterized by price competition.[24]

The combination of the shift in organizational focus to managed care, the enthusiasm for change as change itself, and the move from inpatient to out-patient care strengthened interest in the question of whether there would be a distinct role for hospitals at all in the future, and if so what it would/should be. Does the hospital still exist as an entity, or is it more proper to talk solely about health care. systems? This is not an unreasonable question, given the excursions of hospitals into other fields and their own rush to extend both their functions and their image. The venerable Ohio Hospital Association (formed in 1915) transmuted, for example, into the present OHA: The Association for Hospitals and Health Systems; the journal *Hospitals* became *Hospitals and Health Networks*; and the hospitals' major accrediting agency expanded into the Joint Commission on Accreditation of Healthcare Organizations (JCAHO). Other hospital agencies have followed suit. No one wants to be left isolated, out in the cold, no longer part of the generic health care system. Yet models for this system are slippery and evanescent.

The idea of the hospital's disappearance at the end of the twentieth century presents a tempting, even an aesthetically pleasing theme for the historian, who could cast the twentieth-century history of the American hospital as a simple narrative of rise and fall. The hospital, one might say, rose to prominence at the beginning of the twentieth century, mutated, flowered, declined, and faded, swept away into new types of systems. However there is a warning before we take this route. Hospitals have been tenacious institutions, and one important reason for this is that hospital leaders have long been attuned to changes in rhetoric, language, and self-presentation—using language to position themselves so as to take advantage of new conditions. It is quite possible that the rhetoric of the marketplace and managed care that has distinguished the 1990s will be followed by other organizing slogans in the next few decades.

Hospitals may become more peripheral institutions in the health system but they may also become health care systems themselves.[25] Both sets of moves are evident over the past ten years, creating considerable diversity in the system. The extended role is illustrated, for example, by the University of Pennsylvania Health System, which has been buying up primary care practices to complement its specialist practices and tertiary hospital services. Other hospitals have fol-lowed suit, although the financial results are at best, mixed. Many hospitals are taking a more cautious (or fiscally constrained) approach, working with managed care organizations and extending their outpatient services, often at distant sites, but not attempting to provide comprehensive care. Some hospitals that are not closely affiliated with university medical schools have been billing themselves as "academic" or "university" hospitals, attempting to appeal to patients on grounds of quality and to doctors who avidly seek faculty status. The common wisdom in the late-1990s is that there is so much organizational variation that change can only be properly assessed through case studies at the local level. I would merely observe here that there are still hospitals in the United States, diverse in role and buffeted by change though they may be.

Even a short list of major forces for change in the health care system in the 1990s gives a sense of the upheavals faced by American hospitals, and of the dizzying speed of change. These include:

- the rapid development of managed care as the standard model for health insurance in the United States, now covering three-fourths of all insured workers, employed by both large and small firms;[26]
- a major shift in the locus of financial decision-making away from the traditional providers of health care, notably hospitals and doctors, to those who pay the bills: employers and insurers (including managed care organizations);
- pressures on hospitals to reduce inpatient admissions, length of stay, and costs through the pre-admission review processes of managed care, and through negotiated capitation payments: the level of payment is set by contract between hospitals and managed care firms, with hospitals competing with each other for contracts, often on a lowest-price basis;
- decline in the number of hospitals, hospital beds, admission rates, hospital occupancy rates, and length of stay;
- an accelerated shift of emphasis from inpatient to outpatient care, and the parallel development of free-standing ambulatory surgical centers;
- shifts in organizational arrangements among doctors and between doctors and hospitals, challenging the centrality of the hospital in medicine, and its longtime role as doctors' workshop;
- the rise and fall of interest in national health insurance between 1991, when Harris Wofford swept into the Senate under the banner of national health insurance, and 1994, when the Clinton administration's ambitious health plan was abandoned, joining the dust heap of earlier federal insurance proposals;
- dramatic growth in both for-profit and not-for-profit hospital systems;
- an accelerated move by many hospitals into integrated (or at least extended) health care systems, in part as a move to increase market share in a climate of fierce competition for patients, prestige, power, and income;
- increased political visibility for Medicare and Medicaid at both federal and state levels, accompanied by audits, charges of fraud for hospital billings, and increased financial stringency;
- transfers of patients covered by government programs into privately controlled managed care;
- the financial vulnerability of major teaching hospitals and academic health centers, as high-technology services proliferate in competing

specialist groups and non-teaching hospitals, and as hard-line insurers cut back on the traditionally much higher reimbursements for care in teaching hospitals;

- a steady rise in the number of Americans who are uninsured, and therefore may present themselves to hospitals without means of payment;
- significantly increased erosion of public trust in hospitals and doctors, coupled with criticism in the media and regulatory responses;
- and, partly in response to the criticism, a growing commitment by hospitals and managed care organizations to methods of measuring quality of care.

These pressures on hospitals were mutually reinforcing in the 1990s. The Clinton health reform proposals, though unsuccessful, helped generate first, the development of managed care, integrated delivery systems, and hospital mergers—both as anticipatory devices in case of passage of the program, and as private alternatives to government intervention. Second, after their demise, the proposals directed full political attention to Medicare, which became *the* central focus for federal policymaking in health for the 1990s, particularly after 1994.

Similarly, pressure to bring down the health care costs incurred by employers, the federal government, and the states (via Medicare and Medicaid) put further pressures on the number of people insured and the type of coverage, and increased the amount of out-of-pocket expenses. Traditionally, hospitals have picked up some of the costs of gaps in insurance coverage for individuals via charity care and writing off bad debts, passing along the costs to other patients by cost-shifting. However, although both not-for-profit and for-profit hospitals report a substantial amount of such care, the traditional elasticity of their budgets has been dwindling because of pressures imposed by managed care and other purchasers, responding in turn to the concerns of employers and taxpayers. Eli Ginzberg has described the "limited potential of hospitals to balance their books by expanding their services when the two principal payers—government and employers—are seeking to constrain their outlays," as one of several "warning signs" pointing to dissonance for hospitals in the future.[27] History may well prove him correct.

A key question is whether American hospitals, weighed down as they are by burdens of debt and by the lack of marginal funds for charity, venture capital, and organizational innovation, will lose their flexibility to such an extent that they will no longer be able to act as organizational chameleons. In theory, managed care organizations might take over the hospital's traditional role as centers for technology and health care organization, and as centers, too, for medical education, research, and care of the poor, although these latter functions seem unlikely. Managed care organizations could also acquire the role of community organizations that American hospitals have long claimed, if only partially fulfilled; that is, serve as responsible guardians of the health of communities. At least in theory, managed care organizations are in an excellent position to focus on the successful treatment of chronic conditions, reduction of stress and depression, successful aging, and good deaths. If HMOs focused on healthiness, hospitals might be more clearly delineated as human repair shops. There are obvious caveats to this picture; most notably, the managed care world is currently marked by fiscal instability and stress.

Whatever the inertia of not-for-profit hospitals in the past, there remain advantages in the relative organizational stability of the not-for-profits. The not-for-profit form of organization retains some social capital as an alternative to investor-owned and government institutions, and offers a modicum of stability within a confusing, shifting health care system. The best system for the United States may well be for the different forms of organization to operate in tension.

Stability is important if only because, given the time-honored search for simple solutions to health care policy in the United States, evident throughout the century, there were disorienting changes in direction in the 1990s as one rallying call or buzzword was succeeded by the next. Thus the value of integrated delivery systems, highly touted in the health care literature in the early-1990s, seemed less clear in 1998. The role of the primary care practitioner as "gatekeeper" (rationer or manager) of specialized services in a managed care system seemed an obvious, even inevitable organizational trend in the early-1990s. In contrast, following extensive criticism by doctors, patients, and politicians, direct access to medical specialists was a central credo of the late-1990s, inside and outside managed care. The term "gatekeeper" is more or less dead.

A third example of apparent changes in direction is the credence given to investor-owned health care corporations for much of the 1990s as the innovative leaders of organizational reform. In the ideological arena, the defeat of the Clinton proposals validated marketplace approaches to health system change. Huge investor-owned corporations such as Columbia/HCA exemplified the power, mobility, and superiority of the marketplace as a machine for social engineering. The private hospital/health care corporation, responsible to stockholders and keenly attuned to consumers as well as to the price of its shares, could be set against the seeming irrelevance, and perhaps even the relative lack of accountability, of not-for-profit hospitals in a profit-oriented system. One leader of the not-for-profit sector claimed early in 1997 that the dramatic growth of Columbia/HCA had engendered "enormous fear in the not-for-profit world," because of concern that it would eat up more and more not-for-profit hospitals.[28] Yet later in 1997 Columbia/HCA suffered a dramatic fall, accompanied by cost and management concerns, government charges of fraud in Medicare billings, a sharp drop in the price of its shares, and widespread criticisms of the ethics of fiscal relationships between Columbia doctors and its hospitals that potentially distorted the ability to give the best care to patients.

Continuities and Reappraisals

The historian looking back on our times from the future and looking first at the statistical record, might see little of the turbulence that distinguished hospitals and health care in the 1990s. The number of hospitals had risen and fallen in the prior fifty years, to be sure, but there were still as many hospitals in 1996 as there were in 1946: 6210 compared with 6125, respectively.[29] Despite the intense rhetoric of the for-profit market in the 1980s and 1990s, the great majority of community hospitals (3045 out of 5134 in 1996) continued to be nongovernmental, not-for-profit institutions. In the 1990s as in the 1980s, board members of not-for-profit hospitals talked about whether they had a special role or mission as nonprofit, charitable institutions, distinguishing them from for-profit ventures. The number of investor-owned community hospitals actually declined slightly between 1988 and 1996.

Also suggesting lack of change rather than major systemic upheaval, the volume of inpatient admissions to community hospitals remained quite stable, hovering at about 31 million admissions a year for each year 1988 through 1996. The number of personnel employed by community hospitals seemed on a steady rise, from 3.2 million in 1988 to 3.7 million (full-time equivalents) in 1996. In 1996 hospitals accounted for almost 4 percent of the entire civilian labor force—and these figures exclude doctors and their office staffs and an uncounted number of other health care workers who rely on regular hospital connections.[30] Community hospitals remained major employers. Hospital expenses were also steadily increasing. Community hospitals reported expenses of $169 billion in 1988, $294 billion in 1996.

Hospitals also continued to represent a large chunk of all expenditures for personal health care in the United States through the 1990s, although their relative share was falling as total health expenditures rose. In 1995, Americans allocated almost 40 percent of their entire personal health expenditures to hospital services. Hospitals accounted for almost 5 percent of the country's gross domestic product.[31] Americans spent more on hospitals than on total expenditures for defense.

On the face of it, this might not seem a system in distress or in the midst of massive changes. How, then, can we make sense of the rush of events and the complexity of players: bankers and stockbrokers funding capital acquisitions; hospital board members countering an offer from a hospital system to buy them out; doctors seeking new forms of practice organization, hoping to enhance their ability to negotiate with managed care organizations and employers; managed care organizations seeking to be profitable in a skittish period and to overcome a negative image as they plan extensions and improvements for the future; nurses acquiring status in advanced practice roles (such as a nurse practitioner acting as a primary care giver in managed care) while coping with stresses in hospital nursing, as the intensity of nursing services increases and hospital management reallocates roles to those without the RN in the interests of controlling costs; leaders of academic medicine declaring threats to the research and teaching missions of the academic medical center, as managed care contracts force medical school faculty and their associated hospitals and networks to accept reimbursement for their services at competitive (i.e., lower) community rates; patients concerned about "drive-through" care as the length of hospital stay is cut to the bone and technology switches to outpatient service; employers seeking more informational control over how their health insurance dollars are being spent, and cutting back on coverage to employees; patients and their families troubled by the lack of privacy for medical information, so that it sometimes seems as if employers (and others) know more about their health than they do themselves; policymakers in an era of balanced budgets facing the swelling number of the uninsured—one-seventh of all Americans, mostly workers?

The simple answer to how we can make sense of current events is to say it is impossible. What may seem clear to the historian of the future remains shrouded from us today. We are all too close to the excitement of events not to overstress change in some areas and ignore it in others, and too ill-informed to make considered judgments. But this is an unhelpful and unsatisfactory position for those who seek links between past and future. It is no more difficult to assess the present in 1998 than in 1989—accepting the risk, of course, that future events may prove one wrong, misguided, or naive.

I was clearly wrong in 1989 [in *In Sickness and in Wealth*] about the instrumental role the federal government might play in the 1990s. I then foresaw a swing away from the marketplace toward a renewed focus on collective obligations. Instead, the market has stood in for government action as a more nimble, effective force for a process of reorganization that was long overdue. Medicare's prospective payment system was to have less effect than was generally believed in the late-1980s. I also missed the ambulatory surgery regulations issued in 1982 that contributed to the movement of ambulatory surgery outside of hospitals, a point made to me by David Drake. New roles for government in the health care system were also to appear in the 1990s. Notably, the state legislatures and regulatory agencies became more visible and powerful. The states, rather than the federal government, responded to consumer demands for the regulation of managed care, experimented with broader forms of health insurance, and moved Medicaid programs into managed care systems.

Nevertheless, the federal government remains a powerful player, if only as a silent partner to marketplace initiatives and as a giant purchaser, auditor, and potential regulator of hospital services through Medicare. Medicare and Medicaid together represent more than half of all hospital payments in the United States.[32] Although there has not (yet) been direct exertion of this pressure to plan or regulate hospital or health care services on a grand scale, this force remains as a possibility for the future, should the market fail to deliver. By default, the primary pressure on hospitals in the 1990s has been investor-owned managed care organizations.

The encouragement of Medicare buy-ins to managed care under the Medicare+Choice provision of the Balanced Budget Act of 1997, together with the increased visibility of the Medicare budget and the formation of a presidential Bipartisan Commission on Medicare [which later deadlocked] might lead to a more direct federal role in the future. The sustaining role of government in the twentieth century (sustaining, that is, to the private sector) is clearly demonstrated in the 1990s, though here the private sector represents the purchasers rather than, as in the past, the producers of care.

The not-for-profit sector retreated from its traditional emphasis on voluntarism, charity, and community; the word "voluntary," as in voluntary hospitals, is now rarely used. This may be seen as good survival strategy: The not-for-profits accounted for 73 percent of community hospital outpatient visits, 72 percent of births, 73 percent of hospital personnel, and 74 percent of all hospital expenses in the United States in 1996.[33] American not-for-profit hospitals have acquired the patina of profit-making institutions while residing under the umbrella of nonprofit status, and serving huge numbers of government-sponsored patients. Community commitment by hospitals remains fuzzy, as it has for decades. Hospitals give back largely positive answers to the annual American Hospital Association survey, which asks questions about each hospital's community activities, including what they say in their mission statements and what specific community services they foster and support. The results suggest a stronger role in long-term planning for community health and participation in community health assessments than is apparent on the ground. Hospitals have long been exquisitely attuned to fiscal opportunities, and there are no fiscal incentives, either from the government or the private sector, to push them to become effective leaders in community-building or public health. The tensions between the concept of the hospital as charity and business have never been more visible.

There are some odd juxtapositions in the messages hospitals send out in the late-1990s. Some messages are comfortably traditional. For example, National Hospital Week continues to be held during the week of Florence Nightingale's birthday, May 12. The theme for 1998 was "Health…Caring…Community." The American Hospital Association exhorted its members to spread this message, teaching communities about the "hospital's health agenda and the many ways hospitals benefit them." Specific ideas included offering a health fair with free blood pressure, body fat, and cholesterol screening, asking local merchants to donate door prizes, handing out free coffee mugs and carnations, organizing a name-the-babies contest, offering free aerobics sessions to staff, and sponsoring a community cleanup day.[34] This general message falls directly in line with similar messages sent out to hospitals since the 1920s, designed to create good feelings about the hospital rather than change the community's health. The message also serves to remind us how small many American hospitals continue to be, and how important as centers of local employment, both in rural and urban areas. In 1996, 45 percent of the community hospitals in the United States reported less than 100 beds, and 71 percent less than 200 beds.[35]

Managing the Hospital System

Hospital governance, the changing character of management, and hospital-physician relations were all important themes of the 1990s, with strong historical resonance. The role and effectiveness of hospital boards became more difficult as executives acquired influence as well as expertise in the arcane fiscal, contractual, and regulatory arenas of health care in the 1990s, through executing rapidly-moving business deals; extending the boundaries of the hospital in one direction or another; and orchestrating relationships with systems, networks, and increasingly complicated medical groups. There are still many institutions where board members are selected in the traditional way, for their prominence in the community and/or fundraising ability, rather than for knowledge, statesmanship, and acumen about the health care business. Board members need sufficient expertise and practical entrepreneurialism to advise health care executives, to act strategically, and to carry out their fiduciary responsibilities as board members—whether the hospital is not-for-profit, investor-owned, or public. Although it is not clear in the late-1990s how well these roles are being fulfilled, it is my impression that many boards are dealing from a dangerous base of ignorance, are leaving too much policy decision-making to their executives, and are too readily swayed by them.[36]

Meanwhile, the role of managers is being reassessed. The hard-driving executive, distinguished for pursuing profit (personified by Rick Scott of Columbia/HCA in the mid-1990s), fell into disfavor as a model for management in the late-1990s. The new manager supposedly balances fiscal expertise with ethical institutional objectives and is ideally concerned with the local community. Although the stresses are similar to those of earlier decades, the stress level is more acute than ever before because of the complexity and uncertainty of the environment and the sheer level of financial risk. The 1990s rewarded the understanding and manipulation of power; avoidance where possible of negative risks; sophisticated skills in negotiating with diverse individuals and groups; the ability to make decisions fast in an environment where little has been clear; and the courage to move ahead with plausibility and conviction. The next phase may require, in addition, the wisdom and moral leadership of the statesman.

Physician organizations lurched through uncomfortable changes in the 1990s, as doctors regrouped outside of hospitals, both to deliver out-of-hospital care and to band together for mutual protection. Traditional commitments to open-staff arrangements have largely gone by the board. Little more than one-fifth of community hospitals reported open-staff arrangements in 1996.[37] Physician practice management organizations became a big topic in the 1990s as physicians, after a period of disillusion and loss of confidence, recognized their potential power as providers and as bargainers with hospitals and purchasers. The theme of physician-hospital tensions, a recurring historical theme, demands much more attention that it has yet been given as a contemporary phenomenon in American medicine. As I write this, hospitals and doctors seem to be recognizing their mutual interests as (beleaguered) providers of care.

Are Hospitals Necessary?

I believe hospitals continue to be necessary institutions as centers of medicine, at least in the United States. For all the talk of integrated delivery systems with a marginalized or peripheral role for the hospital, there is no major organizational alternative to hospitals or hospital systems. The adaptability shown by the hospital establishment in the 1990s is at least as impressive as that of earlier decades. The hospital of the early-1990s rose on the banner of surgery (and surgical quality), then at the forefront of medical skill. If medicine continues to be defined by insurers, government, employers, consumers, and taxpayers in terms of advances in, and access to, sophisticated but limited-use technology, then hospitals will continue to be focused factories for technology, rather than centers for comprehensive care of the melioration of chronic illness. The stickability of tax-exempt hospitals (the not-for-profits) reflects a continuing social utility for this form in an environment of mixed messages and ambiguous incentives—standing in a kind of no-man's-land between the supposed commercialization of the investor-owned sector and the supposed inferiority of government-owned institutions. Investors have not wanted to buy them all out, while government has been trying to retreat.

Chapter 17 is an edited version of the preface to *In Sickness and in Wealth: American Hospitals in the Twentieth Century* (1989) on its reissue in 1999 (Baltimore: Johns Hopkins University Press). An adapted version was published as "Hospitals at the End of the Twentieth Century," *The Long Term View*, Fall 1999: 94-106.

Notes

1. For a good review of informed opinion in the late-1990s, see Janet M. Corrigan and Paul B. Ginsburg, "Association Leaders Speak Out on Health Systems Change." *Health Affairs* 11 (1997): 1, 150-157.
2. David F. Drake, author of *Reforming the Health Care Market: An Interpretative Economic History* (Washington, D.C.: Georgetown Press, 1994), personal communication.
3. In 1982, only 18 percent of managed care organizations were for-profit; by 1988, 67 percent. See Daren Davis, Daren Scott Collins, and Cynthia Morris, "Managed Care: Promise and Concerns." *Health Affairs* (Fall 1994): 178-81. Today, insurance is typically in the hands of investor-owned corporations, including those run by major employers. Blue Cross-Blue Shield has also become increasingly profit-oriented.

4. The American Hospital Association defines a PPO as a "pre-set arrangement in which purchasers and providers agree to furnish specified health services to a group of employees/patients." American Hospital Association, *Hospital Statistics 1998 Edition* (Chicago: Healthcare Infosource, 1998) (hereafter AHA, *Hospital Statistics*), Table 3, p. 8.

5. For a good overview, see Chris Ham, ed., *Health Care Reform: Learning from International Experience* (Philadelphia: Open University Press, 1997).

6. Arnold M. Epstein, "U.S. Teaching Hospitals in the Evolving Health Care System." *Journal of the American Medical Association* 273, 15 (1997): 1203-07.

7. See Institute of Medicine, National Academy of Sciences, *On Implementing a National Graduate Medical Education Trust Fund* (Washington D.C.: National Academy Press, 1997); and John K. Iglehart, "Medicare and Graduate Medical Education." *New England Journal of Medicine* 338, 6 (1998): 402-07.

8. Herb McGuire, "Strangers in a Strange Land." *Health Systems Review* (May/June 1996): 31-37.

9. John D. Stoeckle, "The Citadel Cannot Hold: Technologies Go Outside the Hospital, Patients and Doctors Too." *Milbank Quarterly* 73, 1 (1995): 3-17.

10. AHA, *Hospital Statistics*, Table 3, p. 9.

11. Figures are for non-federal short-stay hospitals. *Health United States, 1996-97* (Washington, D.C.: DHSS Publication No. (PHS) 97-1232): 214, 217-19.

12. Eugene Declercq and Diana Simmes, "The Politics of 'Drive Through Deliveries': Putting Early Postpartum Discharge on the Legislative Agenda." *Milbank Quarterly* 75, 2 (1997): 175-202.

13. Eli Ginzberg, *Tomorrow's Hospital: A Look to the Twenty-first Century* (New Haven: Yale University Press, 1996): 43.

14. AHA, *Hospital Statistics*, Table 1, p. 3.

15. Robert M. Wachter, Lee Goldman, "The Emerging Role of 'Hospitalists' in the American Health Care System." *New England Journal of Medicine* 335, 7 (1996): 514-17.

16. Stacey Burling, "A New Breed of Doctors Specializes in Hospital Care," *Philadelphia Inquirer*, Thursday, February 26, 1998, pp. A1, A12.

17. AHA, *Hospital Statistics*, Table 3, p. 8.

18. Bruce Japsen and Lisa Scott, "System Growth a Close Race," *Modern Healthcare*, May 26, 1997, p. 51.

19. Ibid., p. 52.

20. Lucette Lagnado, "Critical Conditions," *Wall Street Journal*, December 10, 1997, pp. A1, A6.

21. Monica Langley, "Money Order: Nuns' Zeal for Profits Shapes Hospital Chain, Wins Wall Street Fans," *Wall Street Journal*, January 7, 1998, pp. A1, A11.

22. Economic and Social Research Institute (ESRI), "A Tale of Two Cities: Hospital Mergers in St. Louis and Philadelphia Not Reducing Excess Capacity," Health Care Financing Administration, *Findings Brief* 2, 2 (April 1998).

23. Bradford H. Gray, *The Profit Motive and Patient Care: The Changing Accountability of Doctors and Hospitals*, A Twentieth Century Fund Report (Cambridge, Massachusetts: Harvard University Press, 1991): ix, 325.

24. James Tallon, "Keynote Address: The Purchaser Revolution," conference on Envisioning Ethical Alternatives in Health Care, 9 December 1996. http://bruno.nccusa. org, Checked on 03-25-98; David F. Drake, personal communication.

25. See especially James C. Robinson, "The Changing Boundaries of the American Hospital." *Milbank Quarterly* 72, 2 (1994): 259-75; and Lawton R. Burns, "The Transformation of the American Hospital: From Community Institution toward Business Enterprise," *Comparative Social Research* 12 (1990): 77-112.

26. According to data from KPMG Peat Marwick's national survey of employers and from the Health Insurance Association of America, 88 percent of small firms and 69 percent of large firms offered conventional (fee-for-service) insurance in 1988; the comparable figures for 1996 were 29 percent and 26 percent. In contrast, 71 percent of small firms and 75 percent of large firms offered employees some form of managed care plan in 1996. "Trends in Managed Care Coverage in Small Firms," Center for Studying Health System Change, *Data Bulletin* 9 (Winter 1998).

27. Eli Ginzberg, *Tomorrow's Hospital*, p. 44.

28. Janet M. Corrigan and Paul B. Ginsburg, "Association Leaders Speak Out on Health System Change," p. 152.

29. AHA, *Hospital Statistics*, Table 1, pp. 2-3.

30. *Health United States*, Table 99, p. 229.

31. *Health Care Financing Review*, Medicare and Medicaid Statistical Supplement, 1997, Table 3, p. 21.

32. U.S. Government, Bureau of the Census, *Statistical Abstract of the United States*, revised December 1997, Table 193, p. 131. www.census.gov/prod/ww/abs/cc97stab/html.

33. AHA, *Hospital Statistics*, Table 1, p. 3.

34. American Hospital Association, "National Hospital Week May 10-16, 1998." www.aha.org/ar/nationalweek/html. Accessed May 6, 1998.

35. AHA, *Hospital Statistics*, Table 3, p. 8.

36. For illustrations of boards that work well, see Hospital Research and Educational Trust and Milbank Memorial Fund, *Governing Health Care Systems: Ten Stories* (New York: Milbank Memorial Fund, 1997).

37. AHA, *Hospital Statistics*, Table 3, p. 8.

Index

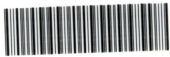